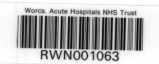

For Baillière Tindall:

Commissioning Editor: Alex Mathieson
Project Manager: Derek Robertson

Essential Science for Nursing Students
An introductory text

Edited by

Roger Watson BSc PhD RGN CBiol MIBiol
Professor of Nursing,
University of Hull, Hull

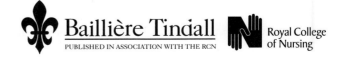

Baillière Tindall
PUBLISHED IN ASSOCIATION WITH THE RCN

Royal College
of Nursing

BAILLIÈRE TINDALL
An imprint of Harcourt Publishers Limited

© Harcourt Publishers Limited 1999

✤ is a registered trademark of Harcourt Publishers Limited

The right of Roger Watson to be identified as editor of this work has been asserted by him in accordance with the Copyright, Designs and Patents Act 1988

First published 1999

ISBN 07020 2126 1

British Library Cataloguing in Publication Data
A catalogue record for this book is available from the British Library

Library of Congress Cataloging in Publication Data
A catalog record for this book is available from the Library of Congress

Note
Medical knowledge is contantly changing. As new information becomes available, changes in treatment, procedures, equipment and the use of drugs become necessary. The editor, contributors and the publishers have, as far as it is possible, taken care to ensure that the information given in this text is accurate and up to date. However, readers are strongly advised to confirm that the information, especially with regard to drug usage, complies with the latest legislation and standards of practice.

The
publisher's
policy is to use
**paper manufactured
from sustainable forests**

Printed in China

Contents

Contributors

Jan S. Gill BSc(Hons) PhD
Honorary Teaching Fellow,
University of Edinburgh, Edinburgh

Dinah Gould BSc MPhil PhD RGN RNT
Professor of Nursing,
South Bank University, London

Sheenan Kindlen MSc LRSC SRD
Visiting Lecturer in Physiology,
Queen Margaret University College, Edinburgh

Jennifer Kelly MSc BA(Hons) RGN DipN DipNEd
Senior Lecturer Practitioner, Wound Care
Addenbrooke's Hospital, Cambridge

Roger Watson BSc PhD RGN CBiol MIBiol
Professor of Nursing,
University of Hull, Hull

Jennie Wilson BSc RGN
Surveillance Coordinator,
Public Health Laboratory Service, London

Introduction

Roger Watson

INTRODUCTION

This book is not complete and, in fact, it never will be. However, it is hoped that it will undergo subsequent editions in which all the aspects of the life sciences that students of nursing struggle to come to terms with are introduced and covered by contemporary experts in the field. Not all of the authors of the present text are nurses. However, all have experience in trying to convey essential aspects of the life sciences to student nurses, all have a passion to instil into nurses an appreciation of the life sciences and the importance of this field of study for practising nurses and each have contributed to areas with which they have found difficulty and where they feel that some success has been achieved in their own teaching.

In this sense, therefore, the book is not comprehensive and it is not meant to be. The current volume does not stand alone; rather, it has to be read in conjunction with any one of the range of major texts in anatomy and physiology with which nurses are familiar. For this reason, references have been kept to an absolute minimum and it is hoped that this book will form a companion to any of these texts and that student nurses will turn to this volume in order to seek clarification of concepts that they find difficult to grasp when first encountered. In this light, the present text is designed to present the main features of a selection of systems, against a background of the highlights of chemistry and cell biology, in such a way that student nurses may understand how these systems work without all the necessary clutter of anatomical detail, extensive physiological interactions and clinical examples that abound in standard comprehensive texts. None of this is meant to demean any of the contemporary texts; it is hoped that the present text can eventually be abandoned by individuals as they become more comfortable with the underlying principles that the various authors have tried to impart.

FROM CELLS TO SYSTEMS

There is an underlying anatomical and physiological logic to the working of the human body and this is best understood by appreciating the various levels of organisation in the body. The lowest level of organisation is the chemical level and, in the human body, this is represented in the biological molecules – the proteins, nucleic acids, lipids and carbohydrates. In order to understand the structure and function of the cell it is necessary to understand the structure and function of these molecules. However, in order to understand the structure and function of these molecules it is vital to grasp some fundamental aspects of chemistry and this is the point at which the present text begins.

To catalogue the intricacies of genetics and the transmission of traits between cells and generations of human beings without, for example, understanding the hydrogen bonding between base pairs in DNA is analogous to understanding how to drive a car without knowing how the internal combustion engine works. Driving a car is perfectly adequate but modern nursing education does not seek to provide practitioners who are merely adequate; it seeks to provide practitioners who are knowledgeable and who can hold their own against the range of well-qualified practitioners in other disciplines alongside whom they work. For example, how much more satisfying it is to administer drugs when you can explain something about their action rather than just the fact that they act in certain conditions.

HOMEOSTASIS

The biological molecules comprise the cells of the body and these are organised into tissues, which are organised as organs and, ultimately, as the systems of the body. The systems of the body are coordinated in such a way that they maintain a constant internal environment and this is under the control of the nervous and endocrine systems. A section of the present text is devoted to control systems because to miss the fundamental importance of homeostasis is to miss the whole point of physiology.

Rather than catalogue all of the systems of the body, several functions have been selected by the present authors based, not only on their own expertise, but through knowledge of the inherent difficulty in understanding the fundamental principles involved. Thus, the chapter on respiration looks at the mechanics of gas exchange and the diffusion of gases at the alveoli and the chapter on the kidneys looks at how the functional units, the nephrons, work to produce urine. In both cases, in common with the other chapters in this section, the student is spared much of the anatomy and incidental physiological functions.

APPLICATIONS

Finally, and probably uniquely for a text on the life sciences, microbiology and pharmacology are included because an understanding of these is intimately related to an understanding of many of the other principles that are related in this text. Protection is placed in the same section as it is, essentially, a response to invasion of the body by microorganisms.

Tables and figures have also been kept to a minimum and are only included where they are considered essential to an understanding of the material in the text. The boxes serve two functions. On the one hand they summarise useful concepts and indicate applications of knowledge. On the other hand, they highlight points that can only be fully understood by studying the text. In all cases, they are considered as signposts to essential knowledge which the student should gain on reading this book.

FURTHER READING

The following textbooks make excellent companions to the present volume:

Cree L, Rischmiller S 1991 *Science in nursing, 3rd edn.* WB Saunders, Sydney

Hinchliff SM, Montague SE, Watson R 1996 *Physiology for nursing practice.* Baillière Tindall, London

McNeill AR 1992 *The human machine.* Natural History Museum, London

Trounce J, Gould D 1997 *Clinical pharmacology for nurses, 15th edn.* Churchill Livingstone, Edinburgh

Walsh M 1997 *Watson's clinical nursing and related sciences.* Baillière Tindall, London

Watson R (1995) *Anatomy and physiology for nurses, 10th edn.* Baillière Tindall, London

Wilson J 1995 *Infection control in clinical practice.* Baillière Tindall, London

1 FROM ATOMS TO CELLS

1 Basic Chemistry

Roger Watson

After reading this chapter you should understand several aspects of basic chemistry including:

- the structure of the atom
- how molecules are formed by different types of bonding including hydrogen bonding
- concentration
- chemical reactions
- acidity and alkalinity
- the behaviour of chemicals in water.

INTRODUCTION

As explained in the introductory chapter, the human body is organised hierarchically with the chemical level of organisation as the simplest. Chemistry is a complex subject, especially for those with no scientific background. However, it is essential to appreciate some of the rudiments of chemistry in order to understand not only the higher levels of organisation in the human body but also some of its functions, such as the breakdown of food and the reproduction of cells.

Chemistry is concerned with matter, in other words, with anything that occupies space. A common term used in chemistry for different types of matter is substances. Matter is familiar in the three states in which it can exist, either as a solid, a liquid or a vapour. Matter can be transformed between states: for example, water in its solid form of ice can be transformed into liquid water and this can be transformed into water vapour. Chemistry is also concerned with the composition of matter, how it is held together and how types of matter can react with one another to give a new type of matter. For example, hydrogen and oxygen can react to form water.

Chemical analysis tells us what matter is composed of: sugars are composed of the elements carbon, hydrogen and oxygen; these elements are held together by covalent bonds and, in the course of being broken down in the body into carbon dioxide and water, that energy is released and used in other bodily processes such as the movement of muscles (Ch. 12).

ELEMENTS

The term 'elements' has been used above and requires definition. Elements are simply chemical substances that cannot be broken down into other substances by ordinary chemical means. Many elements such as those mentioned above and others such as nitrogen and sodium are familiar.

> The most common elements found in the body are carbon, hydrogen, oxygen, nitrogen, sodium, potassium and chloride.

Each element is unique and it is only necessary, for the purpose of understanding the human body, to be familiar with a few, which will be described below. All of the elements, except hydrogen, are composed of subatomic particles called protons, neutrons and electrons. Hydrogen has no neutrons.

A unique atomic number identifies each element and this number is the same as the number of protons it contains. Thus, hydrogen has an atomic number of 1 because it contains one proton and carbon has an atomic number of 6 because it contains six protons.

Each element also has an atomic weight, which is equal to the number of protons and neutrons. Thus, hydrogen has an atomic weight of 1 because it only has one proton and no neutrons, and carbon, which has six protons and six neutrons, has an atomic weight of 12. When different elements are combined in a chemical reaction to form a compound then the compound can be described in terms of its compound or molecular weight, which is simply calculated by adding up all the atomic weights of the element in the compound. This will be discussed in more detail below.

Neutrons, as the name suggests, have no electrical charge. Protons, however, have a positive electrical charge and, because all the elements have an overall neutral charge, the positive charges of the protons are balanced by negative charges, which are found on the electrons. Therefore, in each element, the number of positively charged protons is balanced by the same number of negatively charged electrons. It is easy to calculate the number of electrons in an element from the atomic number, or the number of protons. For example, hydrogen contains one electron and carbon contains six.

ATOMIC STRUCTURE

There is a specific arrangement of protons, neutrons and electrons in each element and the resulting structure is known as an atom. Protons and neutrons are localised at the centre of the atom in the nucleus and the electrons are arranged around the nucleus.

The most convenient way in which to imagine the structure of an atom is to think of the nucleus as a planet with the electrons revolving around it like satellites. Electrons may only occupy certain orbitals around a nucleus and the number of electrons in each orbital is restricted. The orbital closest to the nucleus may contain only two electrons and the next orbital may contain only eight. Very few of the elements relevant to the life sciences contain electrons in the next orbital.

With the above knowledge it is possible, when the atomic number of an element is given, to work out the arrangement of electrons around the nucleus. For example, in hydrogen, which has an atomic number of 1 and therefore one electron, this occupies the orbital closest to the nucleus. In carbon, which has an

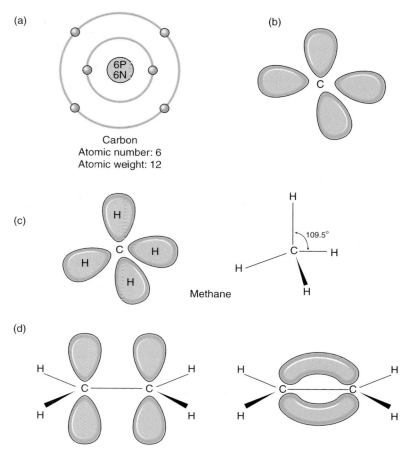

Fig. 1.1 *Orbitals and bonds. (a) Simple representation of the carbon atom. (b) The carbon atom showing second-level orbits (see text for explanation). (c) Covalent bonds between carbon and hydrogen in methane. (d) Formation of a double bond in ethene.*

atomic number of 6 and therefore six electrons, there are two in the orbital closest to the nucleus and four in the next orbital.

The orbital structure described above, however, is a simplification. In organic chemistry, which is concerned with the chemistry of compounds containing carbon and hydrogen and often other elements such as oxygen and nitrogen, it is convenient also to visualise the electrons in the second orbital as occupying their own unique clouds. These clouds, in fact, project away from the nucleus towards the corners of a tetrahedron (Fig. 1.1). As only eight electrons can occupy the second orbital, each of these four clouds can contain a maximum of two electrons, also known as a 'pair of electrons'. If a cloud contains only one electron then it is said to be 'unpaired' and the distribution of electrons in the second orbital is always such that as many of the clouds as possible contain one electron but never more than two. Taking carbon as an example, it has four electrons in its second orbital and each of these occupies one of the clouds. Carbon, therefore, is said to contain four unpaired electrons. The number of unpaired electrons in an atom is referred to as valence and it should be noted that this aspect of the structure of carbon, hydrogen and other organic compounds, which allows them to bond with other elements, is the basis of organic chemistry (Ch. 2). Carbon, therefore, has a valence of 4, hydrogen has a valence of 1 and oxygen and nitrogen have valencies of 2 and 3, respectively. Other elements such as sodium, which have a single electron in their third orbital, can also bond and the nature of chemical bonding will be described below.

> Organic chemicals have electrons in two energy levels with a minimum of one and a maximum of two in the first energy level and a minimum of four and a maximum of eight in the second level.

CHEMICAL BONDING, COMPOUNDS AND MOLECULES

Three types of chemical bonding, which are essential to the structure and function of the human body, will be described. These are covalent bonding, ionic bonding and hydrogen bonding. Covalent and ionic bonding occur between elements and the resulting matter is called a compound. Hydrogen bonds occur between compounds.

When atoms bond to form compounds, the resulting structure is known as a molecule. This applies equally to two different types of atom combining, for example when carbon and oxygen combine to form carbon dioxide, as it does to two atoms of the same element combining, as is the case with molecular oxygen, which is a compound of two oxygen atoms.

Covalent bonding

Covalent bonds are the strongest of the chemical bonds and these bonds hold together familiar materials such as plastics. They also bond the elements in materials such as coal and sugars and the strength of the bonds is demonstrated by the fact that energy in the form of heat is required to break them.

The strength of covalent bonds lies in the fact that they are formed by uniting unpaired electrons, thereby forming very stable compounds. The simplest example of a covalent bond is that between carbon and hydrogen, both of which contain unpaired electrons. Hydrogen contains one unpaired electron in its first orbital and carbon contains four unpaired electrons in its second orbital clouds. The simple organic compound methane is formed when four hydrogen atoms bond to one carbon atom and the four resulting covalent carbon–hydrogen bonds can be visualised as second orbital clouds, each of which contains a pair of electrons (Fig. 1.1). Clearly, once this has happened neither the carbon nor the hydrogen can form further bonds and the compound is said to be saturated.

Variations on the covalent bond are possible where the compounds are not saturated and a good example of this is the oxygen molecule. An oxygen atom has two unpaired electrons in its second orbital and when two oxygen atoms combine they form a double bond whereby both the unpaired electrons become paired (Fig. 1.1). Such compounds are described as being unsaturated. You may already be familiar with the terms saturated and unsaturated when they are applied to the fats in our diet and the use of the terms here means that unsaturated fats contain double bonds and saturated fats contain none.

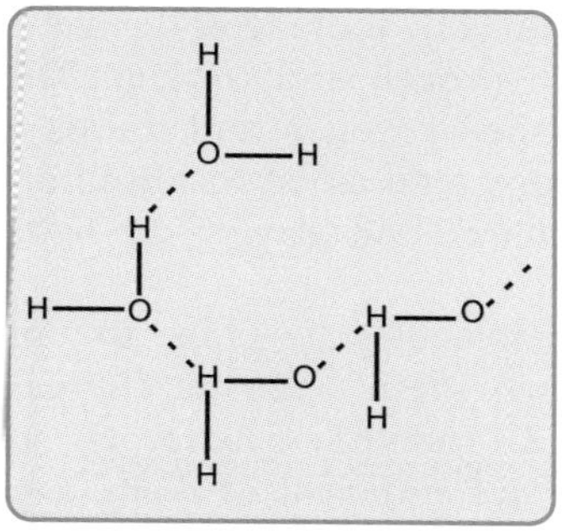

Fig. 1.2 *Diagrammatic representation of hydrogen bonding in water. The broken lines are the weak interactions between the oxygen and hydrogen atoms.*

> Single covalent bonds are more stable, and therefore stronger, than double or triple covalent bonds.

Double covalent bonds are not as stable as single covalent bonds and compounds that contain double bonds are less stable and can form further bonds with other elements. The formation of water from one atom of oxygen and four atoms of hydrogen is a good example (Fig. 1.2).

Ionic bonding

Some elements can lose electrons and others may gain electrons, and this is the basis of ionic bonding. The best example of an ionically bonded substance is common salt, or sodium chloride. Sodium is an element with one electron in its outer orbital and chlorine is an element with seven electrons in its outer shell. Sodium can donate its electron to chlorine in order to 'fill' the outer shell with eight electrons. In this process the sodium atom becomes an ion with a slight positive charge and the chlorine atom becomes a chlorine ion with a slight negative charge. The attraction of the two opposite charges holds the sodium and the chlorine together in an ionic compound. In the solid form of salt the atoms of sodium and chlorine are held together by these opposite charges in a very tight structure known as a crystal.

Ionic bonds are much weaker than covalent bonds and this can be demonstrated by putting salt crystals into water. The salt dissolves and the sodium and chlorine ions go into solution. In this form they are called electrolytes and this is the form in which many elements, among them sodium, chlorine, potassium and magnesium, exist in the fluids of the body such as blood. Solutions and solvents will be considered below.

Hydrogen bonding

Hydrogen bonds exist between covalently bonded compounds, where it is possible for regions of the compounds to have slight positive and negative charges.

This is best explained by looking at the water molecule, which has two covalent bonds between hydrogen and oxygen. The pairs of electrons in the orbital clouds between the hydrogen and the oxygen atoms are not evenly distributed. The electrons tend to be localised around the oxygen atom giving it a slight negative charge and leaving the hydrogen atoms with a slight positive charge (Fig. 1.2).

When water molecules lie close to one another, there is an attraction between these two slight opposite charges and this is known as hydrogen bonding (Fig. 1.2). Individual hydrogen bonds are very weak but, nevertheless, when there are sufficient of them, as seen in water, they are collectively very strong. In fact, if hydrogen bonding did not take place the state of water as a liquid would be impossible and water would only exist as a vapour. Otherwise, hydrogen bonds play a crucial role in biological compounds, as will be described below.

> Hydrogen bonds are very important in biology; they hold water molecules together and stabilise the structures of many biological compounds such as protein and nucleic acid.

EMPIRICAL STRUCTURE

Thus far, elements and compounds have been described in some detail. However, it is inconvenient to describe each element and chemical in this way and chemists have devised a system of abbreviating elements to symbols – usually to single letters – and of describing compounds in a shorthand way known as the empirical structure. Some of the symbols above such as 'H' for hydrogen and 'O' for oxygen have already been used. A complete list can be found in a table called the periodic table of the elements, which gives all of the information needed about an element, including its symbol, atomic number and atomic weight. The atomic numbers are used to arrange the elements in the periodic table. Some common examples of elements, with the information given in the periodic table, are shown in Table 1.1.

TABLE 1.1	**Some Common Elements**		
Name	Symbol	Atomic number	Atomic weight
Carbon	C	6	12
Chlorine	Cl	17	34
Hydrogen	H	1	1
Nitrogen	N	7	14
Oxygen	O	8	16
Sodium	Na	11	22

When elements combine to form compounds, this is known as a chemical reaction and these chemical reactions are represented using the symbols and the empirical structures. For example, when hydrogen and oxygen combine to form water it is represented as $4H + O_2 \rightarrow 2H_2O$. Notice that the equation balances with an equal number of hydrogen and oxygen atoms on both sides of the arrow. Another simple example is the formation of carbon dioxide from carbon and hydrogen, which can be represented as $C + O_2 \rightarrow CO_2$. Some examples of simple organic compounds and their empirical structures are shown in Table 1.2.

TABLE 1.2	Simple Organic Compounds	
Name		Empirical formula
Carbon dioxide		CO_2
Methane		CH_4
Ethanol		C_2H_5OH
Glucose		$C_6H_{12}O_6$

CHEMICAL REACTIONS, EQUILIBRIUM AND CATALYSIS

A chemical reaction takes place when new substances are formed by the rearrangement of atoms. The example of the formation of carbon dioxide from carbon and oxygen has already been described above ($C + O_2 \rightarrow CO_2$). In the case of the above reaction the carbon and the hydrogen are called the reactants and the carbon dioxide is the product. Note that atoms are neither created nor destroyed in a chemical reaction and the number of atoms in the reactants should always be the same as the number of atoms in the product. Such an equation is said to be balanced.

The majority of chemical reactions are reversible and, in fact, because of this reversibility, there is a continuing formation and breakdown of product. When no further net formation of product takes place then the reaction is said to have reached equilibrium. Depending upon the type of reaction, the equilibrium may be such that the majority of the reactants are used in the formation of product or there may be an almost equal amount of substances in the form of reactants and product.

The point at which the equilibrium is reached and, indeed, the ease with which the reaction takes place will depend upon the use of energy or the release of energy in the reaction. The concept of energy will be considered at the end of this chapter but suffice to say here that reactions which release energy (exothermic reactions) will take place more readily than those which consume energy (endothermic reactions). Indeed, exothermic reactions between reactants will often take place spontaneously when the reactants are mixed together. Endothermic reactions, on the other hand, will require the provision of energy, often in the form of heat. An equilibrium reaction may be shifted in either direction either by adding or removing reactants or products. For example, as more reactants (A or B) are added then the reaction shifts to the right and the same effect could be achieved by removing products (C or D) in the reaction $A + B \leftrightarrow C + D$.

Another way in which chemical reactions may be facilitated is by catalysis. A catalyst is a substance which, because of its structure, will reduce the energy required in order for reactants to form products. The catalyst, while it becomes involved in the chemical reaction, does not become changed or reduced in amount in the course of the chemical reaction. Note that the catalyst neither enables nor causes the chemical reaction to take place. By reducing the requirement for energy in the reaction, a catalyst merely accelerates a chemical reaction. Many substances are used in chemistry as catalysts but the catalysts of most interest in the study of the human body are the biological catalysts known as enzymes. Enzymes are protein molecules (to be described in the following chapter) that facilitate specific biochemical reactions to take place in the human body and they are involved in the breakdown of food, the movement of muscle and the synthesis of body materials such as bone and skin.

> A catalyst is a substance that accelerates a chemical reaction without itself being changed in the reaction. Enzymes are biological catalysts.

CHEMICALS IN WATER

The major constituent of the body is water, which is known as the universal solvent. Most chemicals in the body are dissolved in water and it is necessary to understand a little of what happens to chemicals in water. Most of the substances in the body can dissolve in water, with the notable exception of fats. Water is not the only liquid in which other substances can dissolve but, biologically, it is the only example that needs to be considered. As stated above, water is know as the universal solvent and solvent is the general term for any liquid in which other substances can dissolve. A substance that is dissolved in a solvent is known as a solute and the result of dissolving a solute in a solvent is known as a solution.

The process whereby substances spread out through the water in the process of being dissolved is known as diffusion and this takes place until there is an even distribution of the chemical throughout the water. The amount of the chemical dissolved in water is measured by its concentration (see below) and a chemical always diffuses from the region where it is most highly concentrated to the region where it is least concentrated. Once the chemical is evenly distributed in the water the diffusion continues but there is no net movement of the chemical from one area to another. This is most easily demonstrated by dissolving a coloured compound such as copper sulphate, which is blue, in water. If some solid copper sulphate crystals are dropped into the water most of the water is initially clear but there is a region of deep blue around the crystals. After some time the water becomes a deeper shade of blue until all of the copper sulphate has dissolved. The process can be speeded up by stirring or heating the water. Eventually the water remains a uniform shade of blue and it is physically impossible for the crystals to reform unless some change in the volume or temperature of the water takes place either through evaporation or freezing.

A class of molecules that is common in the human body, called lipids, is not soluble in water. Because these are complex biological molecules, their structure and properties will be dealt with below.

MEASUREMENT IN CHEMISTRY

The concept of measurement, in terms of weight, distance, time and temperature as examples, is very familiar. Many of these measures apply to chemistry but there is also a unit of measurement that is unique to chemistry (the mole) which you will encounter and which requires some explanation.

Weight, volume and amount are the key measures to understand in relation to chemistry and SI (International System of Units) units are always used. The measure of weight, therefore, is the kilogram (kg) and the measure of volume is the cubic metre more commonly known as the litre (L). Table 1.3 shows how kilograms, grams (g) and milligrams (mg) are related and also how different expressions of volume are related. The amount of a substance is measured in moles (mol).

TABLE 1.3	Weights, Measures and Volumes			
	Weight (symbol)	Length (symbol)	Volume (symbol)	Relationship
	milligram (mg)	millimetre (mm)	millilitre (ml)	10^{-3} units
	gram (g)	metre (m)	litre (L)	units
	kilograms (kg)	kilometres (km)		10^3 units

NB. $10^3 = \times 1000$; $10^{-3} = \times 1/1000$

Weight is a convenient way in which to measure solid substances and volume is a convenient way in which to measure liquids and vapours. For example, it is possible to measure out, using a weighing scale, an amount of salt or sugar, say 100 g. Likewise it is possible, using a graduated cylinder, to measure out an amount of water, say 100 millilitres (ml).

The mole concept

The mole is a measurement unique to chemistry and it is one which is used for convenience and also one which is rational when carrying out chemical experiments. A mole of any substance, either an elemental substance or a compound, always contains the same number of particles. This number is known as Avogadro's number and is approximately 6×10^{25}. It follows, therefore, that a mole of sodium and a mole of water both contain the same number of particles. In the case of sodium it is 6×10^{25} sodium atoms and in the case of water it is 6×10^{25} water molecules.

In one mole of a substance there are always the same number of particles (atoms or molecules) present.

A mole is either the gram atomic weight or the gram molecular weight of a substance. In order to obtain a mole of an element such as carbon it is necessary to know the atomic weight of carbon, which is 12, and to weigh out 12 g. For molecular substances it is necessary to calculate the molecular weight by summing all of the atomic weights of the constituent elements, according to the empirical structure of the molecule, and weighing out an equivalent number of grams of the substance. Taking the common sugar sucrose as an example, which has the empirical structure $C_6H_{12}O_6$, a molecular weight of 182 is calculated, and therefore 182 g of sucrose contains 1 mol. This is an invaluable concept in chemistry because it allows chemists to measure out equivalent amounts of substances without having to count individual atoms or molecules.

Concentration

When units of weight, or amount, and volume are combined for a measure of a solute dissolved in a solvent then the concept of concentration is introduced. Concentration is an equivalent way of comparing the amounts of dissolved substances regardless of the actual amount of substance present.

If 100 g of salt are dissolved in 1 L of water then the resulting concentration of salt is 100 g/L. Regardless of volume, any amount of a 100 g/L solution will always contain the same concentration of solute but different volumes will contain different amounts of the solute. Therefore, if a sample is removed from a solution the concentration in the sample is the same as in the solution and the concentration of the original solution does not change. If 10 ml of a 100 g/L solution is removed from 100 ml then this small amount contains 100 g/L and so does the remaining 90 ml.

One hundred grams per litre may also be expressed as 10 g/100 ml and in other ways such as 1 g/10 ml. This possibility of expressing the same concentration in different ways can be difficult to grasp but, as a general rule, an effort is made to express a whole number of grams in as small a volume as possible.

Molar concentration is an expression of the number of moles of a dissolved solute. There is a convention in the expression of molar concentrations whereby 1 mol of a substance dissolved in 1 L of water is expressed as a molar solution and this is a common reference for comparison of different molar concentrations. Thus a millimolar solution is one in which there is the equivalent of a thousandth of a mole dissolved in a litre. Note, however, that if 1 ml is removed from a molar solution then this sample is still a molar solution but it contains 1 millimole (mmol) of the substance.

Concentration may be changed by altering either the amount of the dissolved substance or the volume in which it is dissolved. The process of decreasing the concentration of a dissolved substance is known as dilution and the process of increasing the concentration is known simply as concentration. The easiest way in which to dilute a dissolved substance is to add more water. It follows that if the volume of a solution is doubled the concentration is halved. To concentrate a dissolved substance, the easiest way in which to achieve this is to increase the amount of the substance in water and it follows that, if the volume of water remains the same and the amount of the dissolved substance is doubled, then the concentration of the solution is doubled. Another way in which this can be achieved is by reducing the amount of water and this can be achieved by evaporation. Clearly, if the volume of water is halved then the concentration will double.

As the volume in which a substance is dissolved increases, concentration decreases. As amount of a substance in a given volume increases, concentration increases.

For example, if a molar solution of sodium chloride in 1000 ml of water is doubled in volume by adding water to 2000 ml then the resulting solution will be half molar (0.5M). Conversely, if a mole of sodium chloride is added to the solution then the concentration will be doubled to two molar (2M).

OSMOSIS

Osmosis is a property of water that is very important in the human body. Osmosis is the movement of water from a region of high concentration of water to a lower concentration of water across a semipermeable membrane. A semipermeable membrane is one that will allow the passage of some molecules but not of others. Membranes, such as the plasma membrane which surrounds human cells, are semipermeable and osmosis takes place across these membranes in the human body (Ch. 2).

The process of osmosis can be demonstrated if a semipermeable membrane which allows the passage of water but not of other molecules such as salt or sugar is used. If two solutions of salt with different concentrations of salt are separated by a semipermeable membrane then water will move across the membrane from the less concentrated solution to the more concentrated solution – in other words, from the solution in which water is most concentrated to the solution in which water is less concentrated – until the concentration of salt on both sides of the semipermeable membrane is the same (Fig. 1.3). When two solutions separated by a semipermeable membrane are of the same concentration, they are said to be isotonic. The terms hypertonic and hypotonic are used to describe a more concentrated and a less concentrated (in terms of the solute) solution, respectively.

> Osmosis is the movement of water from a region of higher concentration of water to a region of lower concentration of water through a semi-permeable membrane.

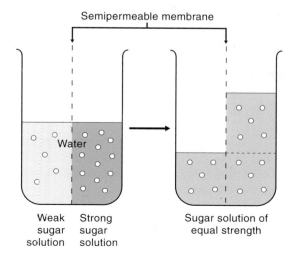

Fig. 1.3   *Osmosis.*

Movement of other substances across membranes in the human body is possible by processes such as diffusion and active transport. These processes will be considered in a later chapter.

ACIDS, BASES AND BUFFERS

An important property of any solution, from chemical and biological perspectives, is its acidity or alkalinity. The human body expends a considerable amount of energy in ensuring that the acidity and alkalinity of its fluids are maintained at a constant level. If either the acidity or the alkalinity of the blood, for instance, increases significantly beyond normal levels then this can have very adverse consequences for body function, including death. In addition to the methods that require expenditure of energy, there are many other systems in the human body that work to maintain a constant acidity/alkalinity in the fluids of the human body (Chs 10 and 11).

A convenient way of measuring and expressing the acidity/alkalinity of a solution is the pH scale and this scale is actually the negative logarithm of the hydrogen ion (H^+) concentration. When the hydrogen ion concentration is expressed in this way the resulting scale of pH extends from 1 to 14 with 1 representing the highest concentration of hydrogen ions and 14 representing the lowest concentration of hydrogen ions. A pH of 7, at the mid-point of this scale, represents neutrality and this is the pH of water. Most body fluids such as blood have a pH that is close to neutrality.

An alternative way of viewing pH is that solutions with a low pH (i.e. high H^+ concentration) have a low concentration of hydroxyl ions (OH^-) and that solutions with a high pH have a high concentration of hydroxyl ions. The concept of pH can be understood by visualising the combination of a hydrogen ion with a hydroxyl ion, which results in the formation of a water molecule ($H^+ + OH^- \rightarrow H_2O$). Where there is an excess of hydrogen ions the solution will be acidic and, alternatively, where there is an excess of hydroxyl ions the solution will be alkaline.

Differences in pH between solutions results in the ability of the compounds dissolved in the solutions to either release hydrogen or hydroxyl ions into the solutions. A strong acid, for example hydrogen chloride (hydrochloric acid), is a compound that easily dissociates into its constituents hydrogen and chloride, thereby releasing hydrogen ions into solution ($HCl \rightarrow H^+ + Cl^-$). A strong alkali, such as sodium hydroxide, is one that will easily dissociate into its constituents, thereby releasing hydroxyl ions into solution ($NaOH \rightarrow Na^+ + OH^-$). Alternatively, weaker acids and alkalis dissociate less easily to release hydrogen and hydroxyl ions, respectively.

Buffers are compounds that resist changes in pH. In addition to physiological mechanisms in the body that help to maintain constant levels of pH, several chemical buffering systems work in conjunction with these and some will be considered in subsequent chapters.

Acetic acid and its acetate ion act as buffers which, respectively, remove hydrogen ions and hydroxyl ions from solution. The reaction involving the acetate ion is $H^+ + CH_3CO_2^- \rightarrow CH_3CO_2H$ and the reaction involving acetic acid is $OH^- + CH_3CO_2H \rightarrow H_2O + CH_3CO_2^-$. One of the most common buffering systems in the human body is that involving carbonic acid/bicarbonate ion

(H_2CO_3/HCO_3^-). Carbonic acid is formed from a reaction between carbon dioxide and water ($CO_2 + H_2O \rightarrow H_2CO_3$) and this reaction is catalysed by an enzyme (described above) which is ubiquitous in the human body called carbonic anhydrase. Carbonic acid can dissociate into bicarbonate ion and hydrogen ions ($H_2CO_3 \rightarrow HCO_3^- + H^+$). Both of the above reactions are reversible and, in conditions where there is an excess of hydrogen ions, carbonic acid is formed and this is broken down into carbon dioxide and water, thereby removing the hydrogen ions from solution and resisting a fall in pH. If the pH rises then the formation of carbonic acid from carbon dioxide and water takes place and, with the dissociation of carbonic acid, hydrogen ions are released into solution thus powering the pH.

> pH is a representation of the concentration of hydrogen ions. A buffer is a substance that resists changes in pH.

ENERGY

The concept of energy has been mentioned several times in this chapter. There are many forms of energy but energy cannot be seen and is only apparent when it is changed from one form into another. Common examples of energy are heat, light and mechanical energy. However, there are less tangible types of energy such as chemical, electrical and electromagnetic radiation.

It is essential to grasp that energy cannot be formed or destroyed, it can merely be transformed from one form into another. The ultimate source of energy in the human body is solar energy. The energy contained in sunshine is used to drive the process of photosynthesis in green plants whereby nutritious substances such as carbohydrates and fats are made. These substances, known as nutrients, contain chemical energy in their covalent bonds, this energy having been derived from solar energy and transformed into chemical energy in the leaves of green plants. When nutrients, such as sucrose or fat, are eaten the human body is capable of breaking down the substances (catabolism) in order to release the chemical energy in the covalent bonds. Some of this energy is released as heat, which is analogous to the process of burning fossil fuels, but most of the energy is trapped in other molecules in the body. The prime example of such a chemical is adenosine triphosphate (ATP), and ATP can subsequently be used to drive other catabolic and synthetic (anabolic) reactions. This process is known as metabolism.

> Energy cannot be created or destroyed but can be changed from one form into another.

The best examples of metabolism are the processes of glycolysis and the Kreb's cycle whereby glucose is broken down into carbon dioxide and water and large amounts of ATP are produced for use in the other metabolic processes of the body. Some of these processes will be described in more detail in other chapters of this book. In order to understand the metabolic processes of the body it is necessary to understand the structure and functions of biological molecules and these are the material of the following chapter.

SUMMARY

This chapter has reviewed the basic principles of chemistry, including the nature of elements and compounds and the range of chemical bonds. The importance of the covalent bond in the formation of organic compounds was covered and the place of the hydrogen bond in water and biological molecules was explained. The issue of measurement in chemistry, particularly the concept of the mole, and some aspects of physical chemistry and the behaviour of chemicals in water such as diffusion and osmosis have been covered. Finally, the concept of energy was considered.

QUESTIONS

1. What is an 'element' and how do elements differ from one another?

2. Can you describe the essential features of a covalent bond and say how it differs from an ionic and a hydrogen bond?

3. How many particles are there in a mole? If you separated two solutions, one with a molar solution of salt and the other with a half molar solution by a semipermeable membrane in which direction would water move and what is this process called?

FURTHER READING

Davis M (1996) The chemistry of living matter. In: Hinchliff S, Montague S, Watson R (eds) *Physiology for nursing practice, 2nd edn*. Baillière Tindall, London, pp 23–48

Watson R (1995) *Anatomy and physiology for nurses, 10th edn*. Baillière Tindall, London

2 Biological Molecules

Roger Watson

> After reading this chapter you should be able to describe the features of the following biological molecules:
> - proteins
> - nucleic acids
> - carbohydrates
> - fats.

INTRODUCTION

Biological molecules are those that are unique to biological systems. They participate in the metabolic reactions of the cells in the human body and they are, thereby, responsible for providing energy in the body and for all of the structural components of the body such as familiar aspects of the body, e.g. skin and hair, and also for the less familiar structures such as the membranes surrounding cells and the lining of the digestive tract. Biological molecules also contain all of the information required to transmit life from one generation to the next and also the inherited traits such as eye colour and intelligence (Ch. 3). The biological molecules that will be covered in this chapter are proteins, nucleic acids, carbohydrates and lipids.

Biological molecules are all organic molecules, containing carbon and hydrogen, and often they contain other elements such as oxygen and nitrogen. Also, biological molecules are all polymers and before looking at biological molecules in more detail a brief review of organic chemistry, including polymers, is presented.

ORGANIC CHEMISTRY

Organic compounds are characterised by the fact that they contain carbon and that the carbon atoms are bonded to one another and often to other types of atoms, principally hydrogen, but also other atoms, the most common being oxygen and nitrogen. As described in Chapter 1, carbon has a valence of 4, meaning that it can form four covalent bonds with other atoms. The simplest organic compound, methane, is the molecule on which the simplest group of organic molecules, the hydrocarbons, is based and it can be used to demonstrate the concept of polymerisation.

Methane is described as a monomer that is simply a single unit from which multi-unit molecules, or polymers, can be built. When a hydrogen atom is removed from a methane molecule this leaves one unpaired electron, which can form another covalent bond. If two such molecules are bonded such that the unpaired electrons become paired then a carbon–carbon bond is formed and a polymer (strictly speaking a dimer because there are two monomers) called ethane is formed. This process can be repeated for longer chains of methane molecules and some examples are given in Table 2.1. This is the basis of hydrocarbon chemistry and these substances, all originally derived from living matter, are familiar to us in the form of fossil fuels.

TABLE 2.1	Simple Hydrocarbon Compounds			
	Group	Name	Empirical formula	Structural formula
	Alkanes	Methane	CH_4	H | H–C–H | H
		Ethane	C_2H_6	H H | | H–C–C–H | | H H
	Alkenes	Ethene	C_2H_4	H H | | C=C | | H H
	Alkynes	Ethelyne	C_2H_2	HC≡CH

The alkanes in Table 2.1 are saturated – in other words, there are only single carbon–carbon and carbon–hydrogen bonds. Note also that all these compounds have the suffix -ane, which indicates that they are saturated. It is possible to form polymers with double carbon–carbon bonds and triple carbon–carbon bonds and these have the suffix -ene and -yne, respectively, as shown in Table 2.1. These hydrocarbons are referred to as alkanes, alkenes and alkynes as shown in Table 2.1.

Conventions in organic chemistry

It is necessary to know a few of the conventions of organic chemistry, some of which were met in the previous chapter, in order to understand the structures of the different types of compound. These conventions are merely convenient shorthand ways of expressing some relatively complex structures.

The concept of empirical structure has already been introduced. For example, the empirical structure of methane is CH_4. An understanding of covalent bonding and valence immediately suggests the structure of methane, as shown in Table 2.1. It is also possible, applying the same principles, to work out the structure of some simply polymers such as ethane from the empirical structure C_2H_6. However, it is clear that the larger the molecule becomes, and when different atoms are introduced, that the empirical structure becomes less helpful in visualising the structure.

The empirical structure of a compound indicates the amount of each constituent atom in the compound.

From the empirical structure C_2H_6O, for instance, it is difficult to know precisely what is the structure of this molecule. If, on the other hand, the structure is written as C_2H_5OH (which is the structure of ethanol, to be discussed below) it is possible to see that the structure is as shown in Table 2.2. With larger molecules with an empirical structure such as $C_6H_{12}O_6$ it is clearly impossible to deduce the structure.

For this reason, classes of molecules have been described and these classes, such as the alcohols and esters, contain particular groups which indicate what are the structures. Also, in representing the structures of organic molecules, it is correct to show all of the covalent bonds by means of short connecting lines between atoms. The carbon–carbon bond, for instance, is represented as C–C. However, when compounds are incorporated into text or into chemical equations there are other shorthand ways of representing them. Thus, the carboxyl group (see Table 2.2), which has a double covalent bond from a carbon atom to an oxygen atom and a single covalent bond from the same carbon atom to a hydroxyl group, is conventionally written as -COOH. Again, knowing to which group the molecules with

TABLE 2.2	Organic Compounds Containing Oxygen and Nitrogen			
	Group	Name	Empirical formula	Structural formula
	Alcohols	Ethanol	C_2H_5OH	H–C–C–OH (with H atoms)
	Aldehydes	Acetaldehyde	C_2H_4O	H–C–C=O (with H atoms)
	Ketones	Acetone	CH_3COCH_3	H–C–C–C–H (with O and H atoms)
	Esters	Methyl acetate	$CH_3CO_2CH_3$	H–C–C–O–C–H (with O and H atoms)
	Carboxylic acids	Formic acid	HCO_2H	H–C–OH (with O double bond)
	Amines	Methylamine	CH_3NH_2	H–C–N (with H atoms)

this particular group belong (the carboxylic acids) and also understanding the rules of valence and covalent bonding, the structure can also be visualised.

A final convention, which will be encountered with the biological molecules, is the use of the 'R' group which, when more than one such group is present, is often also denoted as -R'. This is a particularly shorthand way of representing organic molecules and is commonly applied where a group of molecules, such as the amino acids (to be described below) have a common core structure but where individual molecules within the group are characterised by different, and often large, side groups. From this point onwards these conventions will all be applied without further explanation

Organic compounds containing oxygen and nitrogen

As mentioned previously, oxygen and nitrogen are commonly included in organic compounds. A familiar group of organic compounds containing oxygen are the alcohols, and ethanol is the alcohol that is contained in alcoholic beverages. Its structure is shown in Table 2.2 and it can be seen that its name and structure are related to ethane in that it begins with the prefix ethan- and contains two carbon atoms. Another example, methanol, contains only one carbon atom. Another feature of the alcohols is that their names end with the suffix -ol. The characteristic chemical group in the alcohols is the -OH, or hydroxyl, group and the introduction of this group saturates all the valencies in carbon, oxygen and hydrogen.

The aldehydes and ketones are other groups of closely related organic compounds that contain oxygen. Unlike the alcohols, these are not saturated and they contain a characteristic double bond between carbon and oxygen (C=O) known as a carbonyl group. The aldehydes have hydrogen bonded to the carbonyl group and this is conventionally represented as -CH=O while the ketones have two carbon–carbon bonds attached to the carbonly group.

Finally, the carboxylic acids have a carbonyl group with a hydroxyl attached (-COOH) and these are weak acids because they react sparingly with water to release hydrogen ions (H^+) into solution. Some common examples of aldehydes, ketones and carboxylic acids are shown in Table 2.2.

Esters

An ester is a compound that is formed from a reaction between a carboxylic acid and an alcohol. The reaction is represented in Figure 2.1 and this type of reaction, caused by the removal of water, is known as a condensation reaction. The reverse reaction, whereby water is added to a compound and a covalent bond is broken, is known as a hydrolysis reaction. The resulting covalent carbon–oxygen bond with an adjacent carbonyl group is known as an ester bond. These are important in the human body because these are the bonds that form between fatty acids and glycerol in the formation of triglycerides, which are a lipid component of the diet.

When water is added to a compound to break it into two new compounds this is called a hydrolysis reaction and when water is removed from two compounds to form a new compound this is called a condensation reaction.

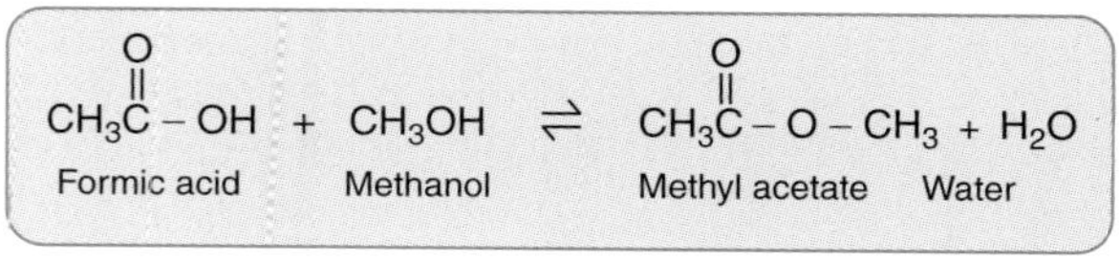

$$CH_3\overset{O}{\overset{\|}{C}}-OH + CH_3OH \rightleftharpoons CH_3\overset{O}{\overset{\|}{C}}-O-CH_3 + H_2O$$

Formic acid　　Methanol　　　Methyl acetate　Water

Fig. 2.1 *Formation of an ester.*

Organic compounds containing nitrogen

Nitrogen has a valence of 3 and exists as a compound with hydrogen, called ammonia (NH_3). Organic compounds containing nitrogen are called amines and, in an amine, one or more of the covalent bonds between nitrogen and hydrogen is replaced by another covalent bond. A simple example of an amine is methylamine, which is shown in Table 2.2. Methylamine is called a primary amide and these compounds, which have an -NH_2 group attached to a carbon atom, are common in biological systems. The amino acids of which proteins are composed (to be discussed below) are common primary amines. All of the amines have the suffix -ine and common examples are the drugs morphine and amphetamine. Amines are weak alkalis because they react sparingly with water to release hydroxyl ions.

PROTEINS

Proteins serve many functions in the human body. They are involved in nutrition both as nutrients and as biological catalysts which help to break down other nutrients. Also, as biological catalysts they control the metabolic pathways whereby other biological molecules, including proteins, are broken down and synthesised. Proteins are also found as structural components of the body in microscopic structures such as the membrane surrounding human cells, where they also have other functions, and in more visible structures such as skin and hair.

Amino acids

Proteins are polymers of amino acids and some understanding of the amino acids is required in order to understand the structure and function of proteins. Amino acids are unique molecules which have both a carboxylic acid group and an amino group (COOHRCHNH$_2$), both of which have been described above. The structure of a typical amino acid is shown in Figure 2.2. When they are dissolved in solution the carboxylic part of the molecule tends to be negatively charged and the amino end tends to have a positive charge. Molecules that have this property of simultaneously displaying different charges are known as amphibolic molecules. Twenty amino acids are found in the human body and some of these are referred to as essential amino acids. This means that they must be taken in the diet because the human body is incapable of making them. There is a shorthand way of writing the amino acids and this is shown in Table 2.3.

Each of the 20 amino acids has, essentially, the same structure with a central

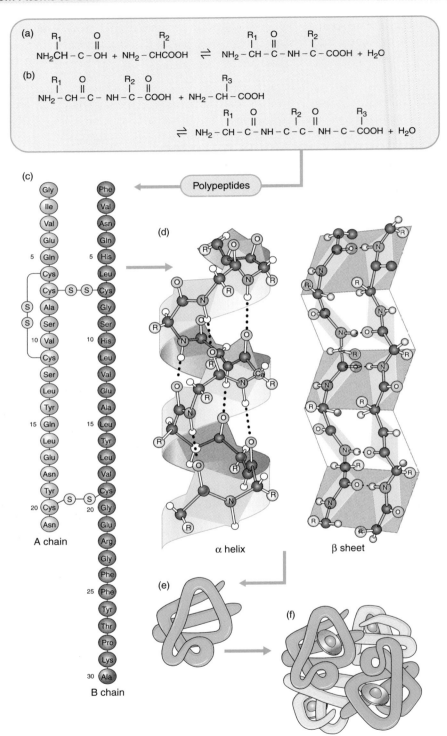

Fig. 2.2 *Amino acids and proteins. (a) Formation of a dipeptide; (b) formation of a tripeptide; (c) primary structure of insulin; (d) features of the secondary structure of a protein; (e) tertiary structure of a protein; (f) quaternary structure of a protein (haemoglobin).*

carbon atom and a hydrogen atom, a carboxylic acid group and an amino acid group covalently bound. The distinguishing features between amino acids is the -R group, which can be a hydrogen atom, in the case of the amino acid glycine, or a very large group containing carbon rings, as in the case of tryptophan. A few common amino acid structures are shown in Table 2.3. The -R groups not only distinguish the amino acids in terms of structure, they also confer unique properties on each. Some have additional amino groups and carboxylic acid groups and these will clearly confer alkaline and acidic properties, respectively.

TABLE 2.3	*Amino Acids*	
Name	*Symbol*	*Empirical structure*
Glycine	Gly	$CH_2(NH_2)CO_2H$
Alanine	Ala	$CH_3CH(NH_2)CO_2H$
Valine	Val	$(CH_3)CHCH(NH_2)CO_2H$
Cysteine	Cys	$HSCH_2CH(NH_2)CO_2H$

The peptide bond

The amphibolic nature of the amino acid confers another property whereby amino acids can form covalent bonds, called peptide bonds, between pairs of amino acids and other amino acids may be added because the new molecule remains amphibolic. The formation of a peptide bond is shown in Figure 2.2. Note that water is removed from the pair of amino acids and this is, therefore, a condensation reaction. Figure 2.2 also shows how further amino acids may be added by subsequent formation of peptide bonds and, in this way, a polymer of amino acids is synthesised. The process of polymerisation through peptide bonding is the chemical basis of protein structure.

> Amino acids all have essentially the same structure with an amino group and a carboxylic acid group at either end of the molecule. The 20 amino acids in the body are characterised by their different side (R) groups. Amino acids form proteins and are held together by covalent bonds called peptide bonds.

Peptides, polypeptides and proteins

The kind of polymer that is formed by the polymerisation of amino acids is known as a peptide. A polymer of two amino acids is called a dipeptide and a polymer of three peptides is known as a tripeptide. Five amino acids form a pentapeptide and up to eight amino acids form an oligopeptide. Longer chains of up to 50 amino acids are known as polypeptides and polymers of greater than 50 amino acids are known as proteins.

As protein polymers are synthesised in the human body, specific amino acids are added at each point. The resulting chain of amino acids has a unique sequence for each type of protein, a process that is determined genetically, and this will be described further below. As a chain of amino acids grows it begins to conform to shapes by bending and twisting according to the sequence of amino acids and each protein has a unique shape. Furthermore, some chains of amino acids come together to form groups and this is particularly the case in many enzymes and in the common blood protein, haemoglobin (Ch. 9). These sequences and shapes are described as the primary, secondary, tertiary and quaternary structures of proteins, which will be described in the following sections.

> Protein molecules all have a primary structure dictated by the sequence of amino acids in the protein chains but can also conform to secondary, tertiary and quaternary structures as explained in the text.

Primary structure of proteins

The primary structure of a protein molecule is the sequence of amino acids in the polypeptide chain. Each protein in the human body has a unique sequence of amino acids, which is genetically determined, and the same proteins in other species often have similar, but not identical, sequences.

The shapes that proteins conform to and the functions which they subsequently serve are dependent on the primary structure. Any alteration in primary structure may result in a change in shape or function or both. Such changes may take place as a result of chemical alteration of amino acids in the polypeptide chain or alternative amino acids may be inserted because of genetic change, which may be the result of a process known as mutation.

The first protein for which the primary sequence was elucidated was the hormone insulin, which has 50 amino acids. Using the shorthand notation for amino acids described above, the structure of insulin is shown in Figure 2.2.

Secondary structure of proteins

The secondary structure of proteins describes two particular types of shape to which the polypeptide chain may conform and these are called α helices and β pleated sheets. Schematic examples are shown in Figure 2.2 and, as indicated in this figure, the forces that hold these two particular types of structure together are hydrogen bonds (Ch. 1).

Clearly, the secondary structure of a protein is dependent upon the primary structure. The secondary structure depends upon amino acids with particular properties, i.e. the ability to hydrogen bond, being situated at particular positions in the polypeptide chain in order for the folding and pleating to take place.

The importance of the hydrogen bond in biological systems is also demonstrated. Because the function of a protein is dependent upon its structure, it is clear that some of the structure and functions would not be possible without hydrogen bonding.

Tertiary structure of proteins

Not every protein has a tertiary structure and it is possible for a protein to have a quaternary structure without having a tertiary structure. Tertiary structure results from folding and twisting of regions of the polypeptide chain giving the protein a unique three-dimensional structure.

Enzymes that have a tertiary structure are called globular proteins and this type of structure is very common in enzymes. The structure of a typical globular protein is shown in Figure 2.2.

Several different forces hold the tertiary structure of proteins together, including hydrogen bonds (Ch. 1) between different regions of the polypeptide chain and, in some cases, covalent bonds between sulphur atoms, which are contained in the amino acid cysteine (Table 2.3). The latter types of bonds are called disulphide bridges. Other regions of the protein chain which are hydrophobic (i.e. repelled by water) are also held together by hydrophobic interactions. The concept of hydrophobic molecules will be considered in more detail in the section below on lipids.

In proteins that are enzymes the tertiary structure brings together particular parts of the polypeptide chain which can catalyse particular reactions. The specific region of an enzyme that can catalyse a chemical reaction is known as its active site. For example, the enzyme glucose-6-phosphate has an active site that can bring together glucose and phosphate and facilitate the covalent bonding of phosphate to glucose at a specific site on the glucose molecule.

Quaternary structure of proteins

Quaternary structure is the highest structure to which a protein can conform and this occurs when more than one protein molecule is brought together. Quaternary structure may offer proteins structural and functional advantages.

An example of a protein where structural advantage is conferred is the protein collagen, which is found in skin and cartilage. Collagen is composed of several strands of protein wound round one another and covalently bonded where hydroxyproline molecules lie next to one another. Hydroxyproline is a form of the amino acid proline, which has a hydroxyl ion attached to it. The quaternary structure lends strength to the collagen molecules, which exist as strands, and it has been observed that, as people age, there are a greater number of covalent bonds between hydroxyproline molecules and this may account for the decreasing flexibility of skin and other tissues containing collagen, such as tendons and ligaments, as people become older. Another example of a protein with a quaternary structure held together by covalent bonds is the keratin in hair where disulphide linkages exist between chains of keratin. The breaking and reformation of the disulphide linkages in the keratin in hair is the basis of perming whereby different shapes are artificially introduced in hair.

Globular proteins can also be brought together to form a quaternary structure and the same forces that hold tertiary structures together hold quaternary structures together, including hydrogen bonding (Ch. 1), hydrophobic interactions and covalent bonding by disulphide bridges. Quaternary structure is common in enzymes where the quaternary structure may confer a functional advantage such that, when one protein molecule binds and catalyses a reaction, a slight change in shape takes place which is transmitted to the other protein molecules and they are prepared to bind and catalyse further reactions. However, one of the best examples of a protein with a quaternary structure is the blood protein haemoglobin, which is composed of four similar, but not identical, globular proteins. Two of the protein molecules are identical as are the other two, as shown in Figure 2.2. Haemoglobin is responsible for binding oxygen molecules in the lungs and delivering them to other tissues where the oxygen molecules are released in order to take part in the metabolic reactions, called respiration, which are essential for life (Ch. 10). The quaternary structure of haemoglobin allows it efficiently to bind oxygen where it is abundant, as in the lungs, and to release it where it is required, for example, in the muscles. The properties of haemoglobin will be described further in a subsequent chapter.

THE NUCLEIC ACIDS

The nucleic acids are possibly the most complex of the biological molecules and they are considered next because of their intimate relationship to protein structure. The nucleic acids are the material from which genes are made; they are polymers of organic molecules called nucleotides, of which there are five types in the genetic material (Ch. 3). Nucleic acids exist as either ribonucleic acid (RNA) or deoxyribonucleic acid (DNA) owing to a small difference in the structure of the nucleotides in each.

The five nucleotides are adenine, guanine, cytosine, thymine and uracil. Adenine and guanine are described as purine bases and the remainder are described as pyrimidine bases. The common feature of the nucleotides is that they all have a ring-like structure containing carbon and nitrogen, as shown in Figure 2.3. The first four (adenine, guanine, cytosine and thymine) are all found in DNA and uracil replaces thymine in RNA.

> The nucleic acids DNA and RNA both contain the nucleotides adenine, guanine and cytosine; DNA contains thymine and RNA contains uracil.
> RNA is a single-stranded molecule and DNA is a double-stranded molecule.

Nucleotides all have the same essential structure containing a base (either a purine or a pyrimidine ring), a carbohydrate (to be considered below) molecule (either ribose or deoxyribose) and a phosphate group. A schematic structure for a nucleotide is shown in Figure 2.3. The polymerisation of nucleic acids takes place by the formation of a covalent bond between the phosphate group and the hydroxyl group of the sugar molecule and this bond is known as a phosphodiester linkage. Similarly to the way in which a long chain of amino acids can form a polypeptide, chains of nucleotides can form polynucleotides.

RNA forms single polynucleotide strands and DNA forms double strands, which have a unique structure called a double helix. The discovery of the double helical structure of DNA in 1953 by James Watson and Francis Crick was a turning point in biological sciences and, arguably, the most important discovery ever. This structure, along with the observation that, in DNA, adenine and thymine are always present in equal amounts and, likewise, guanine and cytosine, led to the elucidation of the mechanism underlying genetics. Genes are unique chemical codes for specific characteristics or traits, and there are mechanisms whereby these codes are passed down through generations in the process of reproduction and maintained in organisms, such as the human body, during

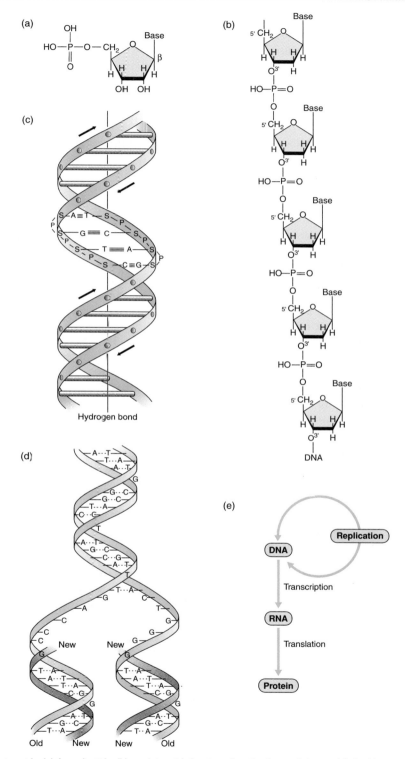

Fig. 2.3 *Nucleic acids. (a) A nucleotide; (b) nucleic acid showing phosphodiester linkages; (c) double-stranded quaternary structure of DNA; (d) unwinding and replication of DNA; (e) the central dogma of genetics.*

the process of cell division. Moreover, the function of RNA, which is to transmit genetic information to the synthesis of protein, was elucidated and the process known as the central dogma (to be described below), whereby genetic information is conserved in cell division and transmitted into protein synthesis, was described.

The double helix

One of the questions answered by the discovery of the double helical structure of DNA was why adenine and thymine, and guanine and cytosine were always present in equal amounts. It was demonstrated that adenine and thymine always form base pairs which lie opposite one another in the double helix, and the same is true for guanine and cytosine. Figure 2.3 shows the structure of a typical region of DNA with the base pairing as described above. One of the reasons why particular bases pair up opposite one another in the strand is that this maximises the number of hydrogen bonds that can be formed between them. In fact, it is hydrogen bonds that hold the double helix together and this is another demonstration of the importance of hydrogen bonds in the human body.

Another question that was answered by the discovery of the double helical structure of DNA was the mechanism whereby the genetic code may be conserved and passed on when cells divide and between generations (Ch. 3). It became immediately apparent that the sequence of bases in DNA may, in fact, constitute a code for the genes that control heredity and development. It also suggested how the code (the genetic code) may be conserved as cells divide with one strand of the double helix acting as a template for the synthesis of the other. For this to happen it would be necessary for the double helix to unwind and this, indeed, has since been demonstrated. Only one of the strands carries the genetic code and this is called the sense strand. The other strand is called the anti-sense strand. However, as shown in Figure 2.3, when a double helix unwinds, two new strands of DNA, each containing a sense strand and an anti-sense strand but both identical to the original strand, are formed. This process is called replication.

The genetic code is not only conserved, when cells divide, by replication of DNA, it is also copied into RNA from the sense strand by a process called transcription. In the process of transcription, regions of DNA unwind and, instead of a DNA molecule being replicated, a single strand of RNA is transcribed. As described above, RNA not only differs in that it contains ribose as opposed to deoxyribose, but it also contains uracil in place of thymine. However, the genetic code contained in DNA is passed on to the RNA by the process of transcription.

In the same way as the two strands of DNA are templates for the replication of DNA and the sense strand of DNA is a template for the transcription of RNA, the single strand of RNA is a template for the synthesis of polypeptide chains and proteins. This process is called translation and the genetic code that is contained in RNA molecules is used to incorporate amino acids into polypeptide chains in the specific sequence referred to above.

The central dogma

The details of how and where the processes of replication, transcription and translation take place in human cells will be described in a subsequent chapter.

In summary, these processes are called the central dogma (of genetics) and this dogma states that information, in the form of the genetic code, always flows in one direction from DNA to protein through the processes of replication, transcription and translation, as shown in Figure 2.3. It should be noted, however, that this dogma does not hold for certain viruses that only contain RNA as their genetic material (for example, the human immunodeficiency virus (HIV) which causes acquired immune deficiency syndrome (AIDS)) and these have the ability to form DNA from RNA, thereby reversing a part of the central dogma.

The genetic code

The existence of a genetic code has already been referred to and the central dogma summarises how the sequence of bases in the nucleic acids codes for the incorporation of amino acids into proteins. There are, however, only four bases in the nucleic acids and 20 amino acids in proteins. Clearly, single bases cannot code for single amino acids and, in fact, it has been established that triplets of bases code for the incorporation of amino acids into proteins. These triplets are referred to as codons and the entire set of codons, which code for the incorporation of all amino acids into protein, has been elucidated; this is what is known as the genetic code. The genetic code for some of the amino acids is shown in Table 2.4.

TABLE 2.4	The Genetic Code for Some Amino Acids
Triplet code	Amino acid
UUU	Phenylalanine
GGG	Glycine
GCU	Alanine
UGU	Cysteine

The genetic code is composed of triplets of nucleotide bases called triplets and these code for the 20 amino acids found in the body.

CARBOHYDRATES

Carbohydrates are more commonly called sugars. The most familiar sugars are glucose, which is the end product of photosynthesis in plants, and also sucrose, which is the form in which carbohydrate is transported and stored in many plants and which we use as a sweetener in drinks and baking. Carbohydrates all contain carbon, hydrogen and oxygen, and the ratio of hydrogen to oxygen in the common sugars is 2:1 (i.e. the same as water) and this is the basis of the name carbohydrate. This ratio can be seen in glucose ($C_6H_{12}O_6$) and also in sucrose ($C_{12}H_{22}O_{11}$). Types of sugars are labelled according to the number of carbon molecules contained; therefore, glucose and fructose are called hexoses because they contain six carbon atoms and the ribose, which is contained in the nucleic acids, is called a pentose because it contains five carbon atoms.

The structure of some common hexose and pentose sugars is shown in Table 2.5. It is clear from the structures shown in the table that carbohydrates contain many hydroxl groups and some have aldehyde and others ketone groups. They are also known as polyhydroxyl aldehydes and polyhydroxyl ketones. The table also shows how the carbohydrates may be represented either as chains or as cyclic forms and this is due to an interaction between either an aldehyde or ketone group and a hydroxyl group further along the chain. In solution an equilibrium exists between the open and the cyclic form of carbohydrates.

TABLE 2.5	Carbohydrates – Monosaccharides		
Type	Name	Empirical formula	Structure
Pentose	Ribose	$C_5H_{10}O_5$	
Hexose	Glucose	$C_6H_{12}O_6$	
	Fructose	$C_6H_{12}O_6$	
	Galactose	$C_6H_{12}O_6$	

Isomers

A feature of organic chemistry that has not been covered thus far is that of isomerisation and this is demonstrated well by the carbohydrates. An isomer is an alternative form of a compound with the same empirical structure. Taking glucose and fructose as examples, which both have the same empirical formula $C_6H_{12}O_6$, it is clear that they have different structures by referring to Table 2.5. This can be demonstrated by tasting glucose and fructose; fructose is a much sweeter sugar. This also demonstrates the limitation in using the empirical formula for an element in order to explain its structure, as discussed above.

Carbohydrate polymers

Single carbohydrate molecules, such as glucose and fructose, are called mono-saccharides. Sugar molecules may form covalent bonds called glycosidic link-ages and, thereby, polymerise to form polysaccharides. Polysaccharides are less complex than proteins and nucleic acids in that they do not have specific sequences of different carbohydrates in the polymers. Polysaccharides are com-posed of the same monosaccharide. For example, the common plant polysac-charide, starch, is composed entirely of glucose molecules as is glycogen in the human body.

There are many different classes of polysaccharides including disaccharides, trisaccharides and oligosaccharides but it is only necessary to consider a few monosaccharides, disaccharides and polysaccharides in order to understand their function in the human body. Table 2.6 shows three common monosaccha-rides and the corresponding disaccharides that can be formed from them. Sucrose is a common form of carbohydrate found in plants, and particular plants such as sugar cane and sugar beet are abundant in sucrose. Lactose is the form of sugar found in milk and maltose is found in cereals. In all cases these disaccharides must be broken down into monosaccharides in order to be absorbed by the human body and used in metabolism, and enzymes that effect this are found in the intestine. Some individuals are unable to break down lac-tose and are thus described as being lactose intolerant. As a result of the process of osmosis, water is retained in the gut and this causes the lactose-intolerant person to feel bloated and to pass watery faeces.

TABLE 2.6	Carbohydrates – Disaccharides	
Constituent monosaccharides	Disaccharide
Glucose and glucose	Maltose
Glucose and fructose	Sucrose
Glucose and galactose	Lactose

Starch

Starch is commonly used in plants as a storage form of carbohydrate; potatoes, for example, are rich in starch. Before this can be used in the human body for nutrition it has to be broken down by enzymes in the mouth and intestine into glucose, which can then be absorbed and used in metabolism. Polysaccharide forms of carbohydrate are required because they are less soluble than monosac-charide or disaccharide forms and they can, therefore, be stored more easily in the cells responsible for their storage.

Starch is a polymer of glucose and exists in two forms: amylose and amylopectin.

Starch exists in two forms called, respectively, amylose and amylopectin. The structures of these two forms of starch are shown in Figure 2.4. It can be seen

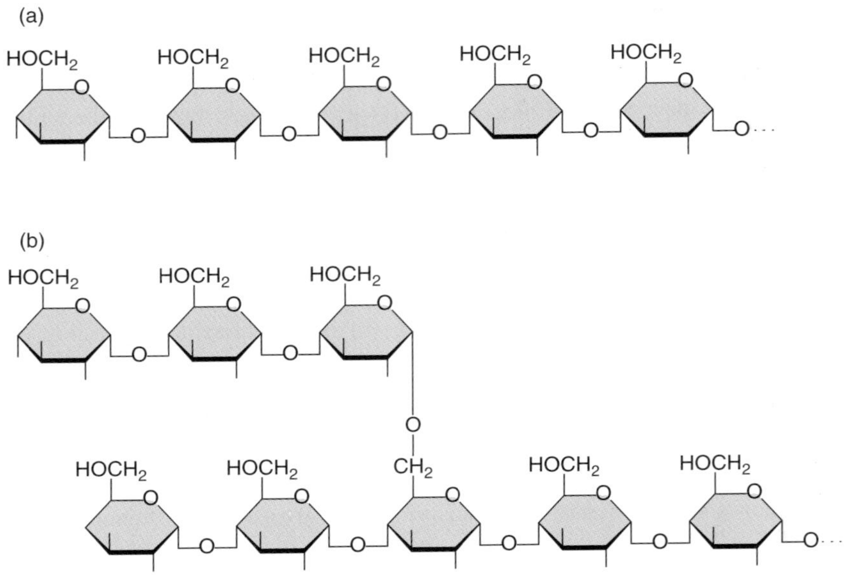

(a)

(b)

Fig. 2.4   *Structure of starch. (a) Amylose; (b) amylopectin.*

that in the branched form of starch two types of glycosidic linkages are formed: those within the chains and those between chains. In the mouth only those within the chains can be broken down and this leaves a substance called limit dextran, which can only be fully broken down in the intestine. The process whereby nutrients such as starch are broken down is called digestion.

LIPIDS

The lipids are a group of organic molecules that are insoluble in water. They are, however, soluble in other substances called organic solvents, of which the liquid hydrocarbons, such as petrol, are examples. A substance that is soluble in water is described as being polar and this indicates that it has small areas of positive and negative charge on it. The concept of polarity was described above in relation to the formation of hydrogen bonds which result from the polarisation of the covalent bond between hydrogen and oxygen in water molecules. These substances can usually be identified from this structure because they contain oxygen atoms and hydroxyl groups and the carbohydrates are common examples.

Substances, such as the lipids, are conversely described as being non-polar and because they do not have areas where polarisation can occur, they are unable to dissolve in water. Polarity and non-polarity may exist in the same molecule giving it interesting properties, which will be described below in a type of lipid called the phospholipids.

Classes of lipids

Two classes of lipids will be described here: the simple and the compound lipids.

Simple lipids are esters (described above) of a molecule with three hydroxyl groups (a tri-alcohol) called glycerol and three molecules of a carboxylic acid attached. These are also known as the triglycerides and these are the form of fat which is taken in the diet. Triglycerides are sometimes referred to as fats, when they are in the solid state, and oils, when they are in the liquid state. The carboxylic acids that form ester bonds with glycerol are described as the fatty acids and these include palmitic acid and stearic acid.

Fatty acids

The features that distinguish fatty acids are the length of the hydrocarbon chain attached to the hydroxyl group and whether or not the molecule is saturated (i.e. contains double bonds) or not. Some common examples of saturated and non-saturated fatty acids are shown in Table 2.7 and the structure of a triglyceride molecule is shown in Figure 2.5.

TABLE 2.7	Fatty Acids		
Type	Name	Empirical formula	
Saturated	Palmitic acid	$CH_3(CH_2)_{14}CO_2H$	
	Stearic acid	$CH_3(CH_2)_{16}CO_2H$	
Unsaturated	Oleic acid	$CH_3(CH_2)_7=CH(CH_2)_7CO_2H$	
	Linoleic acid	$CH_3(CH_2)_4(CH=CHCH_2)_2(CH_2)_6CO_2H$	

Triglycerides in water

Because the triglycerides are not soluble, if they are mixed with water they float to the top and form an oily layer on the surface of the water. If, however, a mixture of triglyceride and water is shaken very vigorously the layer will be broken down into small particles, or globules, of triglyceride, which will spread out through the water and form an emulsion of suspended triglyceride globules. If the emulsion is left to stand, however, the small globules will eventually float to the top and a layer will be formed again.

Detergents

Detergents are molecules that have a polar and a non-polar end; the concept of detergents is familiar from washing powders, which contain these molecules in order to facilitate the removal of oily stains from clothes. Soap molecules also have this property of having both polar and non-polar regions. The polar regions are also described as being hydrophilic (i.e. attracted to water) and the non-polar regions are described as being hydrophobic (i.e. repelled by water).

Detergents are molecules that have an end which is attracted to water (hydrophilic) and an end which is repelled by water (hydrophobic). The phospholipids of which the plasma membrane is formed are detergent molecules.

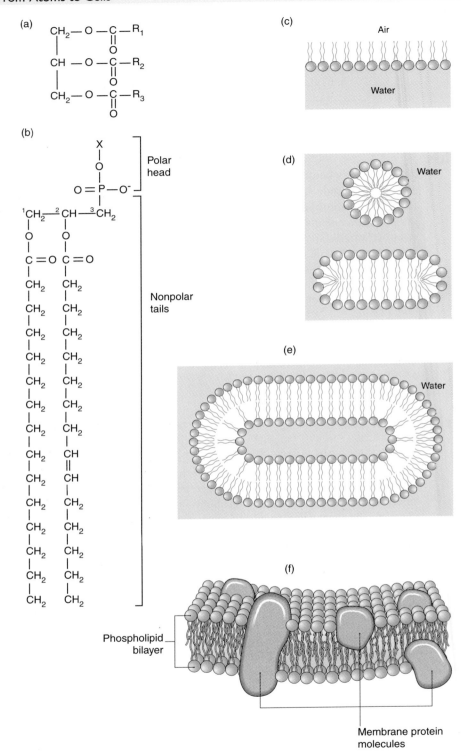

Fig. 2.5   *Lipids. (a) Triglyceride molecule (R = hydrocarbon chain); (b) phospholipid molecule; (c) phospholipid in water; (d) micelles in water; (e) a liposome in water; (f) the plasma membrane.*

If a detergent is added to a mixture of triglyceride and water it encourages the formation of an emulsion and will maintain the emulsion suspension in the water. The detergent is behaving in such a way that the non-polar end is being attracted to the fat globules while the polar head remains in the water, as shown in Figure 2.5. In this way the suspension is maintained and, indeed, detergents encourage the breakdown of triglyceride layers on the surface of water.

Phospholipids

Phospholipids belong to the class of compound lipids because, in addition to a glycerol molecule and two (as opposed to three) fatty acid molecules, they also contain a phosphate group, which is polar. As described above therefore, the phospholipids are essentially detergent molecules with a polar and non-polar region. The structure of a typical phospholipid is shown in Figure 2.5 and this structure gives the molecule properties that are important in the human body where phospholipids are an essential component of the plasma membrane, which surrounds the human cell.

The participation of the phospholipid can be described by considering how phospholipids behave when mixed with water. If a phospholipid is poured into water it behaves like a triglyceride and forms a layer on the top of the water. However, because of the properties of the phospholipid, the molecules orient themselves such that the polar regions, described as the head, of the molecules all remain in the water while the non-polar region, described as the tail, projects out of the water, as shown in Figure 2.5.

Furthermore, if a phospholipid and water mixture is shaken vigorously an emulsion is formed and the phospholipid droplets suspended in the water form micelles, which are spherical groups of molecules with the non-polar tails in the middle and the polar heads on the surface of the sphere. This is shown in Figure 2.5.

Finally, if a phospholipid and water mixture is subjected to high-frequency sound, a process known as sonication, a unique structure called a liposome is formed and this is shown in Figure 2.5. The unique feature of the liposome is that it is composed of a phospholipid bilayer; the bilayer, which is surrounded by water with the hydrophilic heads of the molecules on the surface, also encloses some water and the inner surface of the liposome is also lined by hydrophilic heads. The hydrophobic tails of the phospholipid molecules line up on the inner region of the phospholipid bilayer. The importance of this phenomenon in the human body is that it is the form taken by the plasma membrane. The plasma membrane is, essentially, a phospholipid bilayer with protein molecules embedded in it, as shown in Figure 2.5, and this structure will be considered in more detail in Chapter 4.

SUMMARY

Following the chapter on chemistry, this chapter considered a particular range of molecules involved in the structure and function of the human body. Beginning with a review of organic chemistry the following types of biological molecules were considered: proteins, nucleic acids, carbohydrates and lipids. In each case the unique type of covalent bond between the building blocks of the biological molecules was shown and the place of hydrogen bonding in the structure of proteins and nucleic acids was demonstrated. In each case the particular structural and functional position of the biological molecules in the human body was exemplified: for example, the enzymes, genes, metabolic substrates and the plasma membrane in the case of protein, nucleic acid, carbohydrate and lipid, respectively.

QUESTIONS

1. Can you explain the primary, secondary, tertiary and quaternary structure of proteins?

2. Describe the process whereby genetic information is passed from DNA to proteins.

3. What are the essential features of the phospholipid molecule and how does this type of molecule contribute to the structure of the cell membrane?

FURTHER READING

Montague S, Knight D (1996) Cell structure and function, growth and development. In: Hinchliff S, Montague S, Watson R (eds) *Physiology for nursing practice, 2nd edn.* Baillière Tindall, London, pp 49–69

Watson R (1995) *Anatomy and physiology for nurses, 10th edn.* Baillière Tindall, London

3 Genetics

Jennie Wilson

After reading this chapter you should understand:
- how characteristics are passed down from one generation to the next
- how cells are able to conserve genetic information as they divide
- how gametes (egg and sperm cells) are produced
- what happens at fertilisation.

INTRODUCTION

In order to reproduce, an organism must have a mechanism whereby it can transfer information about how it is constructed to its offspring. Genetics is the study of this inheritance and the transmission of traits or characteristics from one generation to the next. The science of genetics began with a nineteenth century monk called Gregor Mendel who laid the foundations for modern genetics, long before DNA was identified as the means by which the characteristics of an organism are passed to the next generation. The principles of heredity identified by Mendel are still valid, even though we now have a much better understanding of many of the biological processes involved

The genetic makeup of an individual is referred to as their genotype whilst their appearance is called the phenotype. Mendel discovered that it is not possible to know everything about the genotype of an organism by only knowing the phenotype, but that it was possible to have some understanding of the genotype by studying the transmission of phenotypic characteristics from generation to generation.

For thousands of years, people have been taking advantage of the genetic diversity within a species by selectively breeding those animals or crops with desirable characteristics and such experimentation has played an important role in agriculture. For example, dogs were probably derived from wolves and over 10 000 years have been developed, by selective breeding, into the 100 or more contemporary breeds of domestic dog. Although these breeds differ enormously in size and appearance, they all belong to the same species and can therefore interbreed. Likewise, crops such as wheat and maize have been gradually developed from species of wild grass by selecting those which produce the largest grains and highest yields.

The advances in understanding how genetic information is stored, transferred, decoded and expressed have led to another field of genetic study: molecular genetics. Since the 1980s, techniques have been available that enable individual genes to be identified and transferred into other individuals. These techniques have been used to great benefit, for example the artificial production of human insulin has been made possible by inserting the insulin gene into the genome of yeast, but they also have the potential to cause serious adverse environmental and social effects.

The first part of this chapter reviews the molecular processes that are involved in the transfer of genetic information from parent to offspring. The second part looks at the inheritance of genetic traits and genetic disorders.

THE GENOME OF THE CELL

The structure of the proteins required to construct every type of cell in the body is encoded in the DNA, the genome, of every cell (Ch. 2). Each segment of DNA that carries the code for a single protein is called a gene. There are up to 100 000 genes in the whole genome and it is this set of genes which provides the mechanism for the transfer of information. Some of the genes determine structural proteins; others determine transport proteins, membrane receptors and enzymes, which control the activity of the cell. The same set of genes is present in every cell of the body (except mature erythrocytes, which have no nucleus) but, because not all the proteins are required in every cell, some genes will be switched off so that they are not transcribed into their corresponding protein.

> Every cell of the body, except red blood cells which lack a nucleus, contain all of the genetic information of the body. However, not all of this information is expressed by every cell.

Genes are organised into chromosomes. Each chromosome is a single molecule of DNA together with some proteins and RNA. The particular way in which the DNA and proteins are twisted and coiled is probably important in regulating which of the genes are switched on or off. The chromosomes of a cell are only visible during certain stages of cell division.

Humans, like other higher organisms, are diploid, i.e. they carry two copies of each different chromosome in their genome. In a typical human cell, there are 22 different chromosomes, together with another copy of each. These pairs of homologous chromosomes are called autosomes. The genome also contains two sex chromosomes which in the female are homologous, both X chromosomes, but in the male are non-homologous, an X and a Y chromosome. This makes a total of 46 chromosomes in the human cell.

In most circumstances, the organism only needs a single copy of each gene to grow and survive, but carrying two copies can confer considerable benefits. If one gene is damaged by mutation the organism may still be able to survive if the second copy is unaffected. On the other hand, advantageous mutations that may spoil the original function of the gene can be incorporated into the genome because the spare copy of the original gene will still be present. This ability to develop new genes through mutation of the spare copies of existing genes enables diploid organisms to improve and develop their genome.

Even in homologous chromosomes, genes governing a particular characteristic may occur in several different forms. These different versions of the same gene are called alleles. For example, the gene determining eye colour may be for blue eyes or brown eyes. If the two copies of the same gene are identical, i.e. if they are both for blue eyes, they are called homozygous, but if they are different, i.e. if one is for blue eyes and the other brown eyes, then they are heterozygous. Some forms of a gene are dominant, i.e. the trait that they determine will be displayed even if the gene is present on only one of the chromosomes in the pair. Traits dictated by recessive genes will only be displayed if both copies of the gene in the chromosome pair are the same.

> Genes are present in pairs called alleles. The genes are not always the same, e.g. one may be for blue eyes and one may be for brown eyes, and sometimes one allele is dominant, meaning that only its genetic information is expressed.

Some alleles can be co-dominant, which means if they are present together in a chromosome pair they are both expressed, e.g. an AB blood group occurs when a person has both the A blood group gene and the B blood group gene.

The X and Y chromosomes have a small section that contains the same genes, which allows them to pair up during cell division. Because females carry two X chromosomes, all eggs have an X chromosome. The male gamete will determine the sex of the offspring: 50% of the sperm will have a Y chromosome and will form a male offspring after fertilisation with the egg, and the other half will have an X chromosome and will form a female offspring. The Y chromosome is very small and contains very few genes. The X chromosome has many genes that are not related to sexual differentiation, such as aspects of blood grouping, glucose metabolism and the nervous system.

Female cells contain two copies of the X chromosome but, to avoid making twice the amount of X chromosome products, have developed a mechanism of inactivating one copy. The copy is reactivated during the formation of eggs so that the female can pass on either copy of the X chromosome.

Cell division

When cells divide into two, an exact copy of the genetic information is made and one copy is transferred into each daughter cell. This type of cell division is called mitosis and occurs in all types of cells to enable tissue growth and replacement (Fig. 3.1).

The structure of DNA is the key to how this transfer of information can occur. Because the two strands in the double helix of DNA are complementary, both strands carry the same genetic code and one strand can be used to build a copy of the second. The two DNA strands are separated and each acts as a template for the construction of its partner strand, resulting in the production of a duplicate copy of the genetic information. Each copy will consist of one original strand and one newly synthesised strand (Ch. 2).

SEXUAL REPRODUCTION

Sexual reproduction involves the mixing of genomes from two individuals to produce offspring that are genetically different from their parents and from each

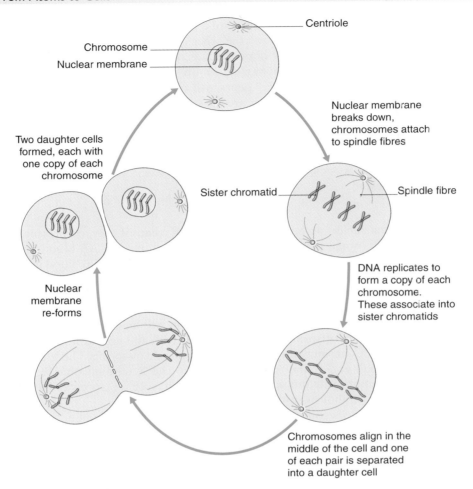

Centriole

Chromosome

Nuclear membrane

Nuclear membrane breaks down, chromosomes attach to spindle fibres

Two daughter cells formed, each with one copy of each chromosome

Sister chromatid

Spindle fibre

DNA replicates to form a copy of each chromosome. These associate into sister chromatids

Nuclear membrane re-forms

Chromosomes align in the middle of the cell and one of each pair is separated into a daughter cell

Fig. 3.1 *Stages in cell division by mitosis.*

other. This is achieved by fusing two cells, one from each parent. To avoid the daughter cell having two sets of chromosomes, the cells which fuse are haploid, i.e. they contain a single set of chromosomes with only one copy of each gene. Haploid cells are made by a special form of cell division called meiosis, which only occurs in the production of eggs or sperm in the gonads. During fertilisation, a sperm cell fuses with an egg, the full complement of chromosomes is restored and the genetic material in the resulting offspring will be a unique mixture of genes from the two parents.

Sexual reproduction is needed to help the chromosome remain diploid in successive generations. If a diploid organism did not reproduce sexually it would not mix genes between individuals, the two copies of each gene could gradually evolve differently and eventually would no longer function as diploid. Because the offspring from sexual reproduction acquire their genome from two individuals, a lethal mutation in a gene from one parent will in most cases be paired with a functional gene from the other parent. Where both parents have the lethal mutation, only one in four of the progeny will have both mutated genes; the other three will have one mutated and one functional gene and therefore will be

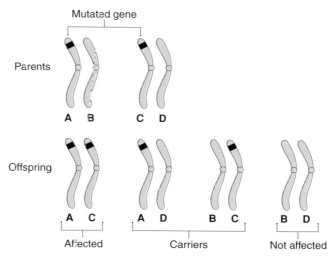

Fig. 3.2 *Inheritance of a lethal mutation. A lethal gene mutation carried on one chromosome of each parent is paired with a functional gene and therefore is not expressed. Offspring will inherit one chromosome from each parent, I in 2 will carry an abnormal gene and I in 4 will inherit two copies of the lethal mutation.*

able to survive (Fig. 3.2). Mixing the genomes of two individuals also provides the opportunity to produce new collections of genes. In a variable and regularly changing environment, some combinations of genes will favour survival over others.

Meiosis

In mitosis the cell divides to produce two identical daughter cells, each with a full complement of chromosomes (Fig. 3.3). In meiosis the chromosomes are divided such that each daughter cell is haploid, containing only one version of each pair of chromosomes. This is one of the principles discovered by Mendel and is called Mendel's law of segregation.

Because the chromosomes in a pair are separated and then randomly assigned to a daughter cell, each will contain one chromosome from each pair and these will be a mixture of paternal and maternal chromosomes. This principle was also described by Mendel and is called Mendel's law of independent assortment.

The haploid cells produced after meiotic division are called gametes and the process by which they are formed is called gametogenesis. Unlike mitosis, in which a single division results in two daughter cells, in meiosis there are two cell divisions resulting in the formation of four daughter cells, each with a haploid number of chromosomes, from a single diploid cell. The stages in meiosis are described in Figure 3.3.

Sex cells, or gametes (eggs and sperm), are produced such that they contain only one of the genes from each allele in the body. Each gamete is unique in terms of the composition of genes it contains.

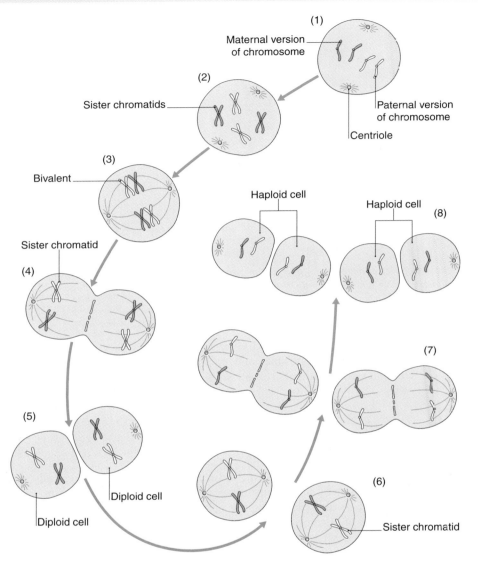

Fig. 3.3   *Stages in cell division by meiosis. (1) The chromosomal DNA is replicated and the two copies remain together as sister chromatids. (2) The sister chromatids associate with those formed from the corresponding chromosome with the same gene set and assemble on the spindle as four chromatid structures, called bivalents. The pairs of chromatids cross-over each other, paternal and maternal chromatids become attached at these points and sections of chromosome are exchanged. (3) Each pair of sister chromatids behaves as a single unit, separating from the bivalent structure together, one pair of chromatids moving to each daughter cell. (4) The cell divides into two. This first meiotic division results in two daughter cells, still with a diploid number of chromosomes. (5) The two copies of each chromosome in these diploid cells are the same, having been derived from either the paternal or maternal chromosome, not one from each parent. This is because the sister chromatids are moved into the daughter cells still in their pairs and not separated into independent chromosomes, as occurs in mitosis. These pairs do not separate into independent chromosomes but remain associated, until the second division of meiosis. (6) In the second meiotic division, a spindle is formed in each of the daughter cells, the sister chromatids line up on the spindle and separate into two more daughter cells. (7) This results in four cells, each with half the number of chromosomes (haploid); they contain one copy of each chromosome, either maternal or paternal, instead of a maternal and paternal copy.*

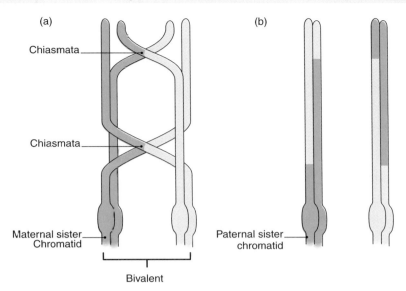

Fig. 3.4 *Crossing-over during meiotic cell division. (a) Four chromatids arranged in two pairs intermingle and become attached at the points where they cross-over. Sections of DNA break off and rejoin a different chromatid at these points. (b) Following crossing-over, each sister chromatid contains a mixture of maternal and paternal genes.*

In addition to mixing of maternal and paternal chromosomes in the daughter cells, genes are also redistributed by genetic recombination, which occurs during a process called chromosomal crossing-over. This process happens during the first meiotic division when the sister chromatids from each pair of chromosomes assemble together as a bivalent structure. The maternal and paternal chromatids intertwine and at the points where the chromatids cross over they become attached. Sections of DNA are exchanged between each chromosome in the pair by breaking off and rejoining at the same point on a different chromatid. Between two and three of these points, called chiasmata, occur on each chromosome so that after meiosis a chromosome will contain a mixture of paternal and maternal genes, rather than only maternal or only paternal genes (Fig. 3.4).

Linked genes

Genes that are in close proximity to each other along the length of the chromosome are less likely to be separated during crossing-over. They will end up in the same gamete and will therefore be inherited together. Such genes are considered as linked and can be useful in the study of genetics.

GAMETE FORMATION

The cells that are destined to become the germ cells are determined early in the development of the embryo. By the third month of gestation these primordial germ cells have migrated to the developing gonads, which are the ovaries in females and testes in males. The two types of gamete need to perform quite different functions. The egg contributes most of the cytoplasm and the organelles to the zygote and needs large reserves of materials to sup-

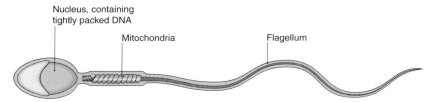

Fig. 3.5   *A human sperm.*

port growth and development; it is therefore a very large cell. On the other hand, the sperm must be able to travel considerable distances very rapidly to deliver its DNA to the egg and is therefore extremely small, has no organelles but is specialised for swimming, with a flagellum powered by mitochondria (Fig. 3.5).

The process by which male and female gametes are generated varies considerably but basically involves an initial multiplication by mitosis followed by meiotic division into gametes with haploid nuclei. In the male, meiosis occurs in the seminiferous tubules of the testes and begins at puberty. Each germ cell produces four sperm. In the female, meiosis occurs in the ovaries. Egg production is initiated during development of the fetus but then remains dormant until about 12 years of age. The meiotic divisions of the female germ cell produce one egg and three polar bodies.

The formation of a female gamete – oogenesis

Eggs have the unique ability to develop from a single cell into a complete new individual, with its multitude of cell types. This process occurs in only a matter of weeks from the point at which the egg is activated by fusion with a sperm.

Eggs vary in size according to species. Where embryo development takes place outside the body of the mother (e.g. birds), the egg must be very large to store enough reserves of nutrients. Even in humans, where embryo development takes place in the mother's body, the egg cell is about five times the size of most other cells in the body.

Development in the embryo

The development of the egg begins in the ovaries of the embryo. Here, the primordial germ cells multiply by mitosis to form oogonia. The oogonia then begin the first division of meiosis and become primary oocytes. By the eighth month of gestation, several million primary oocytes have accumulated in the ovaries, although only a few hundred will eventually mature into eggs. The primary oocytes remain in the first phase of meiosis for many years, until puberty. This stage of cell division has a considerable benefit for the developing egg because the nucleus contains two pairs of every chromosome and this means that twice the normal amount of DNA is available for RNA synthesis, enabling the egg to increase to a significantly greater size than other cells.

The primary oocyte is surrounded by a layer of follicle cells, which help to provide it with nutrients, and is called a primordial follicle. The follicles are stimulated by hormones called gonadotrophins released by the pituitary gland and other hormones, called oestrogens, released by the follicle cells themselves. These hormones trigger the completion of the first meiotic division, the maturation of the oocyte and the multiplication of follicle cells. The first of these gonadotrophins, follicle-stimulating hormone (FSH), stimulates a few primordial follicles to develop into antral follicles by causing the accumulation of several layers of follicle cells and enlargement of their oocytes.

Development at puberty

At puberty, the pituitary gland starts to release a second gonadotrophin, luteinising hormone (LH). This hormone is released once a month, in the middle of the menstrual cycle, and initiates maturation of the oocyte. This hormone affects only 15 to 20 of the developing antral follicles and only one of these will actually continue to mature into a secondary oocyte. LH stimulates the oocyte to complete the first meiotic division, which results in two daughter cells of unequal size but each with half the original number of chromosomes. The large cell is the secondary oocyte and the small cell is the polar body, which eventually degenerates. The follicle containing the secondary oocyte enlarges rapidly and moves to the surface of the ovary where it ruptures to release the secondary oocyte surrounded by a coating of follicle cells (Fig. 3.6). The second division of meiosis is only completed when the egg is fertilised and results in a mature egg (ovum) together with another small polar body.

The duration of reproductive life

Mature eggs are released from the ovary, once a month, from puberty until between 40 and 50 years of age. Because all primary oocytes are made before the fetus is born, towards the end of this reproductive life the secondary oocytes will have been developed from primary oocytes which have been held in the first meiotic division for four or five decades. The damage to the genome caused during this long period may help to explain the increased incidence of genetic abnormality that occurs in children born to older women.

The formation of male gametes – spermatogenesis

In human males, sperm production (spermatogenesis) occurs in the epithelial lining of the seminiferous tubules of the testes. Primordial germ cells are laid down in the lining of the seminiferous tubules during embryo development but spermatogenesis does not commence until puberty, from which point it occurs continuously. Like oogenesis, spermatogenesis is controlled by hormones. At puberty the pituitary gland begins secreting LH, the same gonadotrophin that initiates oogenesis in the female. This hormone stimulates cells in the seminiferous tubules to produce large amounts of another hormone, testosterone. It is the testosterone that initiates spermatogenesis.

Under the influence of testosterone, some of the immature germ cells (spermatogonia) differentiate into primary spermatocytes. These then undergo the first division of meiosis to form two secondary spermatocytes, each with duplicate copies of 22 chromosomes (one from each pair of similar chromosomes)

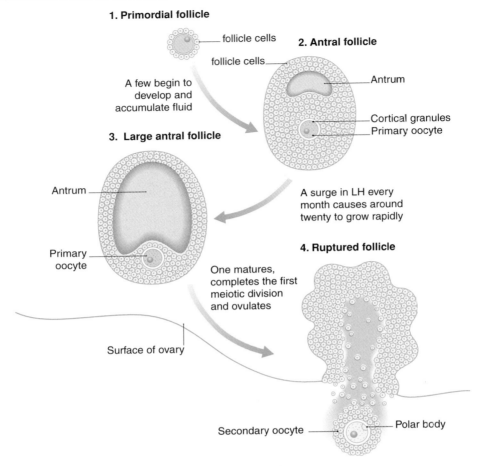

Fig. 3.6   *Stages in oocyte development after puberty. LH, luteinising hormone.*

and duplicate copies of the sex chromosome, either two copies of Y or two copies of X. The secondary spermatocytes then undergo the second meiotic division where the duplicate copies are separated into four haploid spermatids (Fig. 3.7). Conversion from spermatocyte into spermatid takes about 24 days and during this time all the daughter cells are contained within the cytoplasm of the original spermatogonia because only the nucleus and not the cytoplasm divides until the spermatids are formed. This organisation is essential to enable the original, diploid genome of the spermatogonia to direct spermatogenesis and ensure each developing sperm receives all the products of the full genome. Because some of the haploid sperm will not contain an X chromosome, they need to be able to receive the vital products that are encoded on this chromosome, otherwise they would not be able to survive.

The spermatids are then modified over a period of 5 weeks to form spermatozoa before being released into the lumen of the seminiferous tubule. They then pass into the epididymis, a coiled tube above the testes, where they are stored. At this stage the spermatozoa undergo further changes including development of motility, before they become fully mature sperm.

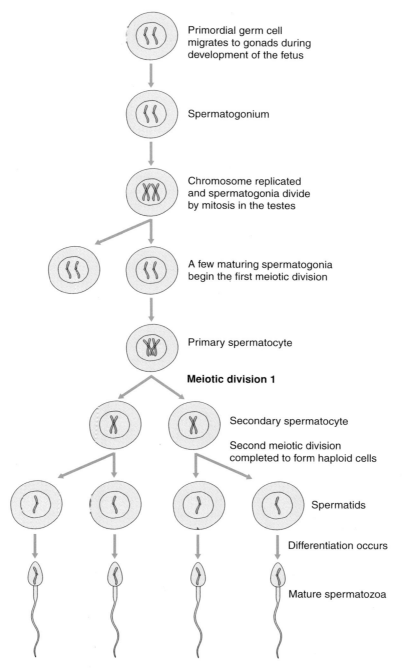

Fig. 3.7   *Stages in spermatogenesis after puberty.*

FERTILISATION

At fertilisation the two haploid gametes, an egg from the female and sperm from a male, fuse and the resulting zygote has the full complement of 23 pairs of chromosomes. One chromosome in each pair will be derived from the egg and one from the sperm.

Fertilisation, the union of a sperm cell and an egg cell, leads to the formation of a cell with two copies of each gene.

The egg has a few secretory vesicles just beneath the plasma membranes and after fusion with the sperm these expel their contents and prevent any more sperm from fusing with the egg. In mammals, structures in the mother that are required to protect the embryo and supply it with nutrients (the amniotic sac and placenta) are derived from the fertilised egg.

Fertilisation initiates an extremely complex process enabling a single, tiny egg to transform into a baby made up of billions of different types of cell. The zygote formed by fertilisation of the egg undergoes a series of mitotic divisions without any growth, dividing it into many small cells. After about 4 days it consists of a ball of 32 cells and is called a morula. After 8 days these cells have separated into two distinct layers: the outer layer of columnar cells called the ectoderm, which eventually forms the skin and nervous system; and the internal layer made of cuboidal cells called the endoderm, which forms the lining of the gut and associated structures. Differentiation into these two types of cell seems to be determined by their relative position, the key factor being the number of contacts they have with other cells. Those with few contacts become ectoderm, whilst those with many contacts become endoderm. After 3 weeks a third layer of cells, the mesoderm, is laid down between the ectoderm and endoderm; this will form the muscles, connective tissue, vascular system and urogenital system.

Many different types of cell are generated from the fertilised egg. Diversification into different types of cell is influenced by the position of the cells and their contacts with other cells. However, these early influences determining how a cell will develop are retained so that even if cells are moved to a different part of the embryo they are already committed to their particular specialised activity and this is inherited by their progeny. For example, the precursors of muscles cells are determined at an early stage; they then move to many different places such as the point of limb formation, where they develop their specialised function by producing large amounts of contractile proteins. This memory is conferred by molecules in the cytoplasm or the activation of master regulatory genes which turn on the specific set of genes required for a particular type of cell. Cells release signalling molecules to communicate their relative position to other cells.

Eventually, most cells become irreversibly differentiated. A few cells can still divide into a variety of cell types according to demand and these are called stem cells, for example the precursors of blood cells in the bone marrow. Many cells such as erythrocytes and nerve cells do not divide at all.

PRINCIPLES OF GENETICS

Several rules govern how particular traits are inherited by subsequent generations and which can be used to determine the probability of a trait being passed on to an offspring. These principles are applied in genetic counselling of couples who have inheritable genetic disorders.

The rules of inheritance were first described by Gregor Mendel in 1865. He drew his conclusions from a series of experiments with garden peas, which he studied over a period of 9 years. The principles he described form the basis for modern genetics and are referred to as Mendel's first law, the law of segregation, and Mendel's second law, the law of independent assortment.

The law of segregation means that each characteristic or trait is determined by a pair of genes (Mendel did not know about genes and referred instead to 'cellular factors'). When the reproductive cells or gametes are formed, the pair of genes are separated such that each egg or sperm cell (or, as in Mendel's experiments, pollen grain) contains only one of the original genes: half the cells will contain one gene and the other half the other gene. When the male and female gametes are fused the offspring will contain a new pair of genes for that trait, one from each parent.

The law of independent assortment means that the genes are separated into the reproductive cells randomly and the way that they are segregated is not influenced by other pairs of genes. This is because the chromosomes in each gamete are made up of a random mixture of both maternal and paternal chromosomes.

Mendel also realised that the appearance of the offspring (its phenotype) could disguise which factors (i.e. genes) it was carrying because, of the two factors determining a particular trait, one would be dominant over the other and would always be expressed. The concept of a dominant and recessive version of a particular gene is conventionally expressed as a capital letter denoting a dominant gene and the same lower-case letter as its recessive pair, 'Aa'.

Mendel was able to establish the principles of heredity because he chose to focus on a few simple, but clearly visible, characteristics such as short or tall, round or wrinkled seeds in one species, the garden pea. He was able to control carefully which types of plants were mated because they would normally reproduce by self-fertilisation. To cross-fertilise he would take out the male parts of a plant and dust the female parts with the pollen from another plant. He would then allow the offspring from a cross-fertilisation to self-fertilise for several generations and carefully record the phenotype of the progeny and the ratio of phenotypes in each generation. He studied one trait at a time and then repeated the set of experiments for each pair of traits (Fig. 3.8).

Mendel realised that he could predict the distribution of the trait in subsequent generations by applying simple mathematical principles of probability, which are explained in Box 3.1.

Genetic disorders

The faithful copying of the genome of a cell is essential to ensure that daughter cells retain the basic characteristics of the organism and the correct genetic information is transferred from parents to offspring.

DNA mutations and how these are repaired

The genetic record needs to be maintained in an accurate form because any errors in the DNA sequence could lead to the inactivation of a crucial protein

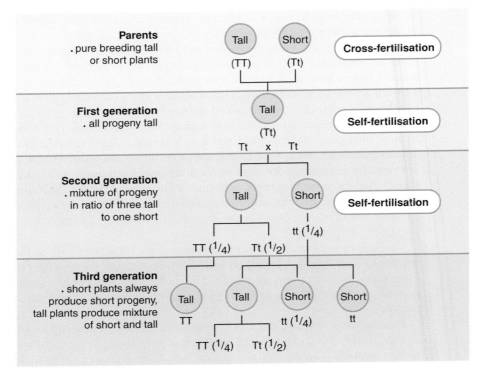

Fig. 3.8   *Mendel's experiments with short and tall garden peas.*

BOX 3.1	*Principles of Probability*

The probability of an event occurring is expressed as a fraction ranging between 0 and 1. If an event is going to occur every time, then the probability of it occurring will be 1, whilst if it is never going to occur its probability of occurring will be 0. For example, the probability of throwing a 3 on a die is 1/6, the probability of throwing a 7 is 0 and the probability of throwing any number up to 6 is 1.

To calculate the probability of either one of two mutually exclusive events occurring, the probability of both events are added together, e.g. the probability of throwing a 1 or 2 on a die is:

1/6 + 1/6 = 1/3.

To calculate the probability of each of a series of events occurring, the probabilities are multiplied together, e.g. the probability of throwing a 1 and 2 on a die is:

1/6 × 1/6 = 1/36.

and such mistakes would be passed on to subsequent generations. Alterations to the DNA sequence can easily occur during copying, but DNA is also susceptible to damage by high-energy metabolites in the cell and exposure to ultraviolet light. In addition, the spontaneous loss of molecules from the base pairs can affect hundreds of bases on a single genome every day. To cope with this problem the cell has an efficient method of DNA repair which immediately recognises and repairs any mistakes or damage to the genome. The process involves a range of enzymes that recognise altered base pairs or distortions in the double helix. Once found, the damaged section is excised and a new section inserted. The repair process is made possible because the DNA is composed of two strands; if one strand is damaged, the piece can be removed and a new section copied from the second strand. Very rarely this process fails and allows a permanent change to be incorporated into the DNA. Studies of mutation rates in animals, such as mice, that breed very rapidly have shown that a protein of average size is likely to be altered by a random mutation once every 200 000 years. Most of these mutations will have a harmful effect on the individual and will therefore be eliminated from the population by natural selection.

Mutations in the genome

These changes can arise spontaneously or may be inherited from a parent. They may affect a large amount of genetic information, such as a chromosomal abnormality, or may just involve the alteration of a few nucleotide bases in the DNA strand. As the nucleotides in the DNA strand are read in series of three, the addition or deletion of a single nucleotide can shift the entire reading frame of the strand. Defective proteins will be produced as a result of altered amino acids in the polypeptide chain or by the chain being shortened or lengthened by misreading of stop codes. Where only one nucleotide base is altered, this is called a point mutation. Because most amino acids have several different three-base codes, a point mutation may not necessarily result in a change to the amino acid translated. This process is shown below.

DNA:	TTT	AGC	CTG	ATT
RNA:	AAA	UCG	GAC	UAA
Amino acid:	Lys	Ser	Asp	Stop

If T is deleted from the first codon:

DNA:	TTA	GCG	TGA	TTA
RNA:	AAT	CGC	ACT	AAT
Amino acid:	Ileu	Leu	Thr	Ileu

there is no stop code, therefore the chain elongates until another stop code is reached.

Somatic cell mutations

If mutations occur in the body, or somatic cells, they will only affect descendants of that cell. If the mutations occur early on in the development of the embryo then the damaged genome will be passed on to a larger number of somatic cells than if the damage occurs late in embryo development.

Germ cell mutations

If gene mutations occur in a gamete that is subsequently fertilised, then the changes to the genome are passed on to the developing offspring and to both its somatic and germ cells. Some mutations may be very minor and have no overt effect on the individual; others result in diseases or deformities in the offspring. These are called congenital disorders. Because the fertilised egg contain two sets of genes in each chromosome, one from each parent, the effect of the mutated gene may be cancelled out by a normal gene from the other parent and the offspring not affected. However, the individual will carry the mutated gene in their genome and will pass it on to subsequent offspring.

Gene mapping

Scientists are able to locate specific genes to particular points on specific chromosomes. The distance between genes on the same chromosome is referred to in map units. Genes that are 50 or less map units apart are considered to be linked. Linked genes are often useful to genetic analysis because if the gene under study cannot be detected by the physical appearance of the individual, a linked gene determining a detectable trait can be looked for instead (Box 3.2).

BOX 3.2	*Human Genome Project*
	This ambitious project was launched in 1990 with the aim of analysing and recording the sequence of DNA on all of the human chromosomes. Whilst the project was conceived in the USA, it has now developed into an international initiative with sequencing being carried out in many countries. So far the genome has been roughly mapped, with easily recognisable sequences recorded at regular intervals along each chromosome. By the year 2005 it is anticipated that the DNA sequence of the whole of the genome will have been recorded. The information obtained by the project is already enabling gene mutations that cause diseases ranging from Alzheimer's disease to cancer to be identified and tests to detect them to be developed. Ultimately, they may give clues towards both prevention and therapy of such conditions.

MEDICAL GENETICS

Medical genetics is the study of genetic disorders and the clinical application of genetics to their management. Advances in techniques of genetic analysis mean that it is now possible to investigate many genetic disorders by looking at the genetic make-up of an affected individual. However, inferring information by outward appearance (phenotype), including clinical history, biochemical tests such as enzyme activity and drawing up a family tree (pedigree) to establish who else in the family may be either affected or a carrier, is still an important part of any investigation and counselling process.

Not all genetic disorders are associated with mutation of a single gene. There are actually five types of genetic disorder.

Chromosomal abnormalities

Chromosomes are sufficiently large to be seen under a light microscope. Each species has a characteristic number of chromosomes with a characteristic appearance. This is the karyotype of the cell. Chromosomal abnormalities that are extensive enough to be seen when viewed under a light microscope are called chromosomal aberrations. Sixty per cent of spontaneous early miscarriages, 5% of late spontaneous miscarriages and 4–5% of live still births are caused by chromosomal aberrations. Chromosomal abnormalities can occur during the formation of the gamete or can be transferred to the gamete from a mutation in the parent or ancestor of the cell. Chromosomal abnormalities can also affect all the other cells of the body (somatic cells) and be transferred to the offspring in the gametes. There are two forms of chromosomal abnormality:

1. Numerical abnormalities occur when there are too many or too few chromosomes. They occur during cell division (either meiosis or mitosis) when pairs of chromosomes fail to separate properly. Where this occurs during meiosis the result is one daughter cell containing an extra copy of a chromosome (a trisomy) and the other a missing copy of the chromosome (a monosomy). Down's syndrome is caused by an extra copy of chromosome 21 and is referred to as trisomy 21. These numerical abnormalities occur with increasing frequency with maternal age, hypothyroidism and possibly after irradiation or viral infection. There is also a familial tendency.
2. Structural abnormalities are caused when the chromosome breaks. These breaks occur spontaneously and are normally repaired immediately, but if more than one break occurs the wrong ends may be rejoined and the sequence of genes carried on the chromosome changed. The normal rate of chromosome breakage is increased by ionising radiation and mutagenic chemicals.

Mitochondrial abnormalities

Mitochondria have their own chromosome containing the DNA necessary to form their structural proteins and to perform their function as the site of energy production in the cell. The genetic information in the mitochondria is transferred from parent to germ cell by the inclusion of mitochondria in the ovum made by the female parent. Mutations in the mitochondrial chromosome are therefore passed only from a mother to her offspring. All the offspring will be affected, but only the female offspring will pass the defect onto their children. An example of a mitochondrial genetic disorder is Leber optic neuropathy where an affected individual suddenly develops blindness in early adulthood.

Multifactorial abnormalities

Multifactorial traits are determined by the interaction of several genes at different sites on the chromosome together with environmental factors. If a trait is determined by multifactorial inheritance then relatives will share a proportion of the genes and will show the trait in proportion to their genetic similarity. Examples of multifactorial traits are height, intelligence and blood pressure.

Cleft lip and palate are congenital malformations that are inherited as a multifactorial trait. The risk of inheritance is higher in an affected family than in the general population but much lower than the risk of inheritance with single gene traits. Multifactorial congenital disorders have a range of effects (in the same way that there is a range of height inheritance). In cleft lip one or both sides of both the lip and palate may be affected. Parents may have no history of the disorder but both must have some defective genes for lip or palate formation. Some multifactorial traits show unequal distribution between the sexes. For example, congenital dislocation of the hip is six times more common in females than males and rheumatoid arthritis three times more common in females.

Somatic cell abnormalities

Most cancers are now recognised to be caused by mutations in the genetic material of cells in the body. Cancer can affect almost any type of tissue in the body and it occurs in more than 100 different forms. A tumour will not develop from a single gene mutation; several different mutations in the genes that control cell growth are necessary before the tumour becomes malignant and it may take three or four decades for these mutations to accumulate.

Specific mutations in the genes that control the growth and division of the cell are required to produce cancers. Normally the cells within a tissue are interdependent; they will only divide in response to growth factors and these growth factors are proteins secreted by one cell which bind to specific receptors on the surface of other cells. When a growth factor binds to the receptor, it stimulates proteins in the cytoplasm and these in turn cause proteins in the nucleus to switch on transcription of the genes necessary to initiate the growth cycle of the cell. Cells also respond to growth-suppressing factors which stop the growth cycle in the cell once sufficient divisions have taken place. This arrangement ensures that the tissue is maintained in the correct size and structure. For a cancer to occur, mutations must develop in at least two genes: the proto-oncogene and the tumour suppressor genes. Proto-oncogenes code for the proteins that respond to the binding of the growth factor; a mutation in this gene can cause them continually to stimulate cell growth and division. Tumour suppressor genes respond to the growth-suppressing signals that would normally switch off the cell growth cycle if it continues abnormally. Sometimes, the receptor genes mutate so that they signal the cell to grow even when they have not been stimulated by growth factors. Some people may inherit a mutation, for example in their tumour suppressor gene, that strongly predisposes them to develop cancer at an early age. Most people inherit genes without such mutations, but they are gradually acquired as the DNA is exposed to carcinogens in the environment, chemicals within the cell or errors during copying.

The mass of cells formed from a cancerous cell can become quite large without causing any damage and this is known as a benign tumour. Normally cells can only survive if they are attached to the extracellular matrix of the tissue and if they are detached they will die. A tumour can become malignant by starting to invade nearby tissue and migrating to other sites in the body (metastasise), but for this to occur the genes that usually tell the cell that it is anchored in the right place must become defective. This then enables the cells to roam away from their tissue and establish elsewhere; when this happens the cancer becomes very difficult to treat because the new tumours can damage other tissues and be impossible to treat surgically (Fig. 3.9).

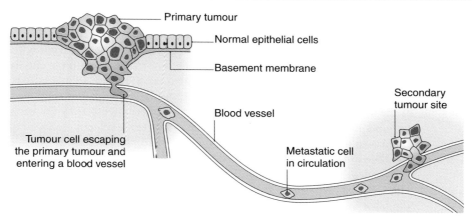

Fig. 3.9   *Metastasis of cancer cells.*

Single gene abnormalities

There are several forms in which single gene abnormalities can be inherited.

Autosomal dominant inheritance

The mutation occurs on a gene that is expressed when only one copy of it is present. One in two of the offspring of an affected parent will develop the disease, although this type of genetic disorder is associated with variable expression so that the time of onset and severity of the condition varies between individuals. The reason for this variation is unclear. Examples of diseases associated with autosomal dominant inheritance include adult polycystic kidney disease and Huntingdon's disease.

Autosomal recessive inheritance

In this type of single gene disorder both copies of the gene must be affected by the same mutation. The parents can carry just one copy of the gene and therefore be clinically normal but able to pass the affected gene on to their offspring. Offspring will only be affected if they inherit mutant genes from both parents although it is possible to have several different variants of the same mutant gene and these may be expressed slightly differently.

   An example of this type of genetic disease is sickle cell disease. In this condition the red blood cells are distorted and survive for a relatively short time, which leads to chronic haemolytic anaemia. Affected individuals need repeated blood transfusions and the misshapen blood cells may block blood vessels, causing infarctions in lung, bone and spleen. The main type of haemoglobin in normal blood is haemoglobin A, each molecule of which is made up of two alpha-globin molecules and two beta-globin polypeptide chains. In sickle cell disease there is a mutation in the beta-globin gene on chromosome 11, which causes the substitution of one amino acid and the formation of haemoglobin S (HbS) in place of haemoglobin A. This change causes the red blood cells to distort, especially at low oxygen concentrations.

   An individual will only be affected if they have two mutant HbS genes inherited from both parents. If both parents are carriers, 1 in 4 of their offspring will be affected and 2 in 4 will become carriers of the mutant gene. If a parent has sickle cell disease and therefore two HbS genes, but has offspring with a carrier, then the risk of the offspring being affected is 1 in 2. If both parents have sickle cell disease then all their offspring will also be affected.

Sickle cell disease affects 1 in 40 African blacks, 1 in 3 of whom are carriers of the mutant gene. In Africa, HbS is resistant to infection by the malaria parasite and therefore sickle cell disease may confer a selective advantage against malaria in areas where this infection is endemic.

Other autosomal recessive disorders include cystic fibrosis (0.5/1000), congenital deafness (0.2/1000) and phenylketonuria (0.1/1000).

X-linked abnormalities

Males only have one copy of the genes located on the X chromosome because this chromosome is partnered with the Y chromosome, which has very few genes on it. In the male, genes carried on the X chromosome will always be expressed because there is no second version. For example, colour blindness is caused by a defective or missing gene on the X chromosome. A male with this gene will therefore be colour-blind whilst a female is likely to have a normal gene on the second X chromosome and will therefore only be colour-blind if the second X chromosome also has a defective or missing gene.

SUMMARY

The genome of each cell contains the set of genes necessary to construct every type of cell in the body. This genome also provides the mechanism by which the information can be transferred to the next generation. The genes are carried on chromosomes which are arranged into pairs. Each chromosome in a pair contains the same set of genes, although they may carry slightly different versions of each gene. When cells divide to replace tissue or enable growth, the genome is copied exactly and one copy transferred into each daughter cell. In sexual reproduction, a special form of cell division called meiosis occurs, to produce gametes, the eggs and sperm. In this type of cell division, the pairs of chromosomes are separated and each daughter cell receives only one chromosome from each pair. At fertilisation, a sperm and egg cell fuse, restoring the full number of chromosomes but with a unique mixture of genes from both parents. Fertilisation initiates a complex process of cell division and differentiation that enables a single cell to develop into a small human.

The inheritance of genes by subsequent generations is governed by the principles of probability. Gregor Mendel was the first to describe simple rules of inheritance in 1865. He realised that each trait was determined by a pair of genes, one derived from each parent, and that one of these genes would be dominant over the other and therefore determine the appearance of the offspring. Genetic disorders can arise when a gene is damaged or mistakes are made in copying. When a mutation occurs in the genome of a sperm or egg cell it will be passed on to the offspring. Because the fertilised egg contains two copies of each gene, the mutated gene may be disguised by a normal gene acquired from the other parent. Mutations can also occur in other cells in the body and, where these affect genes that control cell growth, can result in a tumour. If enough adverse mutations occur, cell division becomes completely uncontrolled and the tumour becomes malignant.

QUESTIONS

1. Where is the genetic material of the cell stored and how is it stored there?

2. Compare and contrast mitosis and meiosis.

3. What is an X-linked genetic abnormality and why are males more likely to display these?

FURTHER READING

Montague S, Knight D (1996) Cell structure and function, growth and development. In: Hinchliff S, Montague S, Watson R (eds) *Physiology for nursing practice, 2nd edn.* Baillière Tindall, London, pp 49–69

Watson R (1995) *Anatomy and physiology for nurses, 10th edn.* Baillière Tindall, London

4 Cell Biology

Jennie Wilson

> After reading this chapter you should be able to:
> - explain how proteins are synthesised using DNA as a template
> - list a range of sub-cellular particles
> - describe the surface of the cell.

WHAT ARE CELLS?

The cell is the smallest unit of living matter capable of independent survival. All cells are similar, and consist of a nucleus and cytoplasm surrounded by a semi-permeable membrane and sometimes an outer cell wall. They all contain genetic information in the form of deoxyribonucleic acid or DNA (Chs 2 and 3). There are two basic types of cell: the eucaryotic cells of higher forms of life such as plants and animals and the more primitive prokaryotic cells of bacteria. The term eucaryotic comes from the Greek word *eu*, meaning true or real, and *karyon*, kernal. This describes the nuclear material, which in 'eucaryotic cells' is contained in a well-defined structure called the nucleus and is surrounded by a nuclear membrane. In prokaryotic (Greek *pro*, primitive) cells the nuclear material is not enclosed within a membrane but is distributed throughout the cytoplasm as long, circular threads of DNA. The most primitive forms of life consist of single cells, which replicate by dividing in two. Higher organisms such as ourselves, consist of millions of cells, grouped to perform specialist functions and linked by complex communication systems.

> Cells are the smallest units of living matter capable of independent survival.

To explain how cells work, this chapter will look at the structure and function of eucaryotic cells. A typical eucaryotic cell is shown in Figure 4.1. Chapter 13 will discuss the structure and function of microorganisms and, in particular, the simple prokaryotic cells of bacteria.

THE STRUCTURE OF THE CELL

Eucaryotic cells consist of a nucleus surrounded by cytoplasm and enclosed by a plasma membrane. The nucleus contains the genome of the cell and is the main site of DNA and RNA synthesis; the cytoplasm consists of a variety of

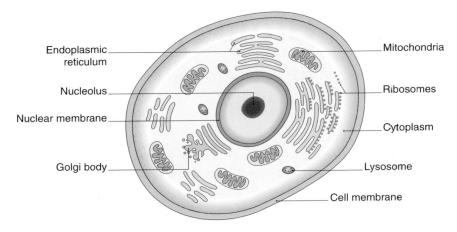

Fig. 4.1 *A eucaryotic cell.*

TABLE 4.1	Cell Organelles and Their Function	
	Organelle	Function
	Nucleus	Contains the genetic information of the cell. Site of DNA synthesis
	Plasma membrane	Controls movement of substances in and out of the cell. Responds to external signals
	Endoplasmic reticulum	Makes lipids. Directs movements of lipids and proteins throughout the cell
	Golgi apparatus	Modifies and sorts lipids and proteins
	Cytoskeleton	Acts as the internal framework of the cell, enabling it to move and to transport substances through it
	Ribosomes	Translates sequences of RNA into the corresponding proteins
	Mitochondria	Oxidises glucose and fatty acids to make energy in the form of ATP
	Lysosomes	Contains enzymes that break down large molecules no longer required by the cell
	Perioxisomes	The site of oxidative reactions used to inactivate toxic molecules

organelles suspended in the cytosol (Table 4.1). The cytosol is the common space surrounding the organelles and it contains a variety of nutrients which are degraded or altered to supply the basic materials necessary for the activity of the cell. Organelles are distinct structures within the cell, each surrounded by a membrane and containing their own set of enzymes and molecules. Products are transported between organelles by transport proteins, which recognise specific molecules and carry them from one destination to another, or by vesicles, bulges in a membrane that trap a cargo of molecules, pinch off and then empty their contents into another structure by fusing with its membrane (Fig. 4.2).

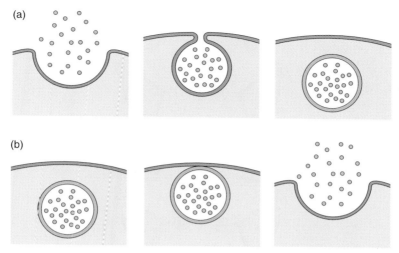

Fig. 4.2 *Transportation of cellular material by vesicles. (a) A section of membrane pinches off, forming a vesicle containing molecules for transport. (b) The vesicle moves to another membrane, fuses with it and empties its contents.*

CELL ORGANELLES AND THEIR FUNCTION

The nucleus and the Genetic Code

Most structures within cells are made from protein and activities within the cell are also regulated by other proteins called enzymes. The genetic information, or genome, dictates which proteins are made by the cell. It is contained in the nucleus in the form of molecules of DNA arranged into one or more chromosomes. Each chromosome comprises a single molecule of DNA. Bacteria such as *Escherichia coli* have one chromosome and the human genome has 24. The length of a DNA molecule varies between different types of cell and, if uncoiled, could be between 2 and 8 centimetres (cm) long. The DNA is enclosed by a nuclear membrane, which has pores to enable small molecules to pass in and out. Large molecules, however, have to be actively transported through the pores as required.

A molecule of DNA is composed of a series of nucleotides. Each nucleotide consists of a sugar and a phosphate molecule attached to one of four bases: adenine, cytosine, guanine and thymine (Ch. 2). Two strands of nucleotides are held together by weak hydrogen bonds between the bases. Adenine always bonds with thymine and guanine always bonds with cytosine (Fig. 4.3). The sequence of bases forms a code of three-letter 'words', with each amino acid corresponding to a particular set of three bases (Table 4.2). An average protein consists of about 400 amino acids and would correspond to 1200 bases along the chain of nucleotides. A section of DNA that codes for a single protein is called a gene. However, by changing the point at which reading starts, several different series of amino acids can be made from a single length of DNA (Fig. 4.4).

Transcription of the Genetic Code

In eucaryotic cells, proteins are synthesised by ribosomes in the cytoplasm and

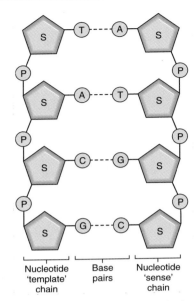

Nucleotide
'template'
chain

Base
pairs

Nucleotide
'sense'
chain

Fig. 4.3   *The structure of deoxyribonucleic acid (DNA). S, sugar molecule; P, phosphate molecule; C, cytosine; G, guanine; A, adenine; T, thymine; ----, hydrogen bond.*

TABLE 4.2	**The Genetic Code**
Sequence of bases on DNA	*Equivalent amino acid*
GCG	Alanine
TTC	Phenylalanine
CGC	Arginine
AAA	Lysine

the cell must therefore have a mechanism to carry the DNA code out of the nucleus. This function is performed by molecules of RNA (Ch. 2). RNA has a similar structure to DNA except that it is made of ribose instead of deoxyribose sugars, has only a single strand of nucleotides, and has the base uracil in place of thymine. Short strands of RNA, corresponding to only a few genes, are copied from the DNA in a process called transcription. The template strand of DNA acts as a pattern against which complementary RNA bases are aligned (Fig. 4.5). Sections of this messenger or mRNA are then completed by enzymes called polymerases before being transported out of the nucleus to ribosomes in the cytoplasm for translation and assembly of the corresponding amino acid chain.

DNA is transcribed into strands of RNA in the nucleus which are transported to ribosomes in the cytoplasm and translated into proteins.

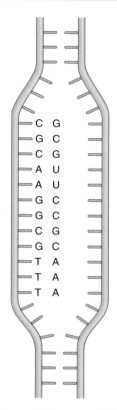

Fig. 4.4 *Transcription and translation of the DNA code. Messenger RNA is copied from the DNA template.*

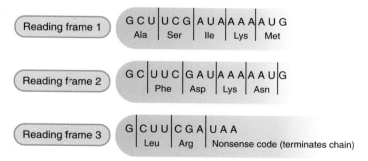

Fig. 4.5 *DNA reading frames. The same sequence of DNA can be used to make more than one protein by altering the frame in which it is read.*

Replication of DNA

When a cell divides, the chromosome of each new cell must contain both strands of DNA. To make an accurate copy of the DNA the two strands are gradually separated and each becomes a pattern against which a new strand is made. The two daughter chromosomes both contain one strand of the parent cell and one newly synthesised strand (Fig. 4.6).

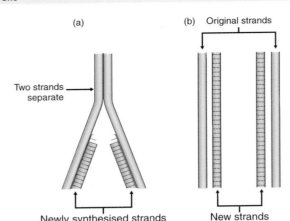

Fig. 4.6 *The copying of a chromosome. (a) The two strands of DNA are separated and a copy made of each half. (b) The two identical chromosomes.*

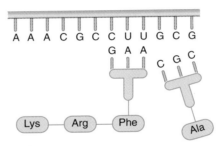

Fig. 4.7 *Translation of RNA into protein. The mRNA moves to a ribosome, where the amino acids corresponding to the code are brought on transfer RNA and assembled into a protein.*

Ribosomes

Ribosomes are made of protein and RNA and have several subunits to their structure. The subunits of all the ribosomes in the cell (except those in the mitochondria) are made in a distinct structure within the nucleus, called the nucleolus, and then transported out into the cytoplasm. Ribosomes are the protein factories of the cell; they translate the genetic code from the RNA, bring together the amino acids specified in the message and enable peptide bonds to form between them (Ch. 2).

The synthesis of protein – translation of RNA

The ribosome finds the correct starting point on the mRNA and this determines the reading frame. It then moves along the mRNA molecule, translating each series of three bases (codons) into the corresponding amino acid. Amino acids are collected from the cytoplasm using another type of RNA molecule called transfer RNA (tRNA). Each different amino acid is recognised by a specific tRNA, which adds their amino acids in turn to the end of the polypeptide chain (Fig. 4.7). The whole process occurs very rapidly with about 20 amino acids being added to the chain every second. A single molecule of mRNA can be processed by more than one ribosome at the same time and in eucaryotic cells the same molecule of mRNA can be translated many times.

Once the polypeptide chain has been assembled, it is released into the cytosol. The proteins fold spontaneously into their correct shape with the direction of the folds being determined by the weak bonds that form between different amino acids in the sequence (Ch. 2). The range of amino acid combinations and folding patterns enables an extremely wide variety of different structures to be formed from proteins.

Some proteins carry a signal at the end of their amino acid chain that causes them to be transported to the specific organelle where they are required, such as the mitochondria, nucleus or perioxisomes. A protein can take as little as a minute to reach an organelle from the time it is released into the cytosol. Most proteins, however, do not carry a signal but are transferred into the endoplasmic reticulum where they are processed and then marked by a sorting signal to indicate their final destination.

Plasma membrane

This is a membrane that encloses the cell and acts as a highly selective filter controlling the entry of nutrients and the exit of waste products to and from the cell. It is able actively to transport ions across the membrane and therefore controls the differences in concentration of ions between the inside and outside of the cell. It also recognises signals from the environment and triggers the cell to respond.

All eucaryotic cell have membranes with the same basic structure. They are composed of two layers of lipid molecules interspersed with protein molecules. The lipids form the basic structure of the membrane and provide an impermeable barrier to most water-soluble molecules. The proteins in the membrane are responsible for most of its functions; they transport specific molecules into or out of the cell, catalyse particular reactions and act as a structural link connecting the plasma membrane to the internal cytoskeleton of the cell or to the membrane of another adjacent cell.

Cell membranes contain three major types of lipid (Ch. 2) – phospholipids, cholesterol and glycolipids – assembled into a bilayer. Phospholipids and glycolipids form a bilayer spontaneously in a solution of water because each has a hydrophilic (water-loving) molecule at one end and hydrophobic (water-hating) molecules at the other end. The hydrophobic ends tend to congregate together so that the molecules are buried inside and protected from the water, leaving the hydrophilic heads to be directed outwards (Fig. 4.8). The free edges of the bilayer will join together to provide a sealed compartment and will reseal themselves if they are torn. Cholesterol molecules are scattered through the membrane and are important for providing its strength and flexibility.

In animal cells, glycolipids expose their sugar molecules on the outer surface of the membrane where they are probably involved in interactions between the cell and its surrounding environment. The type of glycolipid in the membrane varies between species and between different tissues in the same species.

All cells need to take in nutrients and excrete the waste products of their metabolism and must therefore be able to transfer water-soluble molecules

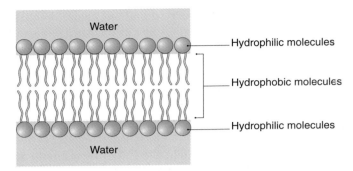

Fig. 4.8   *The lipid bilayer membrane.*

across their membranes. Because lipid bilayers will not allow the passage of such molecules, two types of protein are present in the plasma membrane to perform this function. Carrier proteins bind to a solute and take them across the bilayer. They do this by changing their conformation and in doing so move the site where the solute binds from one side of the membrane to the other side. Some of these proteins act as pumps, transporting solutes against their electrochemical gradient by using adenosine triphosphate (ATP) to drive a series of conformational changes. Channel proteins form a pore across the bilayer and allow the passage of ions of an appropriate size and correct charge to cross the membrane according to their electrochemical gradient. This transfer occurs far more rapidly than by carrier protein. The channels are not usually open all the time but are opened in response to a specific change in the membrane induced, for example, by the binding of a neurotransmitter.

> Substances can be transported across the plasma membrane. Some substances pass freely (diffusion) but others require specific carrier proteins in the membrane (facilitated diffusion) and others require carrier proteins and energy to drive their transport (active transport).

The cytoskeleton

Eucaryotic cells have an internal framework or skeleton made from a network of small protein tubules and filaments. These play an important role in the transportation of substances through the cell, in chromosome separation during cell division and in enabling the cell to change its shape and move.

The cytoskeleton can be formed from combinations of three different types of filament: actin filaments, microtubules and intermediate filaments. Each is made from a different protein, has different properties and can be assembled into a variety of structures.

Actin filaments are contractile, they give cells their strength and enable them to move. In some cell types they have become highly developed and specialised. For example, in muscle cells actin filaments form the bundles of contractile fibres responsible for muscle contraction (Ch. 12).

Microtubules are long hollow tubes made of a protein called tubulin. They radiate out as single filaments from a point near to the nucleus called the centrosome and they provide a system of fibres along which organelles and vesicles can travel. In nerve cells, for example, they provide a channel for neurotransmitters to move along rapidly. They also play an important part in cell division by controlling the point at which the cell divides into two.

Microtubules are also responsible for the movement of cilia such as those lining the respiratory and gastrointestinal tract and the simple flagella of sperm or protozoa. Bundles of tubes slide against each other to cause the whip-like beating movement of cilia.

Intermediate filaments are tough, fibrous proteins that look similar to rope and are thought to be responsible for the tension-bearing properties of the cell. Their structure varies according to the demands of the particular cell. The most resilient form is the keratins, which form a major part of the protective outer layer of skin.

The cytoskeleton does not occur in bacterial cells and therefore may have been crucial in the evolution of higher organisms. Cytoskeleton of one cell can influence that of its neighbours, for example the cooperative working seen in muscles fibres. The ability of cells to communicate with each other is thought to be important in determining the morphology of tissues and organs.

Perioxisomes

These organelles are surrounded by a single membrane and they are able to replicate themselves but, as they do not contain their own DNA or ribosomes, must import the necessary proteins from the cytosol. They use molecular oxygen and hydrogen peroxide to carry out oxidative reactions and are particularly important in liver and kidney cells where they inactivate toxic molecules that enter the bloodstream: for example, alcohol that we drink is oxidised to acetaldehyde.

Endoplasmic reticulum

The endoplasmic reticulum (ER) is a single membrane that extends throughout the cytoplasm like a net and accounts for more than half the total membrane of the cell. The ER is like a factory for the production of lipids and proteins required for the cell organelles, with enzymes on its surface that join together fatty acids from the cytosol to make lipids. It does not make proteins but directs both their movement around the cell and their secretion out of the cell. Proteins and lipids are carried between the ER, plasma membrane, Golgi apparatus and lysosomes in transport vesicles and to mitochondria and perioxisomes by special transfer proteins.

In most cells the majority of the ER has a rough appearance caused by ribosomes bound to the surface. Areas without ribosomes on the surface are called smooth ER. In some specialised cells the smooth ER is used to accommodate enzymes, e.g. cells that synthesise steroid hormones from cholesterol. In the hepatocytes of the liver, smooth ER contains enzymes that degrade lipid-soluble drugs or harmful byproducts of metabolism. The amount of smooth ER in these cells can be rapidly increased in response to large quantities of some drugs, such as phenobarbital.

Golgi apparatus

This structure looks like a stack of plates and is surrounded by a large number of transport and secretory vesicles. It receives newly synthesised proteins and lipids from the ER, modifies and sorts them before distributing them to the plasma membrane, lysosomes or secretory vesicles for excretion from the cell. The number of Golgi apparatus in a cell depends on the cell type and can vary from one large one to hundreds of small ones. Golgi apparatus are particularly important in cells that are specialised for secretion, for example the goblet cells in the lining of the gut which secrete mucus.

> The cytoplasm is not amorphous but contains many particles including cytoskeletal particles and subcellular organelles such as the lysosomes and mitochondria.

Lysosomes

These are bags of enzymes surrounded by a membrane. The proteases, lipases and other enzymes they contain are used to digest large molecules that are no longer required by the cell. The pH inside the lysosome is acid and is maintained by a pump that imports hydrogen ions. The enzymes only work in this acid environment, so that if they leak out of the membrane they are unable to do any damage in the cytosol, which has a pH of around 7. The end products of the digestion are either reused by the cell or excreted.

Mitochondria: the site of energy production

These structures are responsible for respiration: the oxidation of food molecules, in particular glucose and fatty acids. The energy produced during the process is converted into ATP, which can be harnessed and used to drive the activity of the cell. The fuel for these oxidation reactions is stored in the cytoplasm as glycogen and droplets of fat. Glycogen is a large polymer of glucose, which is converted into two pyruvate molecules in a process called glycolysis; fat droplets contain fatty acids in the form of triglycerides. When the cell requires energy, pyruvate and fatty acids are selectively transported into the mitochondria where they are oxidised to form CO_2 and water. The series of chemical reactions that occur during this process are known as the citric acid or Krebs cycle and the energy that they release is converted into molecules of ATP.

Mitochondria have an inner and an outer membrane with a space in between. The outer membrane has a large number of channels, which enable molecules up to the size of a small protein to pass into the inner membrane space (Fig. 4.9). The surface area of the inner membrane is greatly increased by its large number of folds containing many proteins that carry out the oxidation reactions of respiration, enzymes that make ATP and transport proteins that regulate the movement of molecules in and out of the inner membrane. It has to be impermeable to most small ions to enable the oxidation reactions to occur.

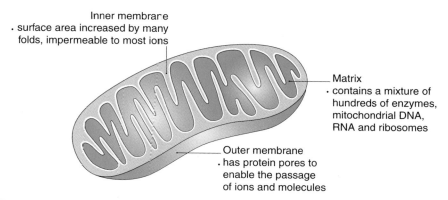

Inner membrane
· surface area increased by many
folds, impermeable to most ions

Matrix
· contains a mixture of
hundreds of enzymes,
mitochondrial DNA,
RNA and ribosomes

Outer membrane
· has protein pores to
enable the passage
of ions and molecules

Fig. 4.9   *A mitochondrion.*

Mitochondria can move around the cytoplasm and change shape. Their position within a cell depends on the function of the cell and its energy demands. In a cardiac muscle cell they will remain fixed next to the muscle fibres where they are needed to supply a constant source of energy. In a sperm cell they will be wrapped around the flagellum, providing the energy necessary for motility.

Fat is the most important source of fuel, releasing six times more energy than glycogen and present in much greater quantities. The human body has enough glycogen to support activity for only about 1 day whereas the fat stores are sufficient for 1 month. Most fat is stored in specialised adipose tissue and released into the bloodstream as required. After a meal most of the fuel used for respiration comes from glucose and any excess is used to replenish glycogen stores or is converted into fats. After a period of not eating, for example overnight, fat has to be mobilised as the source of energy and fatty acids will be used as the main fuel for respiration.

MULTICELLULAR ORGANISMS

In a multicellular organism, cells need to communicate with one another to regulate their development, growth and division, coordinate functions and enable them to organise into tissues. In single cell organisms the rate at which cell division takes place is only limited by the amount of nutrients in the environment and the rate at which the cell can absorb them in order to construct new materials. In a multicellular organism, controls over cell division must be much more complex because different cells will need to divide at a variable rate and may need to change the rate at which they divide at different times. When damage to a tissue occurs, the organism needs to be able to trigger cell division to replace tissue, whilst at other times division need only proceed at a rate sufficient to balance the rate of cell death. It is thought that a range of growth factors stimulate cells to divide; these can be present in the circulation but generally act locally at very low concentrations. They will trigger cell division in those cells that have an appropriate receptor on their plasma membrane. Division is also influenced by the relationship with other cells; a cell that is not attached to other cells will not divide.

THE FORMATION OF TISSUES

Cells have many common aspects of structure and activity, and synthesise a very similar range of proteins. However, different tissues in the body can have widely differing functions dictated by the production of a variety of specialised proteins. For example, haemoglobin is synthesised only in red blood cells (Ch. 2). The body must have some mechanism for coordinating the development of different tissues and assembling them into organs.

The DNA sequences of an organism carry the code for all the protein molecules required to construct its cells. However, it is not possible to construct the organism without knowing which proteins to use and how to use them. Rather than containing different genetic information, different types of cell all contain the same information but express different genes according to their function. In other words, they only transcribe the sections of DNA that correspond to proteins needed to construct the cell and perform its specific functions.

> Cells divide to form specific tissues in the body and this process of differentiation is controlled by turning on and off specific genes in the cells.

The sections of DNA not required by the cell are 'turned off' by special proteins that bind to specific sequences of DNA and prevent them being transcribed. Different cell types have different sets of these gene regulatory proteins and therefore transcribe different genes. By using various combinations of a few regulatory genes, thousands of different cell types can be produced. Some of the regulatory proteins are more powerful; these are called master gene regulatory proteins and regulate large sets of genes, establishing and maintaining the basic plan of a tissue and coordinating its development.

Although the generation of mRNA provides the main control over which sections of DNA are read, other steps in protein synthesis can also be regulated. RNA molecules can be processed by polymerases in different ways, they can be selectively transported out of the nucleus for translation or they may be degraded before they can be translated. Once the protein is made, controls can be used to activate or inactivate them.

Once a specialised cell has become established, its genetic information becomes stable and is inherited when the cell divides. This is why cells grown in tissue culture, away from external influences of the surrounding tissues or blood supply, retain their unique character.

There are two distinct ways in which cells become associated to form tissues. They can form from a 'founder cell', which, as it divides, attaches the progeny cells to an extracellular matrix or to other cells so that they cannot move away. In the developing embryo, epithelial cells form into sheets like this. These are then folded and differentiated to form various tissues and organs. The second method of tissue formation is the migration and assembly of groups of cells to form a tissue made of different cell types. Cells recognise each other by their specific glycoprotein receptors on the cell surface and bind together using special adhesion molecules.

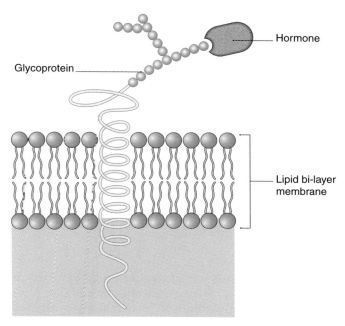

Fig. 4.10 *Cell surface carbohydrate receptors.*

Cell surface receptors

Carbohydrates are present on the surface of all cells, occurring largely as glyco-proteins (linked to proteins) and glycolipids (linked to fats). They provide a structure on the surface of the cell, which can be recognised, for example, by hormones (Fig. 4.10). Unlike the amino acids in proteins, which can only con-nect with each other in one way, carbohydrates can attach to each other in many different ways. This enables them to form thousands of different com-pounds, many with branching structures. As well as providing points of attach-ment for other cells or messengers, surface carbohydrates are involved in mediating the migration of cells during embryo development and also enable harmful agents such as bacteria, viruses and toxins to attach to the cell.

Lectins are proteins that are able to bind rapidly and reversibly with carbohy-drates. They are extremely specific and are able to distinguish between different structures. Frequently found on the surface of cells, they play a role in adhesion of cells by recognising and binding with particular carbohydrates on neighbour-ing cells.

Mechanisms of signalling between cells

In a multicellular organism, cells need to communicate with each other so that they can organise into tissues and regulate their development, function, growth and division. Animal cells can use several different methods of communication. Signal molecules or chemicals, such as hormones, are secreted from a cell and travel through the blood to affect other target cells throughout the body. Specific proteins called receptors on the surface of the target cell bind to the signalling molecule and initiate the response. Some cells secrete chemical mediators with a very localised effect: for example, histamine released by mast cells and the synaptic signals of neurotransmitters which act only on the adjacent postsynaptic cell. A signalling molecule often has different effects on different types of cell because the response to the signal is dependent on the internal machinery of the cell to which the receptor is connected. The plasma membrane can display special signal molecules to influence other cells with which they are in contact, and molecules can also be exchanged in junctions that form between adjacent cells.

> Cells communicate with their external environment and with each other through specific areas on the cell surface (plasma membrane) called receptors.

SUMMARY

All living cells consist of a nucleus containing the genetic information and cytoplasm surrounded by a semipermeable membrane. Higher forms of life are made up of eucaryotic cells, which contain many organelles to help them perform a variety of complex functions. These include the endoplasmic reticulum, which makes lipids and proteins, the Golgi apparatus, which modifies and distributes lipids and proteins, mitochondria, which produce energy by oxidising food molecules, and lysosomes and perioxisomes, which remove unwanted molecules and substances. The entry and exit of nutrients and waste materials is controlled by the plasma membrane and the cytoskeleton is responsible for the transport of substances around the cell.

In multicellular organisms, cells develop specialised functions and form into various tissues and organs. Receptors on the surface of cells enable communication between adjacent cells or with messengers, such as hormones, ensuring that different types of tissue within the organism can cooperate with each other.

QUESTIONS

1. Where do replication, transcription and translation take place?

2. What functions does the cell membrane serve?

3. How are tissues formed?

FURTHER READING

Montague S, Knight D (1996) Cell structure and function, growth and development. In: Hinchliff S, Montague S, Watson R (eds) *Physiology for nursing practice, 2nd edn.* Baillière Tindall, London, pp 49–69

Watson R (1995) *Anatomy and physiology for nurses, 10th edn.* Baillière Tindall, London

2 CONTROL SYSTEMS

5 Autonomic Nervous System

Sheenan Kindlen

After reading this chapter you should be able to:
- understand the functions of the autonomic nervous system
- state the different divisions of the autonomic nervous system
- give some examples of control by the autonomic nervous system.

The activities of many animals are dependent on external conditions. For example, if the weather is cold, they are sluggish and have to wait until the ambient temperature is high enough for them to function. On the other hand, warm-blooded animals such as humans have internalised the climate such that, provided the internal environment is relatively normal, they can function.

The physiological environment is closely monitored and regulated by numerous mechanisms that keep the 'climate' as steady as possible, i.e. to achieve *homeostasis* (Ch. 7). Homeostasis is not, as the name might suggest, a constant state, but a constantly adjusted state. Values for plasma electrolytes, blood pressure or body temperature are not constants; they simply represent the value for that parameter at the time of sampling and are likely to be different if a second measurement is made. There are normal ranges for all homeostatic parameters, with the values constantly being adjusted up and down the range. The aim of the regulatory systems is to use the many mechanisms at the disposal of the body to make sure that the parameter does not move outside its normal range.

The control and regulatory mechanisms of the autonomic nervous system and the endocrine systems are important in the maintenance of homeostasis. The two systems show many similarities. Both respond to incoming signals from the environment they are controlling, both use chemical messengers to make changes in that environment, and both are controlled mainly by the hypothalamus. There are important differences, however, the most obvious being the greater speed of response of the autonomic nervous system. Many aspects of homeostatic control (for example, control of blood pressure and body temperature or the response to stress) are managed cooperatively by the two systems. This widens the range of mechanism available to the body and increases the level of control over the internal environment.

The autonomic nervous system is considered in this chapter and information on endocrine activity is in Chapter 6.

Many of the pathological effects of disease arise from failure of the neural mechanisms or the tissues they supply and much modern drug therapy has stemmed from improved understanding of the autonomic neural mechanisms. In order to understand the workings of the autonomic nervous system, it is useful to be familiar with the way in which neurones themselves work and how they communicate with one another and the tissues they supply.

Anatomically, the nervous system is made up of the central nervous system (the brain and cord) and the peripheral nervous system, which includes all the peripheral nerve fibres going to or coming from the brain and cord. Functionally, the nervous system consists of the somatic nervous system, which is voluntary and conscious, and the autonomic nervous system, which is the unconscious and involuntary system. The underlying principle is that there are afferent or sensory pathways leading into a central or coordinating area with efferent or motor pathways going out to effector tissues.

> Afferent nerve cells take signals to the brain and efferent nerve cells take signals from the brain to organs and tissues.

Nerve communication is achieved when a stimulus activates a first neurone. The signal is transmitted by the first neurone to a second at an area called a synapse, where the two neurones come close together but do not touch. This process is repeated with any subsequent neurones in the pathway until an effect is achieved, for example activity in an effector tissue. The simplest arrangement is that of a reflex arc with only two or three neurones taking part (Fig. 5.1). On the other hand, reflexes involving several separate brain areas may involve uncountable numbers of neurones.

NEURONE STRUCTURE

Neurones are of very different shapes and sizes, but they do have some general characteristic features (Fig. 5.2). The main features are the cell body and the structures that extend from the cell body.

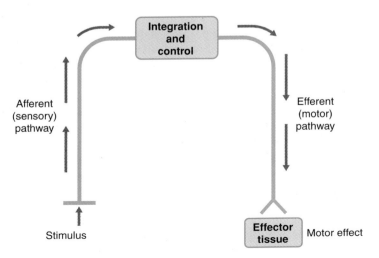

Fig. 5.1 *Reflex arc structure.*

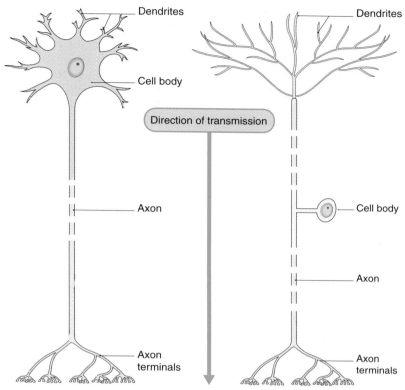

Fig. 5.2   *Generalised sensory and motor neurones.*

Dendrites are the 'receiving end' of the neurone, and are numerous extensions either of the cell body itself or of a longer process leading into the cell body. The stimulus is applied at the dendrites and, if effective, the 'signal' will be transmitted in towards the cell body. Stimuli can take many forms. For example, the stimulus may be chemical, such as a neurotransmitter, electrical, as in the transmission of a nerve impulse, or mechanical, such as compression or stretching of the mechanoreceptors.

The long extension from the cell body is the *axon*. Some neurones have a very long axon; the neurones originating in the cord and supplying the blood vessels in a foot may have an axon length of nearly 1 metre (m). Others can be shorter than the diameter of a red cell. Some neurones have axons sheathed in myelin, which is a thick insulating coating interrupted at intervals down the length of the axon. The gaps in the myelin where the neurone membrane is exposed to extracellular fluid are called the *nodes of Ranvier*. Myelinated axons conduct nerve impulses faster than unmyelinated axons.

NEURONE FUNCTION

All neurones function in a fairly standard way, but the range of stimuli that activate them and the results that they produce allow them to generate a myriad of different results.

The functioning of the nervous system depends on the special properties of the neurone membrane, which give it the property of *electrical excitability*. The molecules in the membrane are arranged so that the membrane is selectively permeable. 'Channels' in the membrane allow the passage of water and some selected ions. Some of the channels show sensitivity to certain chemical triggers, opening or closing in response to the trigger, and this is known as '*chemical gating*'. Other channels open or close at particular values of the voltage across the membrane and these are '*voltage-gated*' channels.

The resting state

When the neurone is not active, it is said to be in a *resting state*. Activity in the neurone, i.e. the generation of a nerve impulse, depends on the disturbance of the resting state followed by its prompt restoration. The term 'resting state' is rather a misnomer; a state of 'dynamic equilibrium' would be a more accurate description.

The migration of ions across the cell membrane is required for both the disturbance and the restoration of the resting state; therefore, the distribution of ions on either side of the membrane is central to the ability of the neurone to generate a nerve impulse. The movement of ions takes place in response to concentration and charge gradients across the membrane and the changes in membrane permeability initiated by a stimulus.

Concentration and charge gradients in the resting state

Intracellular fluid has a high concentration of potassium ions (K^+) and a low concentration of sodium ions (Na^+) (Ch. 1). Extracellular fluid has a low concentration of K^+ and a high concentration of Na^+. There is therefore a concentration gradient for potassium such that potassium ions would flow out from the cell towards extracellular fluid. The concentration gradient for sodium ions would cause them to flow from outside the cell into the intracellular compartment. The membrane has many K^+ channels and is highly permeable to K^+ and these ions can enter the cell easily if the gradients are favourable. The membrane has few open channels for Na^+, which enter the resting cell with difficulty, even when the gradients are in their favour.

The other influence on ion movement across a membrane is the electrical charge gradient. Like charges repel one another, unlike charges attract and the greater the number of charges, the steeper is the gradient. Gradients may 'assist' one another or they may compete. Where there are competing gradients the net effect will depend on the magnitude of the individual gradients.

The cell membrane is impermeable to the protein anions (Pr^-) contained within the neurone. These cannot permeate out of the cell and are referred to as *nondiffusible ions* (Fig. 5.3). The presence of the protein ions close to the membrane on the inside of the neurone produces a state in the resting neurone where the inside of the membrane is more negatively charged than the outside. The difference in charge is called the *electrical potential difference* and it has a value of about 70 millivolts (mV). Because this is always expressed 'inside compared with outside', this potential difference is therefore −70 mV. In electrical terms this is called the *resting membrane potential*. The larger the difference between

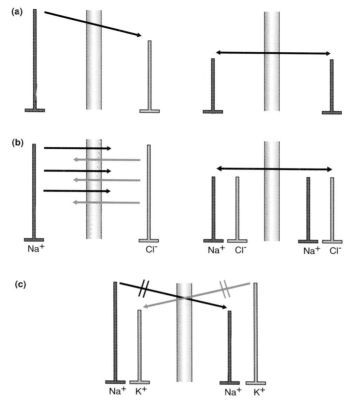

Fig. 5.3 *Gradients and competing gradients. (a) Concentration gradient. The substance moves downhill with the gradient until the concentrations on both sides are equal. (Small shifts continue to take place due to other influences, e.g. osmosis.) (b) Charge gradient – unlike charges attract. (Even at equilibrium, small shifts continue to take place due to other influences, e.g. concentrations and osmosis.) (c) Favourable concentration gradients in competition with unfavourable charge gradients (like charges repel).*

the two sides of the membrane, the larger the potential difference. The electrical charges on the membrane are polarised, more negative on one side, more positive on the other; therefore, in the resting state the membrane is said to be *polarised.*

Sodium/potassium pump

Ions tend to leak in and out of the resting membrane because of the steep concentration gradients and the electrical gradient. In order to maintain the unequal concentrations, the cell membrane incorporates an enzyme system that ejects Na^+ which leaks in and retrieves K^+. This mechanism is called the *sodium/potassium ATPase pump* or sometimes just '*the sodium pump*'. All cells have the sodium pump and it is essential for their survival. Energy is required for the operation of this pump and it has been estimated that it accounts for about 20–30% of total resting energy expenditure. Different cell types have different uses for the pump, but the function of the nervous system depends on the sodium pump to help maintain the very large differences in concentrations inside and outside the neurone membrane that will be required to generate the nerve impulse. The resting state is maintained by the presence of the non-diffusible, mainly protein ions which are negatively charged, the sodium pump and the special characteristics of the membrane.

> At rest there is a charge of approximately 70 mV across a nerve cell. The charge becomes slightly positive when the cell becomes depolarised.

The excited state

The excited state in the neurone is achieved by stimulation. The stimulus can take a variety of forms such as chemical, electrical, mechanical and thermal. It has the effect of changing the degree of selective permeability of the membrane and allowing a small influx of Na^+ along the sodium-specific channels, according to its concentration gradient and attracted by the negative charge inside the membrane. This makes the inside of the membrane less negative than before and therefore a small degree of depolarisation has taken place, i.e. an approach to 0 mV potential difference (see Fig. 5.4). This depolarisation, if large enough, causes the potential difference across the membrane to reach a value at which the voltage-gated Na^+ channels open (this can be equated with *threshold potential*). This greatly increases the membrane permeability to Na^+, which flood in and exceed the capacity of the sodium pump. As the Na^+ accumulate inside the membrane, the inside becomes less and less negatively charged. The difference between the two sides of the membrane gets smaller, then passes through zero. At this point the difference across the membrane is 0 mV and the membrane can be said to be depolarised. Na^+ still enter using the concentration gradient although by this time they are no longer electrically attracted. The potential difference begins to increase towards a positive value, inside compared with outside. This is the *positive overshoot*. The value for membrane potential, which is the maximum positive value that can be reached in the neurone membrane, is referred to as the *action potential*. It is shown on a trace as a spike (Fig 5.4). The action potential is a standard value for any particular neurone and is of the order of +40 mV.

If the stimulus is too small to cause a depolarisation large enough to cross threshold potential, the membrane returns to resting without having achieved an action potential. The membrane therefore responds maximally or not at all, which is the basis for the *all or nothing law*.

As the membrane potential nears the value for an action potential, the membrane begins to change again, becoming increasingly less permeable to Na^+. Lack of concentration and charge gradients in any case reduce the inflow of Na^+ until the influx comes within the capacity of the sodium pump and the accumulated Na^+ are ejected. Once the action potential has been achieved, the membrane potential begins to fall.

Throughout the course of events, K^+ are also involved. K^+ leak out along their concentration gradient, although at threshold potential Na^+ influx exceeds K^+ efflux allowing the positive charges from Na^+ to accumulate rapidly. Near action potential the membrane becomes increasingly permeable to K^+. They now rapidly leak out along their concentration gradient and are repelled by the positive charge inside the membrane. This adds to the loss of positive charges from

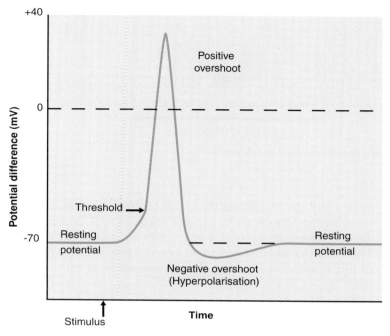

Fig. 5.4   *Nerve action potential/nerve impulse.*

the membrane and the potential drops through 0 mV and becomes increasingly negative (repolarisation). Towards the end of this phase, the action of the sodium pump is increased and the membrane becomes hyperpolarised (*negative overshoot*) before returning to the resting state. During and immediately following the action potential, the membrane is *refractory* and it cannot respond to a stimulus, however large.

This procession of events is referred to as the *nerve impulse* and neurones function by transmitting a train of impulses along their length. (The term action potential is often used to denote the whole nerve impulse; strictly, 'action potential' is the value of the membrane potential when a sign reversal has been achieved.)

When a nerve cell becomes depolarised this generates an action potential which can be transmitted along the nerve cell. The rate of this transmission is accelerated by the presence of a myelin sheath.

Nerve impulse transmission (Fig. 5.5)

The action potential has achieved a sign reversal in a very local area of the membrane. The stimulus is now represented by this 'signal', which must be transmitted along the length of the neurone (see Fig. 5.6).

The positive to negative sign difference on adjacent sections of the membrane has the effect of creating a small electrical circuit with the current flowing from A to B. The small current acts as an electrical stimulus for the membrane at B and results in a new action potential there. In the meantime the impulse at A

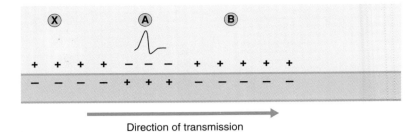

Fig. 5.5   *Nerve impulse transmission in an unmyelinated axon.*

decays and the membrane there will return to resting. In theory there is a current flowing from A to X, but any stimulus at X would be ineffective because the membrane there is still *refractory* following the action potential there. Therefore the transmission of an impulse may radiate outwards from the point of initial stimulus but, once begun, transmission takes place in one direction only.

The action potential lasts for about 0.5 milliseconds (ms) and is repeated down the length of the neurone; therefore, nerve impulse transmission is essentially a wave of electrical activity which travels down the neurone membrane. The step-by-step progression of a nerve impulse along an unmyelinated axon is called *propagation*. A sensory neurone is normally stimulated at the dendrites, at a receptor whose structure is sensitive to changes in its environment. Interneurones and motor neurones are usually stimulated at their dendrites or cell bodies by a chemical transmitter released by another neurone.

Transmission in myelinated neurones

The process of transmission described above is modified in the case of neurones with myelinated axons. Here the membrane is isolated from the extracellular environment by myelin, except at the nodes of Ranvier. Ions cannot pass across the membrane except at the nodes and therefore generation of an action potential can take place only at the nodes. As the current flows along the axon, the impulse appears to leap from node to node. This is *saltatory conduction* (from 'saltare', the Latin word meaning 'to leap') (Fig. 5.6).

This form of conduction is faster than the previous step-by-step propagation, fewer action potentials have to be generated for any length of axon, and because the use of the sodium pump is required only at the exposed node areas, saltatory conduction also uses less energy.

Conduction velocity

Once a neurone reaches its threshold of stimulation, the speed of transmission depends on the type, size and physiological condition of the nerve fibre. Myelinated fibres are faster than non-myelinated fibres and large fibres are faster than small. The fastest fibres are the sensory fibres conveying touch, pressure, temperature and the position of joints, and some of the motor fibres supplying skeletal muscle. Transmission in autonomic neurones is relatively slow.

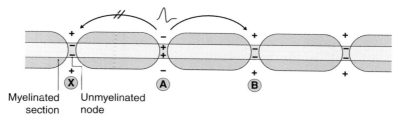

Myelinated   Unmyelinated
section   node

Fig. 5.6   *Nerve impulse transmission in a myelinated axon: saltatory conduction.*

Refractory period

During the time when a membrane is refractory it is incapable of receiving another stimulus and, therefore, incapable of transmitting another impulse. The refractory time depends on the axon diameter; large axons have the briefest refractory time and can repolarise most quickly. The sooner a membrane can repolarise, the sooner it can transmit another impulse. Some large neurones, like the major voluntary motor neurones with thick, myelinated axons, can transmit 2500 impulses per second. Autonomic neurones transmit about 250 impulses per second.

The synapse

Impulses are passed from neurone to neurone in the region called the *synapse* (Fig. 5.7). This is the area where neurones come close to one another but do not touch. Synapses can be excitatory or inhibitory, but at all synapses, conduction can take place in one direction only.

> Transmission between nerve cells takes place at synapses where the electrical impulse in one nerve cell is transmitted chemically to another cell.

Synapses cause a delay in transmission ranging from a few hundred microseconds to tens of milliseconds. No such delay would occur with continuous electrical transmission, therefore it is logical to assume that synaptic transmission takes a different form. The transmission at a synapse is chemical transmission, the diffusion across the synaptic gap of a transmitter substance released by one neurone affecting the state of the next neurone. The neurone on the transmitting side of the synapse is the presynaptic neurone and the receiving neurone is the postsynaptic neurone.

The axon of the presynaptic neurone divides into numerous amyelinated branches, each of which ends in many expanded knobs or *boutons*. These come close to the dendrites of the postsynaptic neurone but not into contact with its surface. One presynaptic neurone may synapse with many postsynaptic neurones or, conversely, one postsynaptic neurone may be synapsed upon by many presynaptic neurones. In the autonomic nervous system, one presynaptic neurone synapses with about 7–10 postsynaptic neurones, giving a diffuse effect.

When the action potential reaches the axon terminal of the presynaptic neurone, it causes the entry of calcium ions into the axon boutons. This in turn

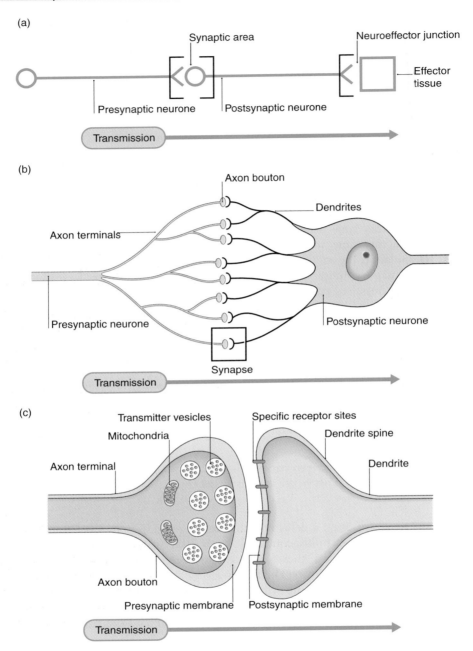

(a)

Synaptic area

Neuroeffector junction

Effector tissue

Presynaptic neurone

Postsynaptic neurone

Transmission

(b)

Axon bouton

Dendrites

Axon terminals

Presynaptic neurone

Postsynaptic neurone

Synapse

Transmission

(c)

Transmitter vesicles

Specific receptor sites

Mitochondria

Dendrite spine

Axon terminal

Dendrite

Axon bouton

Presynaptic membrane   Postsynaptic membrane

Transmission

Fig. 5.7   *The synapse. (a) Pre- and postsynaptic neurones; (b) synaptic area; (c) detail of a synapse.*

causes the migration of the vesicles containing the transmitter towards the presynaptic membrane and the release of their contents into the gap. The transmitter diffuses across the synaptic gap simply by a concentration gradient and makes contact with *specific receptor sites* on the postsynaptic membrane. Receptor sites are protein molecules that are part of the cell membrane. They can bind certain specific substances and the combination of a receptor with its transmitter will cause a change in the cell membrane. A receptor will bind only that chemical for which it is specific. The effect of the transmitter is to increase the membrane permeability at the receptor sites to all small ions and there is consequently a small degree of depolarisation – the *postsynaptic potential* (PSP). The PSP is brief in duration because of the presence, at the synapse, of an enzyme that breaks down the transmitter.

The PSP differs from the action potential in several ways:

- it is a simple depolarisation (below threshold value) rather than a reversal of polarity
- it is a graded response and is related to the amount of transmitter
- it has no refractory period therefore responses may be added to one another until the neurone is activated (summation)
- it is not propagated and decays in intensity with distance from the receptor area.

When the PSP is large enough, i.e. enough terminals are discharging often enough, the local current generated flows into the surrounding membrane, increasing sodium permeability and generating an action potential, which can then be propagated along the postsynaptic neurone.

The postsynaptic potential can be excitatory (EPSP) or inhibitory (IPSP). The EPSP will cause activity in the postsynaptic neurone and the IPSP will prevent any activity. The junction between a motor nerve and an effector tissue is termed the *neuroeffector junction* (the term synapse should be reserved for neural junctions).

The activity at the neuroeffector junction follows a very similar pattern of events to that at the synapse, i.e. production of a transmitter by a neurone and diffusion to specific receptor sites on the effector tissue membrane with the resulting excitation or inhibition of the effector tissue.

AUTONOMIC NERVOUS SYSTEM ACTIVITY

Much of the internal environment is controlled by the autonomic nervous system (ANS). Although the regulation of many homeostatic parameters such as blood pressure, blood gases and gut activity is shared by the ANS and endocrine system, the short term, more immediate control is almost entirely the province of the ANS. The ANS is driven both directly from the higher centres in the brain and reflexly by the lower brain in response to 'body' signals. For example, the sight of blood at a road accident can activate a range of autonomic responses in the bystander just as powerfully as the loss of blood pressure will in the accident victim.

> The autonomic nervous system controls homeostasis along with the endocrine system.

The 'normal' level of homeostatic regulation by ANS, however, is achieved by a series of reflexes (a reflex can be defined as 'the same stimulus always producing the same effect'). Sensory information goes in to the brain (or cord) to be organised by the interneurones in the brain and cord, which in turn stimulate motor activity. The outline organisation is shown in Figure 5.8.

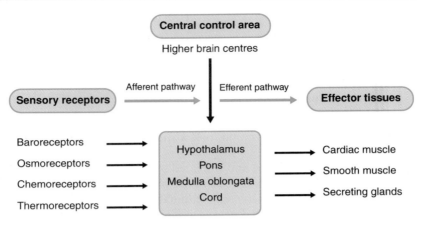

Fig. 5.8   *Outline organisation of the autonomic nervous system.*

The autonomic sensory signals are normally below the conscious level and the motor effect is involuntary. Some of the results of autonomic activity, however, may be felt, or even heard or seen. An increase in heart rate can be felt, increased breathing can be felt and sometimes heard and the effects of vasodilatation may be very visible.

Autonomic central areas

The major central area coordinating and controlling homeostasis is the hypothalamus. Sensory information on all the homeostatic parameters is relayed to the hypothalamus, which can then coordinate the responses that are to be made. It has an important role in coordinating many of the endocrine systems, and it is at this level that many ANS and endocrine activities are integrated.

Other areas with central ANS activity are the pons, medulla oblongata and cord. The medulla oblongata has within it many of the 'operating' centres for ANS controlled mechanisms, such as changing heart rate, vascular capacity and gut function. The activities of these operating centres are integrated by the hypothalamus. It should be remembered that, despite its apparently powerful role, the hypothalamus is not independent. Under certain circumstances, such as the road traffic accident earlier, all its autonomic and endocrine mechanisms can be affected by stimuli from the cerebral cortex.

Autonomic sensory receptors

Sensory receptors of the autonomic afferent nerves include those listed below, with the aspect of the internal environment that they monitor:

- mechanoreceptors
    baroreceptors – blood pressure
    stretch receptors – stretch in gut wall, bladder and respiratory tract
- osmoreceptors – osmotic pressure, concentration of body fluids
- chemoreceptors – many chemicals, e.g. oxygen, carbon dioxide, H^+
- thermoreceptors – core and surface temperature
- nociceptors – tissue damage.

The short list above illustrates the dependence of the internal environment on autonomic mechanisms, with blood pressure, fluid balance, blood gases, body temperature and the presence or absence of tissue damage all within the realm of ANS influence.

Autonomic motor pathways

The motor efferent pathways belong to the *parasympathetic* and *sympathetic* divisions of the ANS. The two divisions often have opposite effects on a tissue, one excitatory and the other inhibitory. The combined effect is to manage tissue activities according to body requirement. The classical phrase describing this was that the effects of the two divisions were antagonistic but synergistic. Many organs such as heart, gut and bladder have both supplies; this is *dual innervation*.

Of the two divisions, the parasympathetic is probably simpler than the sympathetic division. The parasympathetic system is a type of 'in-house maintenance system', running body activities at an economical level, managing digestion and absorption of food and excretion of waste products. The sympathetic system is associated with higher levels of activity, work, exercise or excitement. The phrase used to describe the sympathetic response is 'flight, fight and fright'. This, however, wrongly suggests that the sympathetic system is active only in extreme circumstances; in fact, some measure of sympathetic activity goes on continuously, for example in maintaining blood pressure while just standing upright.

> The autonomic nervous system has two divisions, the sympathetic and the parasympathetic divisions. The sympathetic division can broadly be described as being responsible for keeping the body in a state of readiness (the 'fight or flight' response) and most of its actions are opposite to those of the parasympathetic division.

THE PARASYMPATHETIC DIVISION OF THE ANS

The central or interneurones for efferent parasympathetic nerves lie in the brain and the cord. The outflow is via the cranial and sacral nerves, therefore described as a cranio-sacral outflow. Not all of these nerves carry parasympathetic fibres. The head is supplied by the oculomotor, facial and glossopharyngeal nerves, the thorax and upper abdomen by the vagus and its branches, and the lower gut, bladder and external genitalia by the second to fourth sacral nerves.

Each parasympathetic efferent pathway is composed of two neurones, one presynaptic and one postsynaptic, the presynaptic long and myelinated and the postsynaptic short and unmyelinated (Fig. 5.9). At some tissues the postsynaptic axon is so short that the synapse is almost on the tissue surface.

Although each separate pathway is constructed as in Figure 5.9, the structure of the system consists of numerous pathways running together as nerve tracts. In addition, each presynaptic neurone synapses with several postsynaptic neurones. The synapse regions are located close to one another in the tracts and the

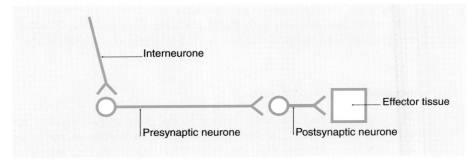

Fig. 5.9   *A typical parasympathetic pathway.*

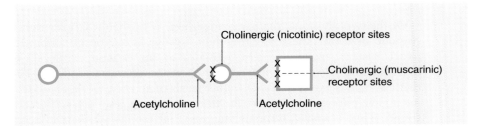

Fig. 5.10   *Transmitters and receptor sites in a parasympathetic pathway.*

presence of the group of cell bodies shows as a lump or small swelling, which has become known as a neural *ganglion*. The terminology was adapted to suit and presynaptic neurones are also known as *preganglionic* and the postsynaptic neurones as *postganglionic* neurones.

Activity in a parasympathetic pathway

The transmitter used by the parasympathetic division is acetylcholine. Acetylcholine is used at the synapse and at the neuroeffector junction; however, the receptor sites are different. Each type is *cholinergic*, i.e. worked by acetylcholine, but on the postsynaptic surface at the ganglion the sites are *nicotinic* and on the tissue surface, at the neuroeffector junction, they are *muscarinic* (Fig. 5.10). The receptor sites are described as cholinergic (nicotinic) and cholinergic (muscarinic).

The adjectives 'nicotinic' and 'muscarinic' originate from the method used to distinguish between the two types of cholinergic receptor. Many subtypes of autonomic receptor have been, and are still being, identified; only the most commonly used are included here.

Tissue responses to parasympathetic activity (Fig. 5.11)

These are shown in Table 5.1 (only selected systems and tissues are listed here as examples).

Transmitter catabolism

In order that any nerve pathway can be kept working, the transmitter, once

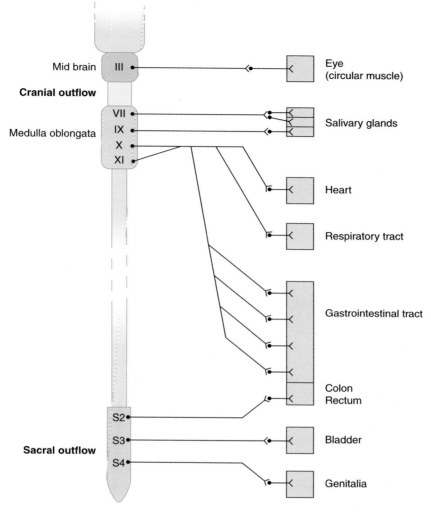

Mid brain

Cranial outflow

Medulla oblongata

III — Eye (circular muscle)

VII
IX — Salivary glands
X
XI

Heart

Respiratory tract

Gastrointestinal tract

Colon
Rectum

S2
S3 — Bladder
Sacral outflow
S4

Genitalia

Fig. 5.11   *Diagrammatic view of parasympathetic outflow.*

released, must be used and then destroyed. If it is allowed to accumulate, a new action potential could not be generated in the postsynaptic neurone and activity in the effector tissue would not take place. The catabolic enzyme acetylcholinesterase is found in both the synaptic and neuroeffector junction gaps and has the effect of breaking down acetylcholine so that it can no longer act as a transmitter.

Pharmacology (see also Ch. 15)

A drug that imitates the parasympathetic nervous system is a *parasympathomimetic* or parasympathetic agonist; it has *cholinergic* effects. Because the effects will be on the tissue rather than at the ganglion, the drug will have muscarinic effects. Drugs such as these are sometimes used to increase motility in

TABLE 5.1	Tissue Effects Produced by Parasympathetic Stimulation	
	System/organ	Tissue effect
	Cardiovascular system	Reduced heart rate
		Vasodilatation at tongue, salivary glands, external sex organs
	Gut	Increased motility, secretions
	Pancreas	Increased exocrine secretion
		Increased insulin release
	Bladder	Contraction of bladder wall
		Relaxation of internal sphincter
	Eye (constrictor (circular) muscle of pupil)	Contraction – pupil constriction

the gut (bethanechol) or the bladder (carbachol). Some drugs, like bethanechol, have very widespread effects because they affect all muscarinic sites, producing many unwanted effects in addition to the effect required. Some are much more specific to certain tissues: for example, carbachol has its main effects on the urinary bladder.

A substance that is similar enough to acetylcholine to occupy the receptor sites but not similar enough to activate them is a blocking agent or parasympathetic antagonist. These would usually be employed at muscarinic sites and would be called antimuscarinic or anticholinergic (muscarinic) drugs or simply muscarinic blockers. Such a drug is atropine, which can be used to block muscarinic sites in the heart and raise heart rate and, consequently, blood pressure. The original use of atropine was as an eye cosmetic. The plant from which it was extracted has the name *belladonna* – beautiful lady. When the extract was used as eye drops it produced pupil dilatation, an effect thought to be attractive. Atropine is still used clinically to dilate the pupil, but it is a long-acting drug and has given way to shorter-acting drugs such as homatropine or tropicamide.

THE SYMPATHETIC DIVISION OF THE ANS

This division has many adaptations, which make it apparently more complex than the parasympathetic division; it can recruit the neurohormones, noradrenaline and adrenaline, to give sympathomedullary or sympathoadrenal effects. The receptor sites have more identified subtypes, one of which provides a negative feedback mechanism. The concentration of the transmitter or neurohormone is also more critical because the sensitivity of the receptor sites varies.

Sympathetic outflow

The interneurones in the cord give rise to efferent pathways emerging from the cord at the thoracic and upper lumbar segments, the system therefore has a *thoraco-lumbar outflow*. Each pathway is, like the parasympathetic outflow, composed of two neurones, one presynaptic, the other postsynaptic.

Pathway structure

The typical sympathetic pathway consists of a short, myelinated preganglionic neurone followed by a long amyelinated postganglionic neurone (Fig. 5.12). The neurones run in tracts, therefore the groups of synapses are marked by ganglia. Most of the ganglia are arranged in chains (the *sympathetic chains*), one on either side of the spinal column. A small number of ganglia are found outside the chain; these are the coeliac and mesenteric ganglia (Fig. 5.13), whose postganglionic neurones supply gut and bladder.

> Tissue receptors which respond to acetylcholine are described as cholinergic and those which respond to noradrenaline and adrenaline are described as adrenergic.

Activity in a sympathetic pathway

The transmitter used at the synapse in sympathetic pathways is acetylcholine; all autonomic ganglia use this transmitter. The receptor sites at the ganglion are, as before, cholinergic and nicotinic. The transmitter released by most sympathetic postganglionic neurones is *noradrenaline*. The receptor sites on the effector tissues are *adrenergic* or *adrenoceptors* (Fig. 5.14).

Adrenoceptors are of different subtypes, α and β, and these are further subdivided into α_1 and α_2 and β_1 and β_2. Each of the subtypes is capable of a different effect and the same subtype may give different effects at different tissues. Noradrenaline, for example, acting on α_1 will cause vasoconstriction at smooth muscle in an arteriole but relaxation at smooth muscle in the gut. The general rules, however, are as follows:

- noradrenaline at α_1 – excitation at blood vessels, relaxation at gut smooth muscle
- noradrenaline at α_2 – reduction in release of noradrenaline (negative feedback mechanism)
- noradrenaline at β_1 – increased rate and force of contraction at heart
- noradrenaline at β_2 – little effect.

> Adrenaline and noradrenaline are able to exert slightly different effects owing to the existence of different types of adrenergic receptors (α, β_1 and β_2). Noradrenaline acts more strongly on α receptors and adrenaline on β receptors.

Sympathomedullary effect

One of the additional aspects of the sympathetic division is its ability to recruit the neurohormones of the adrenal medulla, noradrenaline and adrenaline, jointly called the *catecholamines*. The adrenal medulla is supplied by sympathetic preganglionic nerves (Fig. 5.15) and stimulation causes release of the catecholamines into the general circulation. They are distributed throughout the body and can affect any tissue that has the appropriate adrenoceptor sites; this

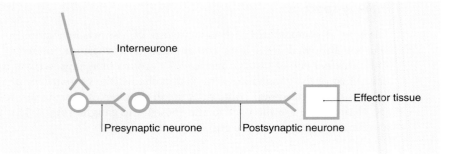

Fig. 5.12   *A typical sympathetic pathway.*

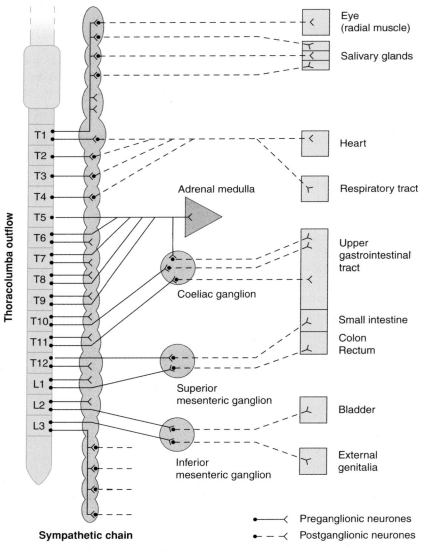

Fig. 5.13   *Diagrammatic view of sympathetic outflow.*

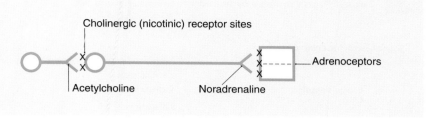

Fig. 5.14   *Transmitters and receptor sites in a typical sympathetic pathway.*

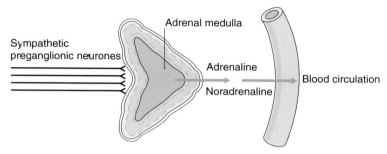

Fig. 5.15   *Sympathetic preganglionic supply to the adrenal medulla (see also Fig. 5.13).*

means that tissues with no direct sympathetic nerve supply can produce a 'sympathetic' response. Where a tissue has a sympathetic nerve supply, the circulating catecholamines will augment the effect of the noradrenaline produced by the nerve.

Effects of adrenaline

Adrenaline and noradrenaline share some effects but there are marked differences between the two catecholamines. Noradrenaline has a more pronounced effect on α receptors, adrenaline on β receptors: for example, noradrenaline causes marked vasoconstriction but has less effect on the heart; adrenaline has a more potent effect on the heart but causes less vasoconstriction. Adrenaline also has a much more potent effect on β_2, particularly in some tissue, for example the smooth muscle of airways and blood vessels. This effect is inhibitory, causing bronchodilatation and vasodilatation, respectively. The evidence can be seen in exercise where the bronchodilator effect allows increased ventilation and the vasodilatation effect allows blood to be quickly diverted to areas such as skeletal muscle.

Adrenaline also has important metabolic effects, e.g. mobilisation of liver glycogen, releasing glucose. Because adrenaline also suppresses insulin release, it plays an important role in the maintenance of blood glucose. This effect assumes great importance in physical stress or injury where a rise in blood glucose is part of the survival strategy of the body.

The tissue effects produced by noradrenaline and adrenaline are shown in Table 5.2 (only selected systems and tissues are listed as examples).

TABLE 5.2	Tissue Effects Produced by Noradrenaline and Adrenaline			
		Adrenoceptor	Tissue effect	Produced by
Cardiovascular system				
	Heart	β_1	Increased rate and force of contraction	Both
	Blood vessels	α_1	Constriction	Noradrenaline
		β_2	Dilatation	Adrenaline
			(Cholinergic dilatation)	(Acetylcholine)
	Bladder wall	β_2	Relaxation	Adrenaline
	Sphincter	α_1	Contraction	Both
	Airways	β_2	Bronchodilatation	Adrenaline
	Gut	α_1, β_2	Tissue dependent	Both
	Eye (radial muscle)	α_1	Contraction, pupil dilatation	Both
	Metabolism		Breakdown of glycogen and fat, insulin suppression of release	Adrenaline

Sympathetic cholinergic effects

The sympathetic system has yet another modification. In some sites (e.g. sweat glands and some skeletal muscle blood vessels) the sympathetic nerves do not release noradrenaline but acetylcholine. The receptor sites are cholinergic and muscarinic, but despite this the mechanism is sympathetic. The effects are production of sweat by the sweat glands and vasodilatation at those particular vessels. The vasodilatation is not a large effect and it may have the effect of reducing afterload on the heart at the beginning of exercise (Ch. 8).

Catabolism of the catecholamines

The catecholamines, like acetylcholine discussed earlier, must be broken down if sympathetic activity is to be maintained. Two main enzymes are involved, one that works outside the cell and can be found in plasma. The other enzyme is an intracellular enzyme and is used to control both the catecholamine level in the cells and any other similar substance that might enter the cells.

The latter enzyme, monoamine oxidase (MAO), is of particular interest because it is found in the cells of the gut where it breaks down monoamines which may be contained in food. These substances, if left intact, can act like the catecholamines and raise blood pressure in some individuals. Inhibitors of MAO (MAOI) can be used clinically as antidepressants and although the drug is aimed at inhibiting MAO in the nervous system, it also inhibits gut MAO. The effect is to allow the absorption of food monoamines with a small risk of acute hypertension. People who take MAOI drugs are warned about the possible risks from foods such as cheese and meat extracts.

Pharmacology (see also Ch. 15)

Drugs that imitate the sympathetic nervous system are *sympathomimetic* drugs, or sympathetic agonists. They may be non-specific, acting at all adrenoceptors, or they may be selective, acting at one or more of the subtypes.

The non-selective drugs, because of the wide range of effects of the sympathetic and sympathomedullary systems, may produce many unwanted effects. A general rule is that the more specific a sympathomimetic is the fewer the side-effects. An important selective agonist is salbutamol, a β_2 agonist used as a bronchodilator in asthma. Although no drug is totally selective, salbutamol can affect the β_2 in the airways without greatly affecting β_1 in the heart and raising heart rate excessively. Antagonists or blockers are similarly either non-selective or relatively site-specific. Beta-blockers are commonly used as antihypertensive agents because they can reduce both heart rate and contractility, so producing a reduction in cardiac output. Those which are non-selective, while they are effective in reducing blood pressure, carry the risk that they will block sympathetic bronchodilatation in the airway, increasing the risk of precipitating an attack in someone who has asthma. In that case it would be much safer to use a cardio-selective antagonist, i.e. one that was specific for β_1 in the heart with little or no effect on β_2 in the airways.

SUMMARY

Much of the complex regulation of body function is autonomic, without the requirement for conscious control. Sensory signals indicating blood pressure, temperature, gut contents, etc., bring about reflex responses in cardiac and smooth muscle and secretory glands. Both divisions of the autonomic nervous system operate to the same pattern. The release of a transmitter is followed by its bonding to specific receptor sites and eventually by either an excitatory or inhibitory effect in the target tissue.

The two divisions of the autonomic outflow have different, often opposite effects on tissues. In some tissues, for example the heart, pacemaker cells are excited by sympathetic activity and inhibited by parasympathetic activity. In the gut, parasympathetic activity is excitatory. The effects of the sympathetic system can be augmented by the release of the catecholamine neurohormones, of which adrenaline, particularly, has additional properties which include its metabolic effects and its ability to cause redirection of blood flow.

The receptor sites, previously regarded as simply cholinergic or adrenergic, actually are of many sub-types, encouraging the development of many autonomic drugs.

Knowledge of the autonomic nervous system allows the understanding, even prediction, of activities of body systems and of the numerous drugs which have autonomic effects.

QUESTIONS

1. Why is necessary to have control systems in the body?

2. How is an action potential generated in a nerve cell?

3. Explain what takes place at a synapse.

FURTHER READING

Allan D, Nie V, Hunter M (1996) Structure and function of nervous tissue. In: Hinchliff S, Montague S, Watson R (eds) *Physiology for nursing practice, 2nd edn.* Ballière Tindall, London, pp 73–99

Watson R (1995) *Anatomy and physiology for nurses, 10th edn.* Baillière Tindall, London

6 Endocrine System

Sheenan Kindlen

After reading this chapter you should be able to:

- outline the main features of the endocrine system
- explain how the endocrine system is controlled
- list the functions of several hormones
- describe some conditions resulting from hormone deficiency or overproduction.

The endocrine system, with its array of hormones, affects all the tissues in the body. The same principles of communication apply as did with the autonomic nervous system (Ch. 5): a chemical messenger is released at the appropriate signal and transferred to a target tissue whose activity is subsequently modified. Some hormones, in association with the autonomic nervous system (ANS), maintain homeostasis; others, again with the ANS, allow the management of stress. The body's size, shape and sexual characteristics, however, are mainly determined hormonally. In view of the number and variety of hormones, this chapter is limited to those that demonstrate the main principles of hormone activity and regulation, and to selected areas of homeostasis.

Hormones are blood-borne chemical messengers that participate in regulating homeostasis.

Simplified definitions are often misleading and this is true in the context of the endocrine system. The classic definition of a hormone as 'a chemical messenger released from one tissue, transported in the blood to a target tissue whose activity it modifies' describes an *endocrine* action; however, some hormones act on cells that are very close to the hormone-producing cells and this should be called a *paracrine* action. The list of endocrine glands, such as the hypothalamus, pituitary, thyroid and so on, has had to be extended to include tissues such as the kidney, gut and heart (Ch. 8), and some hormones may only be steps in pathways that bring about the release of other hormones or agents such as the cytokines (Ch. 14).

Hormones usually act in groups rather than singly: for example, blood glucose is not controlled by insulin or even by insulin and glucagon, but by a larger group of hormones. Body growth, in addition to requiring growth hormone, requires insulin, the thyroid hormones and several other permissive hormones.

General points about endocrine glands and hormones

Release and transport

Because a hormone is usually transferred directly into the blood, an endocrine gland is ductless and must have a good blood supply with many capillaries. The thyroid, for example, has one of the highest perfusion rates per gram of tissue in the body. The hormone, once released, will usually be bound to a protein for transport. The bound form of the hormone is inactive; only the small unbound fraction is active.

Regulation

Hormones are potent chemicals that circulate at very low and carefully regulated concentrations. When the regulation fails, the endocrine disorders provide clear and usually predictable clinical evidence of hormone excess or deficiency. Some hormones are regulated by balancing the factors that stimulate the hormone against the amount of hormone produced (or other hormones produced as a result). This is a negative feedback mechanism (product inhibition) and the hormone would be 'product controlled'. Other hormones are regulated by the parameter they affect, e.g. blood glucose or blood pressure; the hormone in this case would be 'parameter controlled'. Although individual hormones have their own regulating systems, most will be variations on the two broad categories above.

Target cell receptors

The target tissue is identified by the presence of receptor sites that are specific to a particular hormone and the characteristics of the hormone molecule determine where these receptors are. Hormones, such as the steroids, which are lipid soluble, or the thyroid hormones, which are small and carry a metal atom, can penetrate the lipoprotein membrane of target cells (Chs 2 and 4) and have their receptors in the cytoplasm or at the nucleus. Those hormones that are not lipid soluble, e.g. polypeptides such as growth hormone and glucagon, cannot penetrate the membrane and their receptors are therefore on the cell membrane. Because most hormones exert their effect by altering the nuclear activities of the target cell, when a hormone cannot enter a cell a *second messenger* must be used, the hormone being the first messenger. The hormone binds to the membrane receptor and the combination of the two activates an otherwise inactive enzyme, which then goes on to produce a substance that will act as the second messenger. One system used by several hormones is the activation of adenyl cyclase, which can then bring about the formation of cyclic adenosine monophosphate (cAMP) from adenosine triphosphate (ATP). Because ATP is found in all cells, the specificity of the hormone for its target depends on the presence of the membrane receptors. Examples of other second messengers are cyclic guanylyl monophosphate (cGMP) used by antidiuretic hormone (Ch. 11) and glucagon and diacylglycerol (DAG) used by atrial natriuretic peptide (Ch. 8) and noradrenaline (Ch. 5). The second messenger sets in train a series of reactions culminating in the required response from the target cell.

Receptor sites are not fixed in either number or affinity. If the number or affinity increases, this is called up-regulation, the target cell becomes more sensitive to the hormone and better use can be made of the hormone. Conversely, if the tissue cells are down-regulated, the cells can use the hormone less well, i.e. the tissue becomes more resistant to the hormone. This has clinical implications, for example in type II diabetes, where a feature of the condition is insulin resistance due to down-regulation, which can often be attributed to obesity. Glucose tolerance in these individuals can be improved if they lose weight.

Hormone catabolism and excretion

Hormones are metabolised mainly in the liver and are therefore dependent on the health of the liver. Where a liver is damaged, the time taken to metabolise the hormone is increased, i.e. its half-life is increased. The metabolites are excreted mainly in urine and urinalysis may be used either to identify the presence of a hormone by its metabolites or to measure quantitatively its output.

HORMONES AND THE HYPOTHALAMUS

Many hormones are either produced by the hypothalamus or influenced by its activity and it is worth considering this area first.

The hypothalamus is the major control area for the internal environment. As well as controlling the activities of the ANS (Ch. 5), it produces a large number of hormones involved not only in the maintenance of homeostasis but in the management of stress, which constitutes a threat to homeostasis. In addition to this, the hypothalamic hormones are central to establishing and maintaining the body's size, shape and sexual characteristics (morphogenesis).

> The hypothalamus plays a major role in homeostasis and also in growth and development through the hormones that it releases.

Hypothalamic hormones are of two types: those that act as release or inhibitory hormones for the hormones of the anterior pituitary gland, and those that are synthesised in the hypothalamus but released from the posterior pituitary gland. Table 6.1 shows the main hormones produced, the pituitary hormones that result and the area of the body environment affected.

The hypothalamus produces both parameter-controlled hormones and product-controlled hormones, some of which are regulated not by one end product but by several products in an axis. One example of the latter is the regulation of thyroid activity.

The hypothalamo–anterior pituitary–thyroid axis

The thyroid hormones are regulated by the hypothalamo–anterior pituitary–thyroid axis (HPT axis) (Fig. 6.1). The hypothalamus releases thyroid-stimulating hormone releasing hormone (TSHRH), which travels to the anterior pituitary via the small blood supply that runs down the stalk connecting the two

TABLE 6.1   *Hypothalamic Hormonal Regulatory Systems*

Hypothalamic hormone	Anterior pituitary hormone	End organ hormone	Body environment area
*TSHRH or thyrotropin RH	TSH/Thyrotropin	T3/T4	Metabolic rate, heat production, neural development and maintenance
*ACTHRH or corticotropin RH	ACTH/corticotropin	Cortisol	Stress management
*Growth hormone RH and growth hormone inhibitory hormone (somatostatin)	Growth hormone		Body growth
Gonadotropin RH	Follicle-stimulating hormone		Development and maintenance of sexual characteristics, reproduction
	Luteinising hormone		
Prolactin RH	Prolactin		Breast development, milk production
Prolactin inhibitory factor			
Hypothalamic hormone	Posterior pituitary release		
*Antidiuretic hormone →	Antidiuretic hormone		Water conservation/fluid balance/blood pressure
Oxytocin →	Oxytocin		Milk ejection from lactating breast

TSHRH, thyroid-stimulating hormone releasing hormone; RH, releasing hormone; TSH, thyroid-stimulating hormone; ACTHRH, adrenocorticotrophic hormone releasing hormone; ACTH, adrenocorticotrophic hormone.
*Hormone discussed in this chapter.

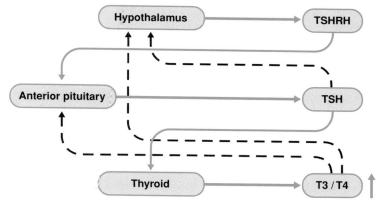

Fig. 6.1   *The hypothalamo–anterior pituitary–thyroid axis. ←--, negative feedback.*

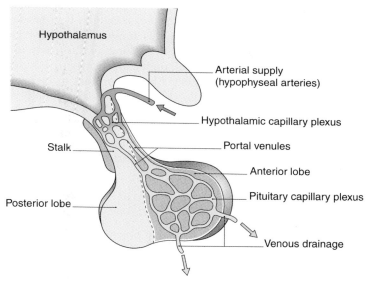

Fig. 6.2   *The hypothalamus and anterior pituitary gland (showing an enlarged and diagrammatic representation of the hypothalamic–anterior pituitary portal blood vessels).*

tissues. There are two capillary beds: one that takes up the released hormone at the hypothalamus and the second at which it is deposited at the anterior lobe (Fig. 6.2). (NB. TSHRH has the alternative name of thyrotropin-releasing hormone (TRH), derived from the alternative name for thyroid-stimulating hormone of thyrotropin.)

In response to TSHRH, the appropriate cells in the anterior pituitary release their hormone, TSH, which is taken up by the second capillary bed and transferred via the general circulation to the thyroid gland. Attachment of TSH to the membrane receptors of the thyroid cells will result in the production and release of the thyroid hormones triiodothyronine (T3) and thyroxine (T4); in the language of the axis system, these are the 'end organ' hormones. T3 and T4 act as a negative feedback on TSH and TSHRH production and, to a lesser extent, TSH acts as negative feedback on TSHRH. At each stage there are also other inhibitors that fine tune the axis and increase the level of control. The axis is stimulated at the hypothalamic level by stimuli from other centres in the hypothalamus itself, e.g. the heat-regulating centre, or from other brain areas.

> A target organ for the hormones of the hypothalamus is the pituitary which, in turn, exerts its effects by releasing pituitary hormones.

The balance between forward stimuli and negative feedback can be illustrated by considering the response to a change in blood temperature. One of the effects of thyroid hormones is to produce an increase in metabolic rate and hence heat production. T3 and T4 are therefore important in the maintenance of temperature homeostasis (Ch. 7). When the blood temperature is reduced, the hypothalamic heat-regulating centre stimulates the centre that produces TSHRH. The increased level of activity in the axis subsequently causes the production of increased T3 and T4, which in turn increase cellular heat production. The rise in blood temperature removes the stimulus at hypothalamic level and the increased T3 and T4 act as negative feedback. As long as the temperature remains low, however, the forward stimulus will outweigh the negative feedback, the T3 and T4 levels will remain high and extra heat continues to be produced. This is an adaptive mechanism, which allows the body to respond to ambient temperature. It takes several weeks to become completely adapted and holidaymakers who go to a warm climate are usually just adapted when they come home, where they find that they feel uncomfortably cold until they (or their thyroid glands) readapt to a lower ambient temperature.

Functions of the HPT axis hormones

Thyroid-stimulating hormone releasing hormone

TSHRH can be considered as a release agent for TSH.

Thyroid-stimulating hormone

TSH has several functions. It is sometimes referred to as a *trophic* hormone; this term means 'nurture' but it can be extended to cover 'growth and development, maintenance and repair', in this case, of the thyroid gland. The thyroid cell size and cell number are therefore dependent on TSH. TSH also increases blood flow to the thyroid, therefore increases the supply of oxygen, iodine and the other substrates required by the thyroid cells. The production and release of T3 and T4 are stimulated by TSH.

Thyroid hormones T3 and T4

The cells producing the hormones are arranged in roughly spherical groups called follicles. T3 and T4 are unusual in being stored within a storage lumen inside the follicles. When the hormones are required, i.e. when signalled by the presence of TSH, they are retrieved from the lumen, stripped of the storage protein (thyroglobulin) in their journey through the follicular cells and released to the circulation. Both hormones circulate bound to a transport protein, e.g. thyroxine-binding globulin.

T4 has a longer half-life and lower biological activity than T3 and is usually regarded as the reservoir form of T3; it can be converted to T3 in the target tissues. A further refinement to the control of the thyroid hormones is at the stage of the conversion of T4 to T3. This conversion yields not only T3 but an inactive version of the molecule, reverse T3 (rT3). The amounts of T3 and rT3 can vary and some conditions such as starvation, some wasting diseases and even some stages of the response to trauma can produce an increase in the proportion of rT3 with a resulting slowing of metabolic rate. This may be an adaptive mechanism, which preserves energy stores in times of shortage. The lumen storage, the binding for transport and the variable conversion of T4 to the much more active T3 all act as modifications that increase control. The thyroid hormones are referred to in the following sections as T3/T4 although the active substance is assumed to be T3.

Functions of T3/T4

The thyroid hormones have a wide range of effects, the most obvious being the effect on the rate of cellular activity. An 'overactive' thyroid can double basal metabolic rate (BMR) and, before sensitive tests of thyroid function were available, BMR was measured as part of the diagnosis of thyroid dysfunction. Heat is generated as a product of this activity and the thyroid hormones are an important part of body temperature regulation in the longer term.

T3/T4 increase the number of adrenoceptors (Ch. 5) and therefore increase the effectiveness of adrenaline and noradrenaline. This becomes evident in thyroid disorders, and tachycardia, even at rest, is a characteristic of thyroid overactivity.

Thyroid hormones have effects on nutrient metabolism mainly by increasing the consumption of stores such as body fat and protein by other hormones. T3/T4 also promote the uptake of carbohydrate from the gut and raise blood glucose during feeding; the overall effect is to raise blood glucose. The hormones are also required for the development and maintenance of the nervous system and even for body growth where they act along with growth hormone and insulin. Some of these effects are best seen when thyroid function is abnormal, as in the examples given below. The use of the HPT axis simplifies the prediction of some of the characteristics of the abnormalities.

Excess and deficiency of T3/T4

T3/T4 excess

If T3/T4 are elevated, whatever the source of the dysfunction, they will give rise to the typical symptoms of hyperthyroidism. Most of the symptoms can be predicted as exaggerations of the normal effects of the hormones:

1. The subject feels hot, looks flushed and feels uncomfortable in warm environments; however, body temperature is likely to be normal because of vasodilatation and sweating, provided hydration is adequate.

2. Heart rate is elevated even at rest and systolic pressure is raised, although diastolic pressure may be significantly lowered by vasodilatation. Pulse pressure is wide (Ch. 8).
3. The subject finds it difficult to rest although easily fatigued; muscle tremor is evident, particularly in outstretched arms.
4. Body weight is lost despite a good appetite and food intake.
5. Tendon reflex time is shortened.
6. There may be metabolic disturbance, e.g. raised blood glucose.

The most common form of overactivity is that seen in Graves' disease. In this condition an antibody is formed to TSH, referred to as thyroid-stimulating immunoglobulin (TSI).

TSI stimulates the thyroid in the same way as TSH, but is outwith normal negative feedback. If hormone levels in the axis are measured, T3/T4 levels are raised, TSH reduced and the presence of TSI is noted. Because TSI has similar properties to TSH, it not only stimulates the production of the thyroid hormones, but also has a trophic action on the thyroid gland, increasing the size and number of the cells and producing the thyroid swelling known as *goitre*. This form of hyperthyroidism is often characterised by retraction of the eyelids and protrusion of the eye (exophthalmos), giving the subject a wide stare.

This condition is treated by removal of part of the thyroid, either by destruction of follicular cells by radioactive iodine or, less usually, by surgery. Drugs such as carbimazole limit the activity of follicular cells and can be used as conservative treatment, but they must be used over a long period of time and their success is somewhat limited. The adverse effects of excess T3/T4 on the heart can be blocked by an adrenoceptor blocker (Ch. 15) and this is useful as an adjunct to other treatment regimes.

Another example of axis abnormality is found in cases of pituitary excess, perhaps due to a functioning tumour of TSH-producing cells. Analysis of the hormone levels in this case would show elevated T3/T4 due to elevated TSH, the presence of goitre (due to the TSH) and if the level of TSHRH were to be measured, one could predict that it would be low. Treatment in this case requires identification and treatment of the pituitary site.

T3/T4 deficiency

Underactivity in the thyroid gland with low levels of T3/T4 shows symptoms many of which are clearly attributable to lack of the normal hormone activity. The condition in its severe form is called myxoedema.

1. The subject is cold and often has a low body temperature. Thyroid function should be considered in patients admitted in a hypothermic state.
2. Heart rate is slow and blood pressure, particularly systolic, is reduced.
3. Tendon reflex time is prolonged.
4. Neural signs such as apathy or forgetfulness may be present.
5. Weight gain without excessive food intake is common.
6. Lack of activity in skin, hair cells, sweat glands and sebaceous glands makes the dry and scaly skin a typical sign.
7. Oedema, particularly facial oedema, is common owing to the deposition of mucopolysaccharides in the tissue spaces.

If the site of dysfunction is the thyroid itself, e.g. if the cells have been destroyed by antibodies or radiotherapy or surgery, the axis would show low levels of T3/T4 but elevated TSH. If the thyroid cells are unresponsive to TSH there may be no goitre.

This condition is treated by lifetime use of thyroxine. The term 'endogenous' is used for a substance that is produced by the body; if that same substance is administered, it would be described as 'exogenous', i.e. hypothyroidism is treated by exogenous thyroxine.

Congenitial hypothyroidism

Congenital hypothyroidism occurs when the thyroid fails to function in the fetal stages. In the uterus, the infant usually develops normally using maternal thyroid hormones; however, after birth, if the condition were to go undetected, neural development and body growth would be impaired. This condition is sometimes known as cretinism. A blood test is carried out on babies soon after birth and if the condition is detected, thyroxine given from then on, and for life, avoids the retardation and damage that would otherwise occur.

Iodine deficiency hypothyroidism

Hypothyroidism such as myxoedema, which is pathological, can be contrasted with the condition known as endemic goitre, which is due to a nutritional deficiency of iodine. Endemic goitre is a world-wide problem with severe consequences. It occurs in areas of the world where soil is poor or leached out by very high rainfall and the food crops produced are deficient in iodine. The prolonged shortage of iodine results in low or barely adequate levels of T3/T4 with elevated TSH due to lack of negative feedback. The enlarged gland may make maximum use of the iodine available and may be able to just maintain normality but at the expense of a large goitre, hence the description endemic goitre. The goitres themselves may be disabling, causing respiratory or feeding difficulties, they are easily damaged and bleed copiously. The possible clinical deficiency of thyroid hormones may lead to an inability to work in a region where there is no support otherwise. An even more serious consequence may be damage to the offspring of the community who may be iodine deficient in the early stages of neural development with consequent permanent impairment. Treatment of nutritional hypothyroidism is by supplementation of iodine, which can be added to a staple food such as flour or salt.

ADRENAL STEROIDS

The adrenal gland

The adrenal gland is made up of two different tissues, the cortex and the medulla. The two are of separate embryological origin: the cortex is an endocrine tissue secreting steroid hormones; the adrenal medulla is supplied by autonomic, sympathetic preganglionic neurones and secretes the neurohormones adrenaline and noradrenaline (Ch. 5).

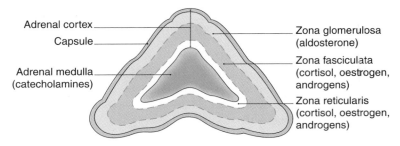

Fig. 6.3   *The adrenal gland.*

The adrenal cortex is made up of three layers: zona glomerulosa, zona reticularis and zona fasciculata (Fig. 6.3).

> The adrenal cortex is also a target organ for hypothalamic hormones and these control the production and release of many of the adrenal cortical hormones.

The adrenal steroids can be subdivided into the following functional types:

- glucocorticoids, e.g. cortisol, produced by zona fasciculata and reticularis
- oestrogens and androgens, produced by zona fasciculata and reticularis
- mineralocorticoids, e.g. aldosterone, produced by zona glomerulosa.

Cortisol and the oestrogens and androgens are axis-regulated from the hypothalamus in a pattern similar to the HPT axis; aldosterone is parameter-regulated with blood pressure and plasma sodium and potassium as the parameters. Only cortisol and aldosterone are considered here.

The hypothalamo–anterior pituitary–adrenocortical axis

The members of the hypothalamo–anterior pituitary–adrenocortical axis (HPA axis) (Fig. 6.4) are adrenocorticotrophic hormone releasing hormone (ACTHRH), adrenocorticotrophic hormone (ACTH) and cortisol. (NB. ACTHRH has the alternative name of corticotropin-releasing hormone (CRH), based on the alternative name for ACTH of corticotropin.)

ACTHRH is the hypothalamic hormone that acts as the release hormone for the anterior pituitary hormone ACTH.

ACTH is produced in the anterior pituitary in response to ACTHRH. It is produced from a much larger precursor molecule pro-opiocortin, which also yields melanocyte-stimulating hormone (MSH) and other neural peptides. As its name suggests, ACTH is a trophic hormone for the adrenal cortex and is required for growth and maintenance, particularly of the two inner zones of the cortex (see Fig. 6.3). If ACTH is withdrawn or suppressed, the cortex will shrink; conversely, if ACTH is present in excess, the cortex will hypertrophy in response. It also promotes the release of cortisol from the adrenal cortex.

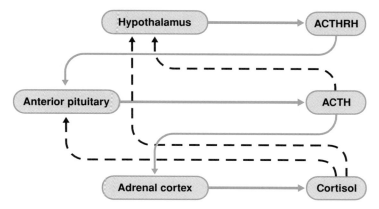

Fig. 6.4   *The hypothalamo–anterior pituitary–adrenal cortical axis. ←--, negative feedback.*

Cortisol

Cortisol is a corticosteroid hormone, described as glucocorticoid. The term refers to the role of cortisol in carbohydrate metabolism. While the term is accurate as far as it goes, it does not take account of the other metabolic actions or the anti-inflammatory properties of cortisol which make it essential for survival. It is regulated by the HPA axis (Fig. 6.4) with cortisol and ACTH acting as inhibitory products or negative feedback. The hypothalamus is affected by activity in higher brain areas and by ascending signals from the body; the stimuli at hypothalamic level are therefore many and various. ACTHRH is stimulated by any form of stress; injury, pain, infection and even severe exercise have large effects, but smaller disturbances in homeostasis, e.g. blood glucose, fluid, electrolytes or body temperature, can also act as stimuli. The greater the stimulus the larger the output of the end organ hormone cortisol; however, the activity in the axis is a balance between the forward stimuli and the negative feedback. Superimposed on this regulation, the HPA axis, and therefore cortisol, has a diurnal rhythm, with the level of cortisol highest early in the morning and lowest about 12 h later.

> Cortisol has widespread effects in the body including suppressing inflammation, controlling blood pressure and increasing the metabolism of protein and fat. Its anti-inflammatory effects are used pharmacologically.

When released, cortisol is bound to a transport protein, e.g. cortisol-binding globulin, and the equilibrium maintained between the bound cortisol and the unbound and active cortisol provides an additional layer of control over plasma levels.

Actions of cortisol

Most body tissues are sensitive to cortisol; it is lipid soluble and capable of passing through cell membranes, therefore receptor sites are to be found in the cytoplasm and at the nucleus of the target cells.

Cortisol is a survival hormone and its actions are such that the parameters important to the survival of the body are promoted. The inflammatory response, which is necessary to combat injury and infection, if left unchecked, might jeopardise blood pressure and survival. Cortisol acts as an anti-inflammatory agent, blood pressure is defended to supply tissue and blood glucose is maintained and allowed to rise in order to ensure a supply to the brain. In extreme circumstance, compromises have to be made: for example, in order to maintain pressure, excess sodium and water may be retained and blood glucose will be maintained at the expense of the body's own tissue.

Anti-inflammatory activity

Cortisol stabilises blood vessel walls making them less sensitive to the chemicals released as a result of injury; the inflammatory substances would otherwise cause vasodilatation and increased permeability, both of which would reduce blood pressure. Cortisol also suppresses immune function, therefore reducing at source the amount of circulating vasodilator chemicals. In doing so, however, cortisol compromises immune defenses making the injured or already sick individual less resistant to infection.

Maintenance of blood pressure

Even in normal health, cortisol is required to maintain blood pressure. In addition to its stabilising effects on blood vessels, it has a minor effect on electrolytes, retaining sodium (therefore water) and excreting potassium.

Metabolic actions of cortisol and maintenance of blood glucose

Cortisol promotes the breakdown of both body protein and fat. Amino acids from the protein can be used as an energy source and some can be used as a source of glucose, fat breakdown products can be used as an energy source and the small amount of glycerol released is used as a source of glucose. Cortisol therefore spares carbohydrate at the expense of protein and fat and raises blood glucose.

Pharmacology

Cortisol, used pharmacologically as an anti-inflammatory substance under the name hydrocortisone, is only one of a large number of steroid anti-inflammatory drugs, many of them more potent than cortisol/hydrocortisone itself. The conditions in which they are used are wide-ranging: asthma, skin disorders, muscle and joint disorders, autoimmune conditions such as systemic lupus where the disordered immune system has attacked host tissue, and even some types of clinical shock where blood vessels have become lax and permeable. While steroid drugs can be life-saving, their use is not without problems – they do after all have the same properties as cortisol. They must be used with care because they are catabolic to protein and fat and may damage vulnerable tissue or may affect blood pressure or blood glucose regulation. Their systemic use may, unless carefully managed, have adverse effects on the user's own HPA axis and put at risk their capacity to deal with stress.

An exogenous steroid will affect the HPA axis in the same way as endogenous cortisol. Prolonged use at high enough levels will inhibit the production of ACTH, the trophic effect on the adrenal cortex will be withdrawn and the cortex will shrink (see Fig. 6.4). If the individual is then subjected to stress such as injury or surgery, the adrenal cortex will be unable to supply the cortisol required to withstand the stress. The exogenous steroid, likely to be at a relatively small fixed dose, is also insufficient and the unchecked inflammatory response may cause a profound drop in blood pressure, i.e. clinical shock. To protect the adrenal cortex and avoid this risk, steroids are usually given at the lowest dose possible and may be intermittent to allow the mass of the cortex to be maintained. Where a patient is using steroids and surgery is elective, higher doses of exogenous steroid are likely to be used over the period of surgery and recovery.

Excess and deficiency of cortisol

Cortisol excess

Excess production of cortisol is called Cushing's syndrome. The dysfunction may be at the adrenal cortex or the pituitary or, unusually, at the hypothalamus; the word 'syndrome' can be used to describe all three. If the dysfunction is pituitary, several hormones and hormonal axes may be involved and the condition would be complicated by excess of all the hormones affected.

Many of the symptoms of excess cortisol can be predicted by exaggerating the effects of cortisol at normal concentrations. The individual loses skeletal muscle mass, especially from the limbs, skin is thinned and loses stretch. Fat is redistributed from limbs to trunk, face and neck. Sodium and water are retained in excess, raising blood pressure and causing oedema, particularly evident in the face. The combination of these effects produces the classic description of 'moon face oedema and large trunk with stick-like limbs.' About 20% of patients with Cushing's syndrome are hyperglycaemic to the point of diabetes.

Cortisol deficiency

Pathological deficiency of cortisol is rare and likely to be combined with a deficiency of aldosterone in Addison's disease; this is covered in the paragraphs on aldosterone. Deficiency of endogenous cortisol as a result of steroid therapy may occur when there is unexpected stress, and it is likely to show itself as an inability to maintain blood pressure and possibly fasting blood glucose.

Aldosterone

Aldosterone is a corticosteroid hormone that shares some of the features of other steroids but it provides useful areas of contrast with cortisol. It is produced by the adrenal cortex from the zona glomerulosa, a zone which, once formed, is relatively independent of the requirement for ACTH for its maintenance. Like all steroids, it can penetrate target cell membranes and therefore occupies intracellular receptor sites.

Aldosterone is classed as a mineralocorticoid because its action is to retain sodium and excrete potassium at the renal tubules (Ch. 11), gut and from sweat and tears. It has no metabolic or anti-inflammatory effects. It is not regulated by the HPA axis but is instead parameter-regulated, the parameters being blood pressure (the renin-dependent mechanism, Ch. 8) and plasma sodium and potassium (the renin-independent mechanism).

> Aldosterone regulates the retention of sodium by the body and diseases leading to either deficiency or excess of aldosterone can be seen in terms of either sodium deficiency or retention by the body.

Regulation of aldosterone release

Regulation by blood pressure

Regulation of aldosterone release in response to blood pressure is achieved using the renin, angiotensin, aldosterone mechanism (Fig. 6.5; see also Ch. 8). A reduction in blood pressure at the kidney causes the release of renin, which acts on the circulating but inactive angiotensinogen to produce angiotensin I, which is converted to angiotensin II by a converting enzyme. Angiotensin II stimulates the adrenal cortex to produce aldosterone. The restoration of blood pressure at the kidney will inhibit the release of renin and act as a negative feedback on aldosterone release (Fig. 6.5).

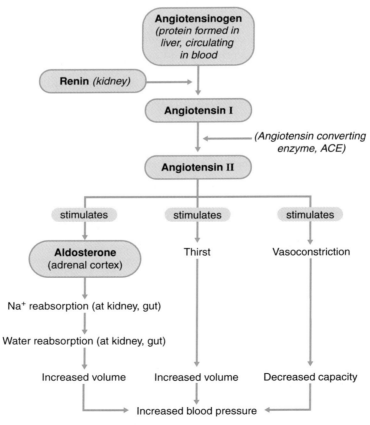

Fig. 6.5 *The renin, angiotensin, aldosterone mechanism.*

Regulation by electrolytes

Regulation of aldosterone in response to plasma sodium and potassium is the 'renin-independent' mechanism. A fall in plasma sodium or a rise in plasma potassium will promote the release of aldosterone by acting directly on the cells of the zona glomerulosa. The restoration of the electrolyte levels acts as a negative feedback on aldosterone and inhibits further release.

Excess and deficiency of aldosterone

Aldosterone excess

Excess aldosterone may be the result of a functioning tumour of the zona glomerulosa (primary aldosteronism) or a response to chronic low blood pressure or fluid shifts to a non-vascular compartment, for example in ascites (secondary aldosteronism). The results are a maintained elevation of blood pressure either to hypertensive levels or to approximately normal in the case of chronic losses of pressure. Elevated blood pressure may be attributable to many different causes but in the case of aldosteronism, the ratio of sodium to potassium is abnormal with hypernatraemia and hypokalaemia.

Aldosterone deficiency

Deficiency of aldosterone occurs in Addison's disease where it is usually accompanied by cortisol deficiency. There is marked sodium loss resulting in water loss, with raised plasma potassium. The subject experiences muscle fatigue (electrolyte imbalance) and inability to maintain blood pressure, sometimes so severe that 'Addisonian crisis' is said to have occurred. If the subject is to survive, exogenous steroids including aldosterone are required.

HYPOTHALAMUS AND POSTERIOR PITUITARY

Anatomical and functional relationship

The relationship of the hypothalamus with the posterior pituitary is different from that with the anterior pituitary. The two main lobes of the pituitary gland are derived from separate embryonic tissue: the posterior lobe is neural in origin, growing down from the brain, and the anterior lobe is endocrine and derived from tissue growing upwards from the roof of the mouth. The two types of tissue become associated in the embryo with the downgrowth having elongated to a stalk from which the posterior lobe is suspended (Fig. 6.6).

The difference in anatomical relationship between the hypothalamus and the two lobes underlies the functional difference between the anterior and posterior lobes. While the link between the hypothalamus and the anterior lobe is a small vascular system, the link with the posterior lobe is via a nerve tract, which begins in the hypothalamus and ends in the posterior lobe. Two hypothalamic hormones, antidiuretic hormone (ADH) and oxytocin, synthesised in the hypothalamus, travel down the axons of the nerve tract and are released into the general circulation at the posterior pituitary.

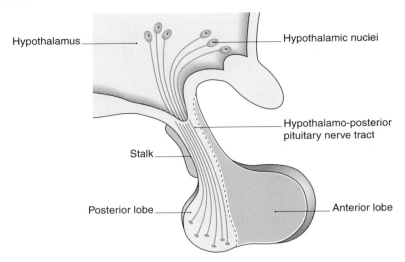

Fig. 6.6   *The hypothalamus and posterior pituitary gland (showing an enlarged and diagrammatic representation of the hypothalamo–posterior pituitary nerve tract).*

Antidiuretic hormone

ADH takes part in the maintenance of blood pressure, fluid balance and osmotic regulation and is central to homeostasis. Its target tissues are the renal tubules (Ch. 11) and blood vessels (Ch. 8). The effects of the hormone are reflected in its alternative names 'antidiuretic hormone' and 'vasopressin'.

> ADH acts along with aldosterone to regulate blood pressure through the combined effects of these hormones on the retention of fluid by the kidney.

It is a peptide hormone unable to penetrate the target cell membrane and therefore requires a second messenger. Unlike many hormones, it travels in the unbound form and has a rapid effect and is rapidly metabolised, i.e. it has a short half-life.

Actions of ADH

At the distal and collecting tubules in the nephron, the effect is to increase the reabsorption of water, which is then taken back into blood, increasing the volume and the hydrostatic pressure. The effect of this dilution is to reduce osmotic pressure (Ch. 1). At blood vessels the hormone acts as a vasoconstrictor, reducing the capacity and increasing blood (hydrostatic) pressure (Ch. 8).

It soon becomes clear that ADH/vasopressin is a parameter-regulated hormone and the parameters are hydrostatic and osmotic pressure. The two parameters are inseparable and are regulated together by several mechanisms of which ADH is only one.

Regulation of ADH by blood pressure

Baroreceptors located in low-pressure circulations such as the pulmonary circuit are stimulated by rises in pressure. Their firing rate increases in response to the pressure rise and the effect is to inhibit the output of ADH. The amount of water reclaimed at the kidney is reduced and blood vessels are less constricted; both actions help to reduce blood pressure. A fall in blood pressure has the opposite effect, the increased output of ADH causing water retention and vaso-constriction and a consequent rise in pressure.

Regulation of ADH by osmotic pressure

Sensory receptors in the hypothalamus, osmoreceptors, are stimulated by a rise in osmotic pressure. These in turn stimulate the area in the hypothalamus producing ADH. The increased ADH retains water, diluting the solutes and reducing osmotic pressure. A fall in osmotic pressure has the opposite effect, resulting in the excretion of water and restoration of normal osmotic pressure.

Deficiency and excess of ADH

Deficiency of ADH

This is the condition diabetes insipidus, which dramatically illustrates the actions of ADH. The subject, unable to regulate water retention, excretes large amounts of dilute urine. As long as a source of drinking water or fluid containing water is available, the subject can usually keep pace with the large loss. However, if water is unavailable, because it cannot be retained as would be the normal response, osmotic pressure rises and blood pressure falls. Other mechanisms, e.g. tachycardia and vasoconstriction by mechanisms other than ADH, compensate (Ch. 8) to some extent but the subject suffers extreme thirst. A water deprivation test is sometimes carried out during the diagnosis of diabetes insipidus and great care must be taken that the test is not overlong otherwise there is a risk of damage arising out of overconcentration of body fluids. The condition is treated by replacement therapy using a synthetic ADH.

Excess ADH

This is found in several primary and secondary forms and is given the overall name of 'syndrome of inappropriate ADH' (SIADH). It can be due to primary causes such as a functioning tumour, but it is more often found in head injury or surgery, or as an unwanted effect of a large variety of drugs. These include the opiates, particularly morphine, tricyclic antidepressants and chlor-propamide.

The most obvious effect is hyponatraemia which cannot be accounted for otherwise (i.e. it must be due to dilution), inappropriate urinary concentrations and low plasma osmolarity. ADH is seldom found to be in excess if measured; in fact, a patient clearly identified as suffering from SIADH may have no detectable ADH in plasma. The cause of the syndrome must be identified and measures taken to excrete the water load without further jeopardising electrolyte levels.

MAINTENANCE OF A HOMEOSTATIC PARAMETER BY A GROUP OF HORMONES

An example that illustrates the complexity of maintaining 'normality' is the maintenance of blood glucose. Blood glucose or plasma glucose is maintained at between 3 and 8 millimoles per litre (mmol/L). These are the extremes of the normal range and blood glucose is more likely to be within the tighter limits of 3.5 to 5.5 or 6 mmol/L, regardless of feeding or fasting. A blood glucose concentration outside the normal range is damaging. Low values (hypoglycaemia) are damaging in the short term because glucose is the major fuel substrate of brain and nervous tissue. The effects of hypoglycaemia can be loss of cognitive function extending to loss of consciousness and, if extreme and prolonged, loss of life. Hyperglycaemia over a long period of time is damaging to all tissues, leading to the complications that can be found in diabetes mellitus. Glucose regulation must therefore be capable of withstanding a large variation of input and expenditure of glucose and constantly maintaining a narrow range of concentration. The hormones involved must be capable of reducing blood glucose during and after feeding and raising blood glucose from a variety of storage substrates over fasting periods that might extend not just for hours but for days or weeks. The following can only be a brief summary of the combined effects of the hormones involved in this complex process.

The hormones involved are insulin, glucagon, adrenaline, growth hormone, cortisol and the thyroid hormones. Of those, only insulin reduces blood glucose; all the others raise blood glucose using a variety of substrates and mechanisms over different time scales (Fig. 6.7). The liver plays a central role in the balancing act; it contains the metabolic pathways that manipulate the nutrient substrates and it is sensitive to the hormones that can selectively stimulate or inhibit the pathways.

> A range of hormones, including insulin, glucagon, adrenaline, growth hormone, cortisol and thyroid hormones, act to regulate blood glucose levels.

The following brief outline of the hormones in the group identifies only the effects of each hormone relevant to glucose regulation and points of principle from earlier in the chapter.

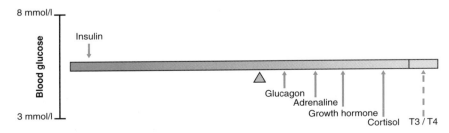

Fig. 6.7 *Glucose balance.*

Insulin

Insulin is a large polypeptide hormone produced by the B cells of the pancreas; the stimulus to its production is rising blood glucose and it is therefore parameter-regulated. The amount of insulin released is modified by many other factors, such as activity in the ANS, where the parasympathetic effect is stimulatory and more insulin is produced for any given amount of glucose. The sympathetic effect is to inhibit insulin release and allow glucose to rise to a higher level before insulin is released. The gut hormones, released during feeding and digestion, increase the insulin response to rising blood glucose giving a larger and more rapid response.

The effect of insulin is to increase the rate of uptake of glucose into skeletal muscle, adipose tissue and liver, referred to as *insulin-sensitive tissues*. It increases the rate of glucose usage by these tissues and the storage of glycogen by liver and skeletal muscle. Insulin also promotes the formation of fat and its deposition in adipose tissue and, with nitrogen available, the formation of protein. These processes all require glucose and it is therefore used or stored and in doing so the blood level is reduced. A useful addition to this is the effect of insulin, which limits the breakdown of stores already formed and avoids adding to the existing glucose. Insulin is therefore a hypoglycaemic hormone. Hypoglycaemia is a dangerous state and to reduce the risk of it happening, it is countered by not one but a group of hormones, each of which has other functions and individual controls adding to the overall complexity.

Hyperglycaemic hormones

Glucagon

Glucagon is a polypeptide hormone using second messengers. It is produced by the A cells of the pancreas in response to falling blood glucose. Its output is increased by sympathetic activity. It is also stimulated by parasympathetic activity and is produced along with insulin during digestion; this has the effect of limiting the reduction in glucose caused by early insulin at the beginning of a meal. It acts early and rapidly when glucose levels begin to fall and its effects are to raise blood glucose by breaking down liver glycogen, from which glucose can be released to the bloodstream. (Muscle glycogen can only be used by muscle; its breakdown products cannot be exported to the blood as glucose.) Glucagon also limits the uptake and storage of glucose by other tissues; it promotes the use of fatty acids so providing an alternative fuel and increases the liver uptake of amino acids, which can be used to provide more glucose (gluconeogenesis).

Adrenaline

Adrenaline is one of the neurohormones secreted by the adrenal medulla. Its effect at the pancreas is to inhibit the release of insulin and allow blood glucose to rise. It also has metabolic effects, working with glucagon to cause the breakdown of liver glycogen. A further effect is to stimulate fat breakdown and, while this contributes little to blood glucose levels, it provides an alternative fuel substrate, which can be used to spare glucose. The overall effect of adrenaline is hyperglycaemic.

Growth hormone or human growth hormone

Growth hormone (GH) is produced by the anterior pituitary gland and its regulation is a complex interplay of hypothalamic-releasing hormones and inhibitory hormones. It is also regulated by factors that are produced in response to it, e.g. insulin-like growth factors (IGF). It is affected not only by blood glucose levels but by the concentration in plasma of specific amino acids. Its effect is to inhibit glucose usage in skeletal muscle and it therefore has a hyperglycaemic effect; however, because GH also increases insulin output, its net effect is to divert glucose from use simply as a source of energy into pathways by which GH and insulin can promote growth. At normal levels of GH and where adequate insulin can be produced, the hyperglycaemic effect of GH is limited.

Cortisol

Cortisol also has hyperglycaemic effects, but the time scale is much longer than the previous hormones and its actions provide glucose from large storage compartments, unlike the glycogen store, which is limited. It has a catabolic effect on protein and promotes liver conversion of the released amino acids to glucose. It also causes the breakdown of adipose tissue, the fat providing some glucose from glycerol but, probably more importantly, a large store of alternative fuel. In normal circumstances, the breakdown of skeletal muscle and adipose tissue is a necessary part of overall tissue turnover; however, as both are very large compartments, in a state of prolonged fasting, they can be used to both provide energy and glucose over a period perhaps of many weeks.

Thyroid hormones T3/T4

The thyroid hormones have metabolic effects that include sparing glucose as a fuel. While they do not normally play a large part in short-term regulation of blood glucose, they do affect the rate at which fuel is consumed and they become significant where conditions are in some way abnormal, for example in trauma or in starvation. In extreme states, thyroid function would be reduced by the formation of more rT3 and the overall effect is hyperglycaemic.

Failure of regulation

Failure of glucose regulation is clinically recognised as diabetes mellitus. Primary diabetes occurs where the fault in the regulatory system is lack of insulin. Where the fault lies in excess of one or more of the hyperglycaemic or counter-regulatory hormones, this would lead to secondary diabetes mellitus: for example, about 20–25% of people who have developed acromegaly (GH excess) or Cushing's syndrome (cortisol excess) will develop diabetes. Steroid therapy may reduce glucose tolerance to a significant degree in some individuals and this must be taken into account when steroids are prescribed.

The effect of trauma, which is to produce increased levels of all the hyperglycaemic hormones, may be enough to produce glucose intolerance in some people. The effect may be mild and temporary, lasting only as long as the early response to the trauma and due mainly to insulin suppression by the catecholamines. Where the injury is large and the response prolonged, for example where there are extensive burns, the suppression of insulin in the early stages, followed by its antagonism by the hyperglycaemic hormones, may be enough to produce a diabetic state that requires treatment.

SUMMARY

The chemical messengers of the endocrine system, the hormones, affect homeostasis, morphogenesis and the ability to resist stress. It is a hugely complex system and this chapter considers only a limited number of hormones which illustrate either particular aspects of homeostasis and its disturbance, or particular methods of hormone regulation. Hormones released into the bloodstream may act close to the endocrine gland or may travel some distance before binding with the receptor sites at the target tissue. Hormones are extremely potent substances and many safety measures have been evolved such as the complex regulation of hormone release. The chapter considers control by homeostatic parameters such as hydrostatic or osmotic pressure and control by product inhibition. Other safety measures include reversible inactivation by binding of the hormone and regulation of receptor site number or affinity.

The properties of hormones are numerous, some may affect membrane permeability, others may affect transcription in the target cell nucleus or some other process within the cell. The evidence for the activity of a hormone is often most clearly seen where there is clinical deficiency or excess and an endocrine disorder becomes manifest. This, however, is complicated by the fact that many biological activities are controlled, not by a single hormone, but by a group of hormones in concert.

QUESTIONS

1. What are the two parts of the pituitary gland and which hormones do they produce?

2. Describe the signs of an excess of thyroid hormones.

3. Give two examples of steroid hormones and state their actions.

FURTHER READING

Boore J (1996) Endocrine function. In: Hinchliff S, Montague S, Watson R (eds) *Physiology for nursing practice, 2nd edn.* Baillière Tindall, London, pp 202–244

Watson R (1995) *Anatomy and physiology for nurses, 10th edn.* Baillière Tindall, London

7 Homeostasis

Dinah Gould

After reading this chapter you should be able to:
- describe the process of homeostasis
- list the component parts of a homeostatic system
- give some examples of homeostatic systems and their component parts.

INTRODUCTION: THE DEFINITION OF HOMEOSTASIS

Every living organism, from the most simple to the most complex, exists in an environment that is subject to change. Fluctuations in the outside world may range from minor alterations in temperature or humidity to dramatic shifts sufficient to alter the integrity of the organism and to disrupt its physiological functioning. In extreme cases, sudden and dramatic alterations in the outside world may not be compatible with life. To combat marked, unpredictable variations in their surroundings, all living organisms have developed the capacity to resist change through the activity of their internal autoregulatory mechanisms. This ability to maintain a stable physiological state in an environment subject to change is called homeostasis, a term first adopted by the American physiologist Walter Cannon. The word homeostasis is rather misleading as its literal meaning is 'unchanging'. However, when referring to physiological systems, the term homeostasis is used to imply not that living organisms are unchanging, but to indicate that they are in a state of dynamic equilibrium. Although the internal environment of an individual will respond to fluctuations in the world outside, its response is always within a narrow range. Individual cells function as homeostatic units, as do all the cells of a complex multicellular organism operating together. Some examples of typical homeostatic control systems are shown in Box 7.1.

BOX 7.1	*Homeostatic Systems: Examples*
	Blood pressure
	Temperature control
	Rate and depth of respiration
	Plasma glucose levels
	Levels of hormones in the blood (e.g. insulin, thyroxine)
	Fluid balance
	Electrolyte levels (e.g. sodium, chloride, potassium)

The breakdown of homeostasis results in imbalance and ultimately in disease. For example, an individual subjected to harsh conditions in the heat of the desert will lose large quantities of water as sweat, which, if not replaced, would result in dehydration and collapse.

THE CONDITIONS REQUIRED FOR HOMEOSTASIS

Several conditions must be fulfilled in order for homeostasis to be possible. Firstly, interactions between the anatomical structures making up the different parts of the body must be highly coordinated. Secondly, the body must have a sufficient supply of energy (Ch. 1) to fuel its many complex physiological functions. Providing these conditions are adequately met, homeostasis is possible at several different levels:

1. The whole organism.
2. Organ systems: for example, the cardiovascular system (heart and blood vessels) controls blood pressure (Ch. 8).
3. Organ systems working together in an integrated manner. Both the cardiovascular system and the respiratory system (Ch. 10) operate together to control blood pressure.
4. Individual cells function as homeostatic units. This is possible because the cell membrane (Ch. 2) separates the internal and external environments and helps to control materials moving in and out of the cell.

THE CONTROL OF HOMEOSTASIS

All basic homeostatic mechanisms include three components: a receptor, a control centre and an effector.

> A homeostatic system requires a receptor, a control centre and an effector. For many homeostatic systems the control centre is either the hypothalamus or the medulla oblongata.

Receptors

Receptors operate as sensory devices. Their function is to sample the external environment for fluctuations and feed information continuously to the control centre. Most receptors consist of nervous tissue (Ch. 5): for example, nerve endings in the skin continuously monitor the temperature of the surrounding environment. The stimuli picked up by the receptors may be physical or chemical. Temperature and blood pressure are both examples of physical variables monitored by different types of receptors in homeostatic systems. However, most receptors relay chemical information such as the concentration of different hormones or electrolytes present in the body fluids.

The control centre

The control centre receives the information relayed from the receptors. Its function is to compare this information with the normal value for the specific physical or chemical entity that it directs, to interpret the information and to initiate the appropriate response. The control centre for many homeostatic mechanisms is either the medulla oblongata at the base of the brain or a small area of tissue called the hypothalamus (Ch. 5) also at the base of the brain, near the pituitary gland.

Effectors

Effectors are the organs that bring about the required change necessary to achieve a constant internal environment. The kidneys (Ch. 11), glands and the muscular layers in the walls of blood vessels all operate as effectors.

Communication in homeostatic systems

Communication in homeostatic systems occurs via nerves or hormones secreted by the various endocrine glands and transported in the blood (Ch. 6):

1. The *afferent pathway* (a nerve or hormone) carries information from the receptor to the control centre.
2. The *efferent pathway* (a nerve or hormone) carries information in the opposite direction, to the effector from the control centre.

TYPES OF CONTROL SYSTEMS

In general, homeostatic control systems fall into one of two broad categories: they are either negative or positive feedback systems.

Negative feedback systems

Most homeostatic systems fall into this category. Here an increase in the level of the product from the process that is being monitored results in the process itself slowing down or ceasing altogether. In other words, these homeostatic mechanisms cause the variable being monitored to fluctuate in the opposite direction to the initial change. For example, if the receptors on the surface of the skin indicate a rise in temperature, nervous impulses are relayed to the temperature control centre within the hypothalamus. Measures are then taken to promote loss of heat, such as sweating. Figure 7.1 shows a typical homeostatic negative feedback system.

Positive feedback systems

In a positive feedback system the initial change leads to a second change, then a third and yet further changes in a cascade of irreversible reactions. In contrast to the situation in negative feedback systems, the change in a positive feedback system always proceeds in the same direction as the original response. Positive feedback systems are far less common than negative feedback systems. They promote infrequent physiological events, which, once stimulated, tend to be

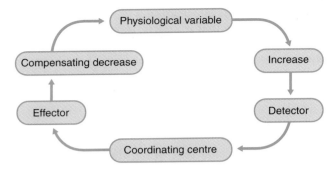

Fig. 7.1   *A typical negative feedback homeostatic system.*

dramatic and self-perpetuating. Examples include parturition (childbirth) and the chain of events set in motion when damage to a blood vessel results in bleeding. Trauma to a blood vessel triggers a chain of events that eventually lead to the formation of a blood clot. This seals the damaged blood vessel, preventing further haemorrhage.

> Most homeostatic systems work by negative feedback, where the initial stimulus leads to a decrease in that stimulus. Some systems work through positive feedback.

Understanding negative and positive feedback systems

A few selected examples of negative and positive feedback systems will now be discussed in greater depth to aid understanding of the fundamental homeostatic systems operating within the human body.

NEGATIVE FEEDBACK: TEMPERATURE REGULATION

Heat is lost continually from the surface of the body by conduction, convection, the evaporation of sweat and, to a much smaller extent, in faeces, urine and expired air. The degree of heat loss is heavily influenced by the temperature and humidity in the surrounding atmosphere. If the air is laden with moisture, water molecules will cling to the surface of the skin and the cooling effect of evaporating sweat is lost. On a dry, windy day convection currents cause sweat to evaporate rapidly so cooling occurs swiftly. Heat is continually generated through metabolic activity, physical exercise, radiation and, to a smaller extent, by eating hot food and taking warm drinks (Table 7.1). Dynamic equilibrium is achieved when the amount of heat lost by the body is equal to the amount of heat gained.

The skin in temperature regulation

The effectors in this system are blood vessels in the subcutaneous tissues of the

TABLE 7.1	Mechanisms of Temperature Regulation	
	Heat gain	Heat loss
	Metabolic activity	Conduction
	Physical exercise	Convection
	Shivering	Perspiration
	Radiation	Expiration
	Hot food and fluids	Excretion

skin, which control heat loss and gain by constricting or dilating according to the needs of the body. In a cold environment the blood vessels constrict so the flow of blood to the skin is reduced and heat is retained. In a warm environment blood vessels in the subcutaneous tissues dilate, blood flow to the surface increases and heat loss is increased. In the typical damp, cool British climate, conduction and convection account for about 70% of the daily heat loss from the body, while the evaporation of sweat accounts for between 3 and 30% of daily loss. Clearly these figures are approximations only: our climate is very variable and in recent years (1994–1996) during our intensely hot summers, remaining cool, dry and comfortable throughout the day has been a problem for many people. From your own experience you will probably be aware that temperature can vary considerably on different occasions and also between different points on the skin of the same individual at the same moment in time: on a cold day it is possible to be warmly wrapped but to have a cold face or ears. This local variation is perfectly normal and is compatible with health. However, deep in the body the tissues are kept at a remarkably constant temperature despite extreme and rapid environmental fluctuations.

The control system in temperature regulation

For temperature regulation the control centre is in the hypothalamus. An area in the anterior hypothalamus controls heat loss and a second area in the posterior hypothalamus controls heat gain. The hypothalamus operates like a thermostat used to control the temperature in a room (Fig. 7.2). In health the thermostat is set at around 37°C. If the temperature of the blood flowing through the hypothalamus is lower than the set point, heat-generating mechanisms will be switched on. Conversely, if the temperature of the blood flowing through the hypothalamus is lower than the set point, mechanisms to promote heat loss will be activated. There are two types of detectors (thermoreceptors) in the temperature control system: peripheral thermoreceptors in the skin, which respond slowly to temperature change in the external environment; and central thermoreceptors within the hypothalamus itself, which respond more rapidly to temperature changes in the deep internal environment of the body. Under normal circumstances the deep tissues are protected from sudden fluctuations in temperature, but should these occur, they will jeopardise health to a far greater extent and more swiftly than variations on the skin.

Exposure to a cold environment establishes a temperature gradient between the body core and the surface, and this is detected by the peripheral thermo-

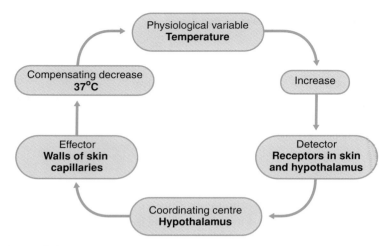

Fig. 7.2   *Temperature control.*

receptors. Information is then relayed via nervous impulses to the blood vessels in the skin. Vasoconstriction (tightening of the blood vessel walls to reduce blood flow) is stimulated to conserve heat. Several other heat conservation mechanisms may also come into play. Hairs on the skin may stand on end, trapping a warm layer of air next to the body. This response, called pilo-erection, is brought about by contraction of the tiny muscles at the base of each hair shaft. It is of minor importance in human beings compared with most other mammals and birds, which often appear visibly larger in cold weather when they fluff up their fur or feathers. In a very cold environment shivering may occur. Large groups of muscles contract and relax rapidly in succession to generate heat. This process uses a considerable amount of the energy reserves of the body and is not, therefore, very efficient. The physiologist Scholander suggested that human beings must be adapted to life in hot rather than cold conditions because our heat conservation mechanisms are less efficient than those intended to promote heat loss. This is supported by the findings of archaeologists which indicate that our ancestors probably evolved in hot countries.

Exposure to a hot environment establishes a temperature gradient between the body core and the surface. This is detected by the peripheral thermoreceptors and the information is relayed via nervous impulses to the blood vessels in the skin. Vasodilatation is stimulated, allowing increased blood flow close to the surface of the skin, and heat loss is promoted.

Behavioural responses to heat and cold

All the changes discussed above form part of the autoregulatory mechanisms of the body and take place without our conscious effort. However, no account of temperature control would be complete without a mention of our very deliberate behavioural responses to heat and cold. In a hot environment we move slowly, shed clothing and stretch out when at rest (look at people on a beach in the sun). In a cold environment people huddle up to reduce the surface area exposed to the external environment, add layers of clothing and may generate heat through movement (stamping feet, clapping hands together).

Temperature control is a good example of a homeostatic system where physiological and behavioural effects act to maintain the core body temperature within a narrow range.

Breakdown of the temperature control mechanism

Hypothermia

Breakdown of homeostasis occurs if the body core temperature falls to 35°C or below. At temperatures between 35°C and 32.2°C the normal responses of vasoconstriction and shivering are still possible, but if the core temperature drops further, tissue metabolism becomes altered and the protective mechanisms of heat conservation are lost. Below 24°C heat is lost passively to the environment and the heart can no longer function properly. If the victim is found in time, gradual rewarming will permit recovery without lasting ill-effect. Hypothermia is a major risk in the elderly and infants because homeostatic mechanisms tend to be less efficient at the extremes of life. In addition, these individuals are less able to make the appropriate behavioural responses when exposed to low temperatures. An elderly person who has sustained a fall may be unable to summon help either because they cannot get up (after a fracture) or because they lack coordinated movement and speech (after a cerebrovascular accident, 'stroke'), while a baby may kick off its wrappings as it moves about in an effort to generate heat.

Hyperthermia

Although probably adapted to life in a hot country, there are limits to human tolerance. Tolerance varies considerably between individuals and appears to be related to the previous degree of exposure to heat and acclimatisation. Those who are unaccustomed to life in hot conditions develop problems if they undertake only a modest degree of exercise during intense heat (Fig. 7.3). An individual who is acclimatised will have an increased blood volume compared with someone who is not acclimatised and is therefore in a better position to lose heat through increased perspiration. Inability to lose heat via the evaporation of sweat causes a breakdown in homeostasis and the body core temperature begins to rise. Once it reaches 42°C the ability to sweat is lost altogether and heat begins to be absorbed passively from the environment. Because metabolic processes generate heat, the body core temperature continues to increase. Irreversible damage to the body's cellular and enzyme systems occurs at 43°C.

Infection and temperature control

Many bacteria and viruses release toxins when they invade the body (Ch. 13). These cause the thermostat in the hypothalamus to become reset at a higher level.

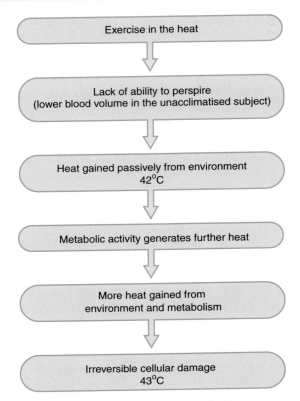

Fig. 7.3 *Effect of high environmental temperature on the unacclimatised subject.*

Temperature is maintained at this new level until the foreign antigens have been neutralised and eliminated. Vasoconstriction and shivering are accompanied by an increase in metabolic rate. The patient feels cold and huddles up irrespective of the number of blankets provided. Pyrexia (fever) is believed to be of value in that it may operate by speeding metabolism so that bacteria and their toxins are more rapidly eliminated from the body. However, pyrexia has disadvantages as well as benefits. The experience of pyrexia is unpleasant as it is usually associated with feeling ill. It can be exhausting and, if the fever is high or prolonged, may drain the body of energy reserves at a time when the individual is not eating properly and nutrients are unlikely to be replenished adequately. Other complications include uncontrollable attacks of violent shivering (rigors) and febrile convulsions in young children (6 months to 5 years of age). These are frightening and may be dangerous, for example the child may sustain an injury or inhale vomit and asphyxiate.

Temperature control is a good example of the control of a physical variable by negative feedback. However, most of the variables monitored by negative feedback mechanisms are chemical, and before we leave this section we will examine a further example of control by negative feedback, this time involving the control of a chemical substance vital in body function – the control of plasma glucose levels.

NEGATIVE FEEDBACK: CONTROL OF PLASMA GLUCOSE LEVELS

In contrast to the temperature control system, which is regulated by the nervous system, plasma glucose levels are controlled by the endocrine system. The endocrine organs are ductless glands that empty their secretions, called hormones, directly into the blood. The actions of individual hormones are highly specific but collectively they exert important effects on general metabolism. Plasma glucose levels are controlled by two hormones, insulin and glucagon, both secreted by the pancreas.

> Two hormones, insulin and glucagon, act antagonistically to regulate blood glucose levels.

To perform their normal metabolic processes, all cells must have continuous access to glucose, a simple sugar derived from starch in the diet, which the body uses as its major source of energy. Plasma glucose levels are maintained within a relatively narrow range: between 3.5 and 8 millimoles per litre (mmol/L) despite fluctuations in the amount of sugar or starch consumed and the amount of energy expended. The normal fasting plasma glucose level (between meals) is 3.5–5.5 mmol/L, rising to 7–9 mmol/L after a meal. It returns to the fasting level approximately 2 h later. If you consume a surfeit of sugar (e.g. in a sugary drink or sweets) the glucose is rapidly absorbed from the digestive tract and floods into the bloodstream. This elevated glucose level stimulates the release of insulin from endocrine cells in the pancreas called the islets of Langerhans. Insulin accelerates the uptake of glucose by most of the cells in the body and promotes the conversion of glucose to a storage form of carbohydrate called glycogen. As a result plasma glucose levels return toward the normal set point of 3.5–5.5 mmol/L and the stimulus for insulin release gradually diminishes. Glycogen is reserved in the liver and muscle ready to convert back into glucose at times of high energy expenditure, such as exercise.

Glucagon has the opposite effect to insulin and is said to have an antagonistic effect upon it. The release of glucagon from the islets of Langerhans is triggered when plasma levels of glucose decline below the set point. This might occur if a meal is missed or if the amount of carbohydrate in the diet is reduced. Glucagon stimulates the liver to convert its reserves of glycogen back into glucose, which is then released into the plasma, restoring dynamic equilibrium.

Disturbances in plasma glucose control

People with diabetes mellitus are either unable to secrete any insulin or are unable to secrete sufficient amounts to meet the needs of the tissues. As a result the concentration of glucose in the plasma builds up and it is excreted via the kidneys (Ch. 11). The individual loses weight because the body converts its stores of fat into glucose in an attempt to recompense the apparent lack of an energy supply. The presence of glucose in urine can be detected by a simple test but more accurate results are obtained by measuring the levels of glucose in the blood. Today this is a straightforward procedure, which can be performed in the home or health centre and which diabetics can use to monitor their own plasma glucose levels as part of their normal routine. People with diabetes mellitus fall into two broad groups:

1. Individuals with insulin-dependent diabetes. These people are generally diagnosed in childhood or early adulthood, must follow a diet and require injections of insulin all their lives. Unfortunately insulin cannot be taken orally because it is a protein (Ch. 2) and would be broken down during digestion.

2. Individuals with non-insulin-dependent diabetes. This condition develops gradually in middle life and may remain undetected for years. Typically the individual is overweight and it is possible in many cases to control their condition by diet alone. Drugs to control non-insulin-dependent diabetes are available, but have several unpleasant side-effects. Control by diet is therefore the treatment of choice.

Both types of diabetes mellitus have serious side-effects if not controlled and those affected must understand the important role of diet in the control of their condition. The modern diabetic diet is high in complex carbohydrate such as starch (Ch. 2) and fibre, and low in fats and the simple sugars such as glucose, which are found in extremely high concentrations in sweets and sugary drinks. Simple sugars are absorbed rapidly from the digestive tract and this has three important effects which are not beneficial to the health of the individual. Firstly, simple sugars provide no bulk in the diet so the individual rapidly becomes hungry and eats again. Secondly, they contain a high proportion of calories but no other useful nutrients. Under these conditions the risk of becoming over-weight is considerable. Finally, a big surge of glucose into the blood causes plasma glucose levels to rise upwards sharply. Therefore the release of insulin has to be swift and in sufficient amounts to promote efficient absorption of all the surplus glucose into the cells. This excess glucose is converted to glycogen in the liver and ultimately to fat, which is stored beneath the skin. The individual who cannot secrete optimal amounts of insulin, but is still consuming large amounts of sugar, will develop both problems of obesity and plasma glucose control. The same low fat diet, high in complex carbohydrate and fibre, is regarded as the most healthy diet for all members of the population.

POSITIVE FEEDBACK: CHILDBIRTH

In this type of system the physiological activity under control is stimulated by its own product, generating an irreversible change. Parturition (childbirth) is one of the few examples of positive feedback that occurs in health. As pregnancy advances, the uterus is stimulated to contract, because the growing fetus stretches its muscular walls. This effect is enhanced by high concentrations of the female hormone oestrogen present in the bloodstream in advanced pregnancy. During the last few weeks before birth the woman becomes aware of regular uterine contractions. As the date of delivery draws near she will notice that they become more frequent and painful. Once labour is established the contractions follow one another in succession and become coordinated while the cervix dilates. Each contraction commences at the top of the uterus (fundus), sweeping downwards so the infant's head becomes pressed against the cervix at the lowest point of the uterus. Increasing pressure causes the rupture of the surrounding membranes, releasing the amniotic fluid which cushioned and protected the baby throughout pregnancy (the 'waters break'). As a result the baby's head is able to push down directly onto the cervix. This stimulates the pressure receptors that it contains to initiate the release of a hormone called oxytocin from the posterior pituitary gland. Oxytocin is an extremely powerful uterine stimulant, making the intensity of the contractions even more powerful, causing further cervical dilatation. Eventually the baby is pushed into the vagina and the woman experiences an irresistible desire to push downwards until it is delivered safely.

> Childbirth is a good example of positive feedback where the pressing of the baby's head on the cervix leads to stronger contractions of the uterus until the baby is born.

Of the examples of homeostasis discussed above, the most typical is perhaps plasma glucose control. This is because it is an example of the control of a chemical substance by a negative feedback system. Like all chemicals in the body, glucose must be present in an aqueous solution before it can undergo chemical reactions. Thus water is a vital ingredient in most homeostatic control systems.

THE ROLE OF WATER IN HOMEOSTASIS

All living organisms have several fundamental requirements if they are to function as healthy, homeostatic units, performing metabolic reactions, growing and ultimately reproducing to give rise to the next generation (Box 7.2). Of these requirements, water is unique. It is essential to life because all the chemical reactions that take place in a living system will do so only if the reacting substances are dissolved in an aqueous solution. Throughout the body, water operates as a universal solvent in which a range of different substances (solutes) are dissolved (Ch. 1). Water also forms a high percentage of the tissues: in a healthy young adult water accounts for 60% of lean body mass. A young male adult weighing 70 kg contains 40 L of water. The amount of water is always a little higher in males than females of the same overall body weight because the female body contains proportionally more adipose (fatty) tissue for the same weight and fat has a low water content. Similarly fat people always contain less water than thin ones. Infants contain more water – approximately 73% – than adults because of their low body fat and low bone mass. The body water content declines with advancing years so that an elderly person contains only about 43% water.

BODY FLUID COMPARTMENTS

The fluid content is named according to its location (compartment) in the body. There are two major locations: the intracellular and the extracellular body fluid compartments (Table 7.2):

BOX 7.2	The Requirements of Living Organisms
	Oxygen Water A supply of nutrients A suitable temperature A suitable pH range Prompt removal of metabolic wastes

TABLE 7.2	The Major Fluid Compartments		
		Volume (L)	% of body weight
	Total body water volume	40	60
	Intracellular fluid	25	40
	Extracellular fluid	15	20
	Plasma	3	20

1. The intracellular compartment (ICF) contains two-thirds of the water in the body, located inside the cells. In the typical young man weighing 70 kg, 40% of the body weight (25 L) is present in the ICF.
2. The extracellular fluid compartment (ECF) consists of the remaining third of the water in the body, present outside the cells. Its key role in homeostasis was first recognised by the French physiologist Claude Bernard during the nineteenth century. Since this time the ECF has become known as the 'internal environment' of the body. It is further divided into two important compartments: the plasma and the interstitial fluid.

Plasma is the aqueous portion of the blood. Its function is to transport materials around the body (e.g. red blood cells carrying oxygen, nutrients, waste products to be filtered and excreted by the kidney).

Interstitial fluid, sometimes known as tissue fluid, is the water present in the microscopic spaces between the cells. Interstitial fluid also has a vital role in transport. It provides a medium allowing the movement of oxygen and nutrients from the plasma to the cells. Waste materials such as carbon dioxide produced during tissue metabolism move in the opposite direction and are removed by the plasma. In the typical young man weighing 70 kg, 20% of the body weight (15 L) consists of water in the ECF. Twelve litres of this water is present as interstitial fluid and the remaining 3 L are present as plasma.

Several other aqueous solutions are included in the ECF. These are listed in Box 7.3.

The ECF operates as a pool for the exchange of water and other substances between the cells and their surrounding environment. It is the source of all the materials required by actively metabolising cells – water, electrolytes, nutrients – which are relinquished to the tissues on demand and returned when they are no longer required. Net gain of materials into the ECF is from nutrients entering the digestive tract, materials that the body has manufactured from these nutrients (e.g. carbohydrates, fats, proteins) and oxygen via the lungs (Ch. 10). Net

BOX 7.3	The Extracellular Fluid Compartment

Plasma – aqueous part of the blood
Interstitial fluid – fluid in the microscopic spaces between the cells
Lymph – fluid in the lymphatic vessels and lymph nodes
Cerebrospinal fluid – fluid filling the ventricles of the brain and the spinal canal
Secretions from the gastrointestinal tract – digestive enzymes, bile
Synovial fluid – secretion of the membranes lining joint cavities
Humors in the eye – the aqueous and vitreous humors
Pleural fluid – secretion of the pleural membranes surrounding the lungs

loss from the ECF occurs via faeces, urine, expired air, sweat and from old, dead cells sloughed from the external and internal surfaces of the body: the skin and the lining of the gut. Materials can also leave the ECF to be stored. For example, an excess intake of carbohydrate in the diet may be stored as fat in adipose tissue beneath the skin. Homeostatic balance is achieved when the net gain of a particular substance in the ECF is in equilibrium with its net loss. However, the composition of the ECF also depends on the shift of water and other materials between the different body fluid compartments. Three potential situations exist:

- negative balance – loss exceeds gain
- positive balance – gain exceeds loss
- equilibrium – loss and gain equate.

FLUID BALANCE

For the individual to remain in fluid balance, water intake must be equal to water loss. In health a typical intake is 1.5 L/24 h. However, this varies considerably between individuals and is to a large extent determined by habit. The chief sources of fluid gain (Table 7.3) are:

- water ingested – 60%
- moist food – 30%
- water produced through cellular metabolism – 10%.

TABLE 7.3	Sources of Water Acquisition and Loss

Average daily intake		Average daily output	
Metabolism	250 ml	Sweat	90 ml
Moist food	750 ml	Faeces	10 ml
Oral fluids	1600 ml	Insensible loss (skin and lungs)	700 ml
		Urine	1500 ml
Total	2600 ml	Total	2300 ml

The chief sources of fluid loss are:

- urine – 60%
- in expired air via the lungs – 28%
- perspiration – 8%
- faeces – 4%.

Healthy individuals are able to maintain the concentration of their body fluids within a very narrow range. A negative fluid balance (dehydration) will stimulate the kidneys to conserve water and concentrated urine will be excreted (Ch. 11). Dehydration occurs when fluid intake is severely curtailed. There is considerable potential for this situation in hospital where patients frequently have to fast before undergoing surgery and may be unable to eat or drink for hours or days afterwards. Dehydration is avoided by the administration of intravenous fluids. Dehydration is also possible when excess water is lost from the body, e.g. severe diarrhoea or vomiting. People who have been badly burned are also at risk because they often lose large amounts of fluid from the surface of the raw, damaged area. Again, intravenous fluids can be life-saving.

> The maintenance of body water level is under strict homeostatic control and this is achieved in several ways, including the exchange of water between body compartments, behavioural responses such as drinking and also through the action of the kidneys.

What the nurse can do

The nurse has a vital role to play in monitoring the fluid balance of patients. In the case of elderly people who may be reluctant to drink adequately through the fear of urinary incontinence or a desire to avoid inconvenience, a simple chart depicting fluid input and output may be all that is required. For the more acutely ill patient, including any who have recently undergone a surgical procedure, monitoring fluid balance will be more elaborate because it will involve continually assessing the input from one or possibly more intravenous lines. Such patients are likely to be sedated or recovering from the effects of anaesthesia. In this condition they will be unable to take fluids orally and unable to communicate their needs. However, they may still experience thirst and a dry, sore mouth. Such patients require regular cleaning of the oral cavity to remove debris and to stimulate the flow of saliva to promote comfort and decrease the risk of infection. Other complications arising from lack of adequate hydration include dry skin, which is prone to the effects of tearing and laceration when the patient's position is altered, and constipation. Again, the nurse must be aware of these complications and take the appropriate preventative measures.

The role of electrolytes in fluid balance

Both the ECF and the ICF contain a range of dissolved solutes that are under homeostatic control. It is essential to understand their properties and distribution because they determine the movement of water across cell membranes and have important implications for the normal functioning of the individual and thus for health.

MOVEMENT OF MATERIALS BETWEEN BODY FLUID COMPARTMENTS

Solutes present within the body's aqueous solutions fall into two broad categories: electrolytes (ions) and non-electrolytes:

1. *Electrolytes* are chemical compounds containing ionic bonds (Ch. 1). They dissociate in water to form electrically charged particles called ions. Because they are charged they are able to conduct an electrical current. Anions carry a negative charge and cations carry a positive charge. Electrolytes include inorganic salts (e.g. sodium and chloride), inorganic and organic acids and bases and many proteins.
2. *Non-electrolytes* are chemical compounds containing covalent bonds. They do not dissociate in water and thus do not carry an electrical charge. Most non-electrolytes are organic molecules. Examples include glucose, lipids, creatinine and urea.

Several different electrolytes essential for homeostatic function are present in the body fluids (Box 7.4). In health the concentration of each is maintained within narrow limits by the kidneys. For example, in healthy people the plasma concentration of sodium is maintained at 135–145 mmol/L. The concentration of potassium in the plasma is maintained at 3.5–5.2 mmol/L despite wide variations in dietary intake. Several hormones are involved in these control mechanisms. For example, the parathyroid hormones control the levels of calcium and phosphate in the body (Ch. 6).

BOX 7.4	*Key Electrolytes in Homeostatic Function*
	Calcium
	Chloride
	Hydrogen carbonate
	Magnesium
	Potassium
	Sodium

Antidiuretic hormone (ADH) secreted from the posterior pituitary gland (Ch. 6) and aldosterone from the adrenal cortex are important in the control of salt (sodium chloride) and water balance. Sodium and water homeostasis are inextricably linked because the osmotic effect of sodium determines the volume of the ECF. Under normal circumstances small quantities of ADH are continuously released into the plasma, but the rate of secretion may be reduced or increased according to the amount of water entering or leaving the ECF and its osmotic pressure. When the amount of fluid in the ECF falls, the relative concentration of solutes, principally sodium, increases (Fig. 7.4). The osmotic pressure of the plasma rises and this change is detected by osmoreceptor cells in the hypothalamus and the great veins in the neck. As a result, ADH is rapidly released from the posterior pituitary gland. It travels in the plasma to its target cells in the kidney tubules and they respond by reabsorbing more of the water they are filtering from the plasma into the urine (Ch. 11). Water is thus retained, the concentration of solutes in the plasma falls and small amounts of concen-

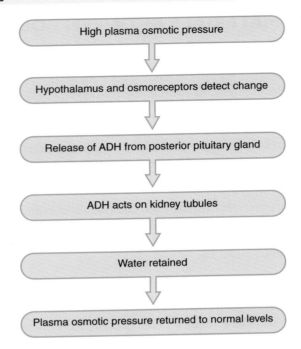

Fig. 7.4   *ADH and fluid balance.*

trated urine are passed. The osmotic pressure of the plasma is reduced and homeostasis is restored.

Conversely, if a large volume of fluid is ingested, the secretion of ADH will fall below its baseline level, stimulating water loss. Large amounts of dilute urine are produced. From this account it will be apparent that we can obtain a fairly good idea of a patient's level of hydration simply by visual inspection of the urine. Other signs of dehydration include a dry mouth with a furred, sore tongue and wrinkled, inelastic skin. These are valuable indicators of dehydration in the patient who is too ill or too confused to complain of thirst.

The adrenal glands, two small glands positioned at the upper end of each kidney, are responsible for the secretion of aldosterone (Ch. 6). This hormone plays an important role in the regulation of sodium and potassium balance. It is released from the cortex (outer part) of the adrenals. The stimulus for the release of aldosterone is provided by a fall in the concentration of sodium in the plasma or an increase in potassium levels. Aldosterone stimulates the kidney tubules to reabsorb sodium from the plasma they are filtering at a faster rate. The resultant drop in the concentration of sodium in the filtrate sets up an electric imbalance because the filtrate now contains a high proportion of negative ions to positive ions. This imbalance is restored by increased diffusion of potassium into the filtrate. Thus, the release of aldosterone not only increases sodium retention; it also stimulates the loss of potassium from the body in urine. However, as the plasma contains more sodium than potassium ions there is still a net uptake of solutes from the plasma. Water is therefore drawn osmotically from the filtrate and retained in the plasma.

Aldosterone release is also stimulated by a reduction in blood volume (e.g. through haemorrhage or loss of large fluid volumes in severe diarrhoea).

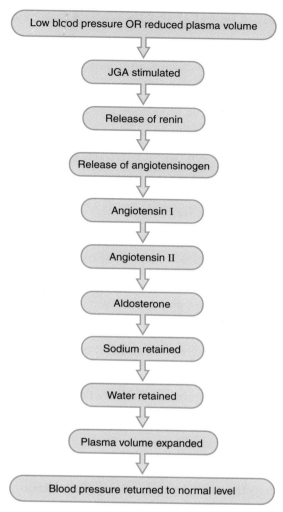

Fig. 7.5 *Aldosterone, salt and fluid balance. JGA, juxtaglomerular apparatus.*

A reduction in the flow of blood to the kidneys is detected by specialised cells called the juxtaglomerular apparatus (JGA). These cells are sensitive to stretch and as reduction in blood volume causes a reduction in blood pressure, the JGA responds, releasing a hormone called renin into the plasma. Renin catalyses the conversion of a plasma protein called angiotensinogen to angiotensin I. Angiotensin I is in turn converted by enzymes in the plasma to angiotensin II. Angiotensin II causes vasoconstriction, helping to increase blood pressure (Ch. 8). It also stimulates the release of aldosterone from the adrenal cortex. Thus sodium and, ultimately, water retention are stimulated, increasing blood volume and blood pressure. These changes are shown in Fig. 7.5.

THE DISRUPTION OF HOMEOSTASIS AND DISEASE

Throughout this chapter the vital role of homeostasis in maintaining normal function and its tremendous contribution to the health of the individual have been emphasised in every control system discussed. The result of homeostatic imbalance – disease – has been pointed out each time. Several situations contribute to homeostatic imbalance and have the potential to contribute to ill-health. This chapter will conclude by summarising the types of individual and situations in which homeostasis is particularly likely to be disrupted. Loss of dynamic equilibrium is particularly likely to occur in the following:

1. Infants in which a high concentration of their lean body mass consists of water. Thus loss of body fluids and the solutes they contain is particularly detrimental to the very young.
2. The elderly. The control systems of the body become less efficient with advancing years. As a result the internal environment becomes less stable, placing the individual at increasing risk of illness.
3. Individuals who have developed pathological conditions in which the usual negative feedback systems operating in health have become overwhelmed. Instead, destructive positive feedback mechanisms come into play. The effect of exercise under hot conditions to the individual who is not acclimatised is an example. The normal negative feedback system controlling thermoregulation is lost because the individual cannot respond by sweating sufficiently to effect temperature loss. Instead, more heat is absorbed passively from the environment, leading to a further rise in temperature. As the normal metabolic activity of the body generates heat, the temperature rises yet again, eventually culminating in irreversible damage to the cells (see Fig. 7.3). Similarly, the administration of excess intravenous fluid will result in overload of the plasma and cause an increase in blood pressure, which will put stress on the heart. Many other cellular mechanisms will be simultaneously affected. One of the most striking effects will be on breathing. Respiration will be affected through the accumulation of excess interstitial fluid in the lungs.
4. Stress. Both the effects of acute and longer-term physical or psychological stress are detrimental to physical and psychological well-being.

SUMMARY

This chapter opened by explaining the concept of homeostasis crucial to understanding physiological functioning. The conditions necessary to maintain homeostasis were given and the manner in which typical homeostatic systems are controlled was discussed. Most physiological systems are controlled by negative feedback mechanisms and this was illustrated using the examples of temperature control and the control of plasma glucose levels. In both cases the events set in train when homeostasis breaks down were explored. Positive feedback systems are less frequently encountered. The example used in this chapter was parturition. The chapter ended with a consideration of the role played by water and the body's fluid compartments in maintaining homeostasis. The implications for nursing practice in maintaining fluid balance were provided.

QUESTIONS

1. What is negative feedback? Give two examples of systems which are controlled by negative feedback.

2. What is the control centre for temperature regulation and how does it achieve this?

3. What are the fluid compartments of the body?

FURTHER READING

Montague S, Herbert R, Watson R (eds) (1996) The human body: a framework for understanding. In: Hinchliff S, Montague S, Watson R (eds) *Physiology for nursing practice, 2nd edn*. Baillière Tindall, London, pp 3–22

Watson R (1995) *Anatomy and physiology for nurses, 10th edn*. Baillière Tindall, London

SELECTED SYSTEMS

8 Cardiovascular System

Sheenan Kindlen

> After reading this chapter you should be able to:
> - list the components of the cardiovascular system
> - explain how the heart pumps blood through the circulation
> - outline the control mechanisms in the cardiovascular system
> - understand the need for the continual regulation of blood pressure.

Body cells need a constant supply of water, oxygen, nutrients and the regulatory factors that control their activities. They must also be able to get rid of waste products and the cells that produce materials used by other tissues must have a means of exporting them. Any transport system must, therefore, be rapid, direct and capable of two-way exchange. This is the function of blood and the cardiovascular system carrying it (Fig. 8.1).

In order that the transport system can meet the requirements, there must be a pump (the heart) to generate the head of pressure required and vessels to act as fast transport routes, and one type of vessel (the capillary) must be permeable to a wide variety of substances.

> Arteries carry blood away from the heart and veins carry blood back to the heart.

Blood vessels are of different types, each type fulfilling a particular role. Blood flows out of the heart into arteries, then arterioles, capillaries and venules, and finally comes back to the heart via the veins. The arteries, which are large, thick-walled and elastic, are the pressure vessels into which the heart ejects blood. Pressure is at its highest here and the vessels must be strong enough to withstand the effects of the high pressure. Blood then flows into many smaller, thick-walled arterioles. These are the resistance vessels, moderating pressure and capable of redirecting blood flow from one area to another. Capillaries are the exchange vessels and are the link between the blood and the tissues. The venules, small veins, collect up the blood from the capillary beds and lead it into the larger veins, which empty the blood into the heart (Fig. 8.2). More detailed information about blood vessels is given on pages 158–165.

The purpose of the cardiovascular system is to supply the tissue cells with requirements which meet their needs at any particular time. The control of the system is aimed at maintaining the correct rate of exchange with the tissue cells.

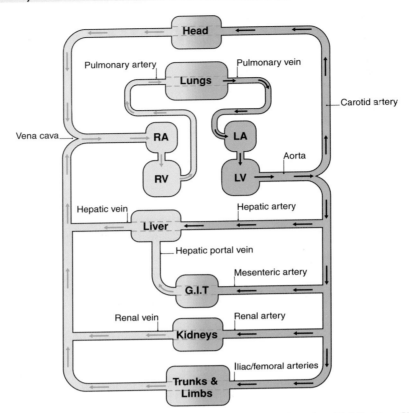

Fig. 8.1   *Diagrammatic view of circulation in the cardiovascular system. RA, right atrium; LA, left atrium; RV, right ventricle; LV, left ventricle; GIT, gastrointestinal tract.*

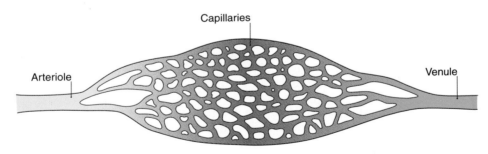

Fig. 8.2   *The microvascular bed.*

The principles of exchange are that there must be enough pressure to force fluid out of the vessels at one end of the capillary bed, enough pressure to pull fluid back in at the other end, and the permeability of the capillary membrane must be such that fluid can pass through. Most of the substances exchanged are in solution and therefore are contained in the 'tissue fluid' that passes out of the vessels. Cells and large molecules such as plasma proteins usually cannot leave the vessels and are retained in the blood. Intermediate-sized molecules may be able to get through some capillary membranes but not others. The process of exchange is shown in Figure 8.3.

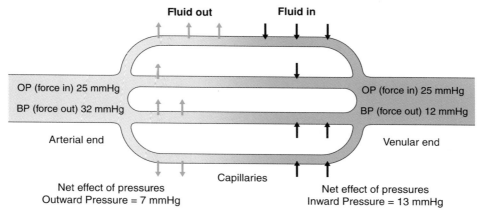

Fig. 8.3   *Fluid exchange at the capillaries. OP, osmotic pressure; BP, blood (hydrostatic) pressure.*

Terms used about pressures

1. *Hydrostatic pressure*. This literally means the pressure of a liquid against a surface and refers to the pressure of the blood in the vessels against the vessel walls. 'Blood pressure' is therefore hydrostatic pressure. The effect of hydrostatic or blood pressure is to push fluid along a vessel if the wall is impermeable, or out of the vessel where the wall is permeable.
2. *Osmotic pressure* is the pressure that retains water. In blood all the substances in solution contribute to the osmotic pressure but the colloid osmotic pressure provided by the plasma proteins is an important contributor. Because osmotic pressure retains water, its effect is to pull fluid into the vessel. At the arteriolar end of the capillary bed, blood pressure (hydrostatic pressure) is higher than colloid osmotic pressure, therefore the tendency is for fluid to move out of the vessel into the tissue.

Each arteriole supplies several capillaries and, as blood flows from one stream (the arteriole) into many streams (the capillaries), the hydrostatic pressure and the flow rate are reduced. This is a law of physics and is an important factor in capillary exchange. It not only reduces the hydrostatic pressure along the length of the capillary bed, it also slows the flow rate to give more time for exchange.

> **Fluid is exchanged between the vascular system and the tissues at the capillaries.**

At the venular end of the capillary bed, the hydrostatic pressure has dropped below the osmotic pressure and the direction of flow of fluid will therefore be into the vessel. The difference between the two pressures is the pressure gradient and the steeper the gradient, the greater the movement of fluid (Fig. 8.4).

The evidence for this system of exchange becomes obvious when there is something wrong. If the blood pressure (hydrostatic pressure) is too high, more fluid moves out into the tissue, less is reclaimed and the tissue becomes overloaded with fluid, i.e. oedema is formed. If the osmotic pressure is reduced, for example where the liver cannot produce enough plasma protein, the pressure

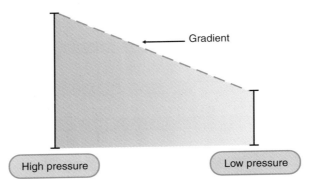

Fig. 8.4   *The principle of a pressure gradient.*

gradient becomes steeper, again more fluid enters the tissue and less is reclaimed, i.e. oedema but for a different reason. If the hydrostatic pressure falls very low, fluid, and the substances it carries, cannot reach the tissue, which may not survive the subsequent lack of oxygen, water or nutrient such as glucose. Not all the fluid is reclaimed at the venular end of the capillary bed. Some is drained off by the lymphatic vessels and returned to the bloodstream at the thoracic duct.

> The exchange of fluid between the vascular system and the tissues is influenced by the hydrostatic pressure which pushes fluid out of the vascular system and the osmotic pressure which draws fluid back in.

Lymphatic drainage

The volume of fluid leaving blood vessels is always more than can be recovered by them. The difference is drained into the lymphatic vessels which run close to the vascular system throughout the tissues. Although both the vascular and lymphatic systems act as fluid distribution systems, there are marked differences in structure, in the mechanics by which they function and the fluids that they carry. The composition and characteristics of blood and lymph (Ch. 9) are considered elsewhere.

The small lymphatic vessels are within tissues and, close to the capillaries, are closed-ended like the fingers of a glove. These run into larger and larger lymphatic vessels ending in the large ducts in the thoracic region; here the lymphatic fluid is emptied into the great veins. Because there is no pump action of the heart driving the lymph, the hydrostatic pressure is lower even than that in tissue. Flow is achieved by the milking movements of muscle near the lymphatic vessels, by the rapid emptying into the great veins and, probably to the largest extent, by the rhythmic contractions of the walls of the large ducts.

The smallest lymphatic vessels are very permeable and allow the entry of large protein molecules, particularly in the area of the liver. The movement of protein into lymph is substantial and may amount daily to about a third of the total circulating plasma protein. The effect of the protein content is to give lymph an osmotic pressure that, although lower than that of blood, is higher than that of tissue fluid. The combination of a hydrostatic pressure lower than in tissue fluid and a colloid osmotic pressure that is higher makes lymphatic drainage effective. In an adult, about 3 litres (L) of fluid is exchanged daily and an obstruction in a lymphatic vessel leads rapidly to tissue swelling around the site.

Blood pressure is clearly central to the exchange of materials with the tissues and it follows that blood pressure is central to the health and even survival of those tissues. Blood pressure is usually measured in an artery but the importance of the measure is that it gives an indication of the pressures at the capillaries and normality of exchange.

Principle of pressure regulation

There are three main routes by which blood pressure can be regulated: cardiac output (or pump output), vessel capacity and intravascular volume (Fig. 8.5).

1. Cardiac output is the volume of blood pumped out of the ventricles per minute and it represents the head of pressure that can then be altered to suit requirements. Changes in cardiac output affect *systolic pressure*, which is the pressure generated when the heart contracts.
2. Vessel capacity determines the size or capacity of the system by altering the diameter of the vessels. In addition to being used to alter the overall pressure, control of vessel diameter can be used to redirect flow of blood from one area to another or to control the rate of flow to a particular tissue. Changes in vessel capacity are likely to affect *diastolic pressure*, which is the pressure of the blood against the vessel walls when the heart is not contracting. If the capacity is reduced, pressure will increase and vice versa.
3. Intravascular volume is the volume of blood within the vessels. If the volume is reduced, pressure will decrease and vice versa. Because volume takes longer to alter than cardiac output or vessel capacity, control of volume provides a stabilising influence over pressure regulation. Changes in volume will affect *both systolic and diastolic pressures*.

REGULATION OF PRESSURE BY CARDIAC OUTPUT

Cardiac output – the volume of blood pumped out by the ventricles per unit time (usually 1 min) – is sometimes shown as:

Cardiac output = heart rate × stroke volume.

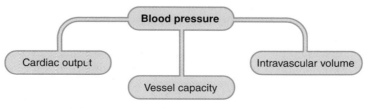

Fig. 8.5 *The major components of blood pressure regulation.*

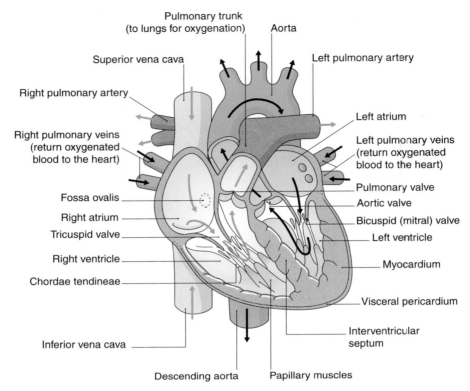

Pulmonary trunk
(to lungs for oxygenation)

Aorta

Superior vena cava

Left pulmonary artery

Right pulmonary artery

Left atrium

Right pulmonary veins
(return oxygenated
blood to the heart)

Left pulmonary veins
(return oxygenated
blood to the heart)

Pulmonary valve

Fossa ovalis

Aortic valve

Right atrium

Bicuspid (mitral) valve

Tricuspid valve

Left ventricle

Right ventricle

Myocardium

Chordae tendineae

Visceral pericardium

Interventricular
septum

Inferior vena cava

Descending aorta

Papillary muscles

Fig. 8.6 *The anatomical heart.*

Stroke volume is the volume pumped out by the heart at one contraction. In an adult at rest this is about 70 millilitres (ml). The resting heart rate is about 70 beats per minute, therefore cardiac output at rest is 70 ml × 70 beats per minute = 4900 ml/min (about 5 L/min). At the other extreme, an athlete may achieve a cardiac output of 30 L/min by increasing both heart rate and stroke volume.

Cardiac output = heart rate × stroke volume.

Heart pump action

The heart is a four-chambered pump. The two smaller chambers are the atria and the two larger are the ventricles. The chambers work in two pairs, one atrium with one ventricle with the atrium acting as a priming pump and the ventricle as the ejection chamber. Blood enters at the right atrium and passes through to the right ventricle from which it is ejected, i.e. the first pump or right heart pump. The blood then passes through the pulmonary circuit where it takes up oxygen and gives up carbon dioxide. It then moves into the second pump or the left heart pump, where it enters at the left atrium and passes into the left ventricle, to be ejected into the general vascular system. The two pumps, right and left, are synchronised so that the effect appears to be from one pump. The

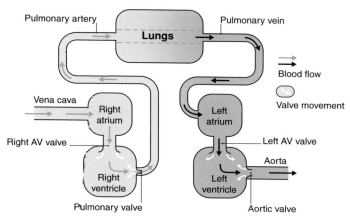

Fig. 8.7   *The heart as a four-chambered pump. AV, atrioventricular.*

anatomical diagram is shown in Figure 8.6, however, the workings of the pump are more easily visualised using the pump diagram shown in Figure 8.7.

The movement of blood from chamber to chamber is controlled by pressure gradients and the valves in the heart. Pressure is generated when the muscular wall of a chamber contracts, reducing the size of the chamber and raising the pressure. Fluid moves from an area of higher pressure to an area of lower pressure and so blood moves from the contracting chamber to the next chamber, not yet contracting, where pressure is lower.

The valves between the atria and ventricles are pushed open when the atria are filling and atrial pressure is higher than ventricular pressure. They are pushed closed when the ventricles contract and ventricular pressure rises above atrial pressure. The atrio-ventricular (AV) valves are the tricuspid in the right heart and the bicuspid in the left heart. The semilunar valves, which guard the entrances to the pulmonary artery and the aorta, are opened when, at ventricular contraction, ventricular pressure rises above the pressure in the vessel outside. They close again when the ventricles relax and ventricular pressure drops below vessel pressure.

The cardiac cycle

The events that make up the cycle of filling, ejection and refilling are called 'the cardiac cycle'. The following is a simple version of the cycle and the description can begin at any point in the cycle, but it is simplest to start when the heart is completely relaxed at total diastole. A complete cycle takes about 1 s at a resting rate of 60 beats per minute. If the rate is greatly increased, rest time between contractions will be reduced and the time for filling the chambers will be less.

Total diastole

All chambers are relaxed, pressure is low in all chambers, and blood is flowing from the great veins into the right atrium and from the pulmonary circuit into the left atrium. The left and right AV valves are open and blood flows through the open valves into the ventricles. Blood pressure recorded at this point, with the heart completely relaxed, would be *diastolic pressure*.

Atrial systole

The atria contract, their capacity is reduced and the pressure inside rises. Blood moves under pressure from the atria through the AV valves, completing the filling of the ventricles. About 75% of ventricular filling is completed before the atria contract.

Ventricular systole

The ventricles contract, ventricular capacity is reduced and the pressure inside increases. When ventricular pressure rises above the pressure in the atria, which have by this time begun to relax again, the AV valves close. They balloon back slightly into the atria but do not leak because the flaps of the valves are tethered by cords of tissue attached to the papillary muscles in the walls of the ventricles. As the ventricles contract, so do the papillary muscles, tightening the cords and preventing backflow of blood into the atria.

The ventricles continue to contract and pressure continues to rise until the pressure inside the ventricle is above the pressure outside in the vessel. At that point, the semilunar valves open, like swing doors when pushed, and blood is ejected from the ventricles. This is the *stroke volume*, being ejected at *ejection pressure* during *ventricular systole*. Blood pressure recorded at this point would be *systolic pressure*.

Ventricular diastole

The pump now has to be refilled. The ventricles begin to relax and enlarge, and pressure is reduced. When pressure is below that in the vessels outside, the semilunar valves close again, pushed closed by the higher pressure in the vessels on the outside of the heart. The ventricles are now closed chambers with the AV valves still closed and the semilunar valves having just closed. The atria have been in diastole and are being filled from the veins. Atrial pressure has been rising and when the pressure is greater than that in the ventricles, the AV valves are opened by the pressure gradient, blood flows through to the ventricles and the cycle begins again.

> Diastole describes the situation when the heart is fully relaxed and systole describes the condition when the heart is fully contracted.

The sounds made by the heart when it beats are sometimes described as *lubb–dup, lubb–dup. Lubb* is the sound of the AV valves closing and the sharper sound *dup* is the sound of the semilunar valves closing.

Blood pressure measured as systolic/diastolic, e.g. 120/80 mmHg, gives information about the force generated when the heart contracts (systolic) and the background pressure of the blood in the vessels (diastolic); the difference between the two (pulse pressure) is a useful indication of the overall state of the pressure.

Heart tissue

The heart tissue is of two main types. One type consists of the contractile cells of the myocardium (Ch. 12) and the other consists of the electrically excitable cells, which act as pacemakers or which carry neural signals from the atria to the ventricles and up the walls of the ventricles. Myocardial cells can contract even when isolated, a property called *intrinsic myogenicity*, but the role of the pacemaker cells is to organise the contractile activity so that the chambers contract in an organised way, and at a controlled rate.

Myocardial tissue sometimes acts independently and out of the control of the pacemaker cells. When this happens, contraction becomes disorganised and cardiac output is jeopardised. The out-of-control tissue is an *ectopic focus* and is often therapeutically controlled by suppressing its activity with lignocaine. If the tissue of a ventricle were to become totally disorganised, ejection of stroke volume could not be achieved and blood pressure could not be maintained. This widespread disorganisation of the ventricle is *ventricular fibrillation*.

Pacemaker cells are located in the sino-atrial node (SA node). The impulses from the node are strong enough to suppress the intrinsic activity of the myocardial cells and therefore the node can regulate their rate and rhythm of contraction. Impulses spread across the atria from cell to cell. This is more rapid than might be anticipated because myocardial cells have modifications that allow ions to pass readily across the cell membrane. This allows them to communicate with one another and act as a tissue unit.

All of the heart muscle is capable of contracting spontaneously but contraction of the healthy heart is initiated and controlled by the pacemaker at the sino-atrial node.

The impulse cannot pass directly from atria to ventricles because of a ring of fibrous tissue separating the chambers. At the junction of the atrium and ventricle, the impulse activates the AV node, then it is passed to a bundle of nerve fibres, the bundle of His or AV bundle, and then to the Purkinje fibres, which are nerve fibres supplying the apex and walls of the ventricles. Activation of the AV node allows the introduction of a small delay in transmission, which allows the atria to complete their contraction before the beginning of ventricular contraction.

BLOOD PRESSURE AND CARDIAC OUTPUT

Arterial blood pressure is proportional to cardiac output. Cardiac output equals heart rate multiplied by stroke volume, therefore blood pressure can be affected by changes in either heart rate or stroke volume. Changes in cardiac output have a direct effect on the systolic pressure.

Blood pressure and heart rate

The SA node is supplied by nerve fibres of the parasympathetic and sympathetic divisions of the autonomic nervous system.

Parasympathetic fibres supplying the heart travel to the SA and AV nodes via the vagus nerve. The transmitter is acetylcholine and the receptor sites on the nodes are of the cholinergic, muscarinic type (see section on the autonomic nervous system). The effect is inhibitory and parasympathetic activity will slow the heart rate. The effect will be to reduce cardiac output and, in turn, reduce arterial blood pressure. The heart rate is under some parasympathetic influence most of the time and this has the effect of reducing the overall workload of the heart and maintaining a moderate blood pressure. The reduction in blood pressure produced by a slower heart rate may be compensated to some extent by increased filling time and a larger stroke volume.

The sympathetic division supplies the SA and AV nodes and the myocardium itself (Ch. 5). The transmitter is noradrenaline, the receptor site type is β_1 and the effect is excitatory. Sympathetic stimulation will therefore increase both the heart rate and the force of contraction, producing a rise in cardiac output and arterial blood pressure. Sympathetic stimulation can considerably increase the systolic pressure.

Sympathetic stimulation of the adrenal medulla brings about the release of the neurohormones adrenaline and noradrenaline, which circulate to the heart and augment the effects of the noradrenaline produced by the sympathetic endings. This effect on the adrenal medulla is the *sympathomedullary effect*. Like the sympathetic effects, by increasing heart rate, it increases cardiac output and systolic pressure. There is a limit to the effectiveness of raising the heart rate in order to raise the blood pressure, because, if the heart rate increases to the point where the chambers do not have enough time to fill, cardiac output will not be increased.

Although heart rate is often measured, it is not of prime interest to the body. The factor that does matter is blood pressure and heart rate changes are only a physiological means of regulating blood pressure.

Regulation of heart rate

Regulation of heart rate is carried out by a series of autonomic reflexes. These are feedback loops which are continually sensitive to changes in blood pressure and continually adjust the blood pressure to meet changing demands while staying within safe limits (Ch. 7).

The baroreceptors are sensory nerve endings that respond to increased stretching of the vessel wall (which would indicate increased blood pressure) by increasing their firing rate. Their effect on the control centres in the brain stem is inhibitory and the result is a reduction in heart rate and force of contraction, so lowering cardiac output. A fall in blood pressure would have the opposite effect, resulting in a rise in heart rate and force of contraction, which would raise the blood pressure.

These baroreceptors are located in the carotid arteries, where they monitor the pressure of blood entering the brain, and in the aortic arch, which carries the blood supply for the whole body. Their role is to act as rapid-response, short-term regulators of blood pressure.

Factors affecting heart rate

Temperature

Other factors that affect heart rate are, for example, heat and cold. If the blood temperature rises, the heart rate increases; an increase of 1°C will raise the heart rate by about 10 beats per minute and, conversely, a fall in blood temperature will reduce the heart rate. If the blood temperature falls sufficiently low, the heart will no longer beat and this can be used clinically to carry out surgery on a heart. Blood temperature has a direct effect on the excitability of the pacemaker cells. The autonomic reflexes, however, will compensate for the direct effects brought about by changes in temperature. If a rise in blood temperature is enough to cause vasodilatation, resulting in a fall in blood pressure, there will be a reflex rise in heart rate in addition to any effect brought about by the increased temperature at the SA node.

Hormones

In addition to the neurohormones adrenaline and noradrenaline, other hormones can change the heart rate. The thyroid hormones, for example, increase the heart rate by increasing the effectiveness of adrenaline and noradrenaline. One of the characteristic features of overactivity of the thyroid gland is a rapid heart rate (tachycardia) even at rest and a slow heart rate (bradycardia) typifies the underactive thyroid.

Blood pressure and stroke volume

Stroke volume is the volume ejected by the heart at each beat. Because the stroke volume affects cardiac output, it also affects arterial blood pressure.

Ventricular capacity in an adult is about 120 ml, and, at the end of the filling period (i.e. at the end of diastole), the volume of blood in the ventricles is called the *end-diastolic volume*. Stroke volume at rest is about 70 ml and the blood remaining in the ventricles after ejection is called the cardiac reserve. The fraction that has been ejected is called the *ejection fraction*. If the ventricle contracts more forcibly, the stroke volume can be increased by expelling some of the cardiac reserve volume, and the ejection fraction will be increased. This happens in exercise when increased sympathetic stimulation increases contractility and it is one of the mechanisms that provide the increased blood pressure necessary in any form of physical activity.

Stroke volume is affected by several factors, each of which will in turn affect blood pressure.

Ventricular contractility

- Increased by sympathetic stimulation, as described above.
- Increased by stretching the ventricular muscle during filling. The physiologist Starling gave his name to a law which says that 'the more the heart is stretched in diastole, the stronger is the following contraction'. This is one of the mechanisms allowing the heart to match input with output.
- Increased by stretching of the atrial muscle. This is a short-lived effect, lasting for only 10–20 beats, produced by overfilling the atria perhaps by a long filling period or infusion of fluid. This is called the Bainbridge effect after the physiologist who first recorded it, and it is another mechanism allowing the heart to manage a change in input.

Altered ventricular volume

This may be an effect of exercise training when, like all muscles, the heart muscle enlarges. As stroke volume increases, a higher cardiac output can be achieved without a large increase in heart rate and many highly trained athletes show evidence of this by their low resting heart rate. There is a limit to the benefit achieved by enlarging the heart, because when the walls of the chambers are overthickened they become more difficult to contract.

Venous return

Venous return is the blood returning to the right atrium via the great veins. This returning blood will be used to fill the heart ready for the next ejection, therefore cardiac output is greatly dependent on venous return.

> The venous return is the amount of blood returned to the right atrium from the peripheral circulation and this is enhanced by the action of skeletal muscle pumps and the respiratory pump.

When standing up, blood must return to the heart from the lower body for a distance of perhaps over a metre. Hydrostatic pressure in veins is low, the driving force is much reduced and the effect of gravity is to oppose the upward flow of blood to the heart. Venous return is very good when lying down, but in the upright position it has to be assisted by several mechanisms and one of the reasons for the variability of heart rate is that it is used to compensate for changes in venous return (Fig. 8.8).

The factors that compensate for the upright posture and improve venous return include the muscle and respiratory pumps, and venous tone (Figs 8.9 and 8.10).

Muscle pump

As skeletal muscles contract, pressure is increased on the veins running through them, forcing blood up through the veins. When the muscles relax, venous pressure drops, but the blood, which would otherwise drop back down the vessel, recedes only as far as the nearest of the valves, which are found in limb veins. The lower pressure allows the vein to refill and the next muscle contraction

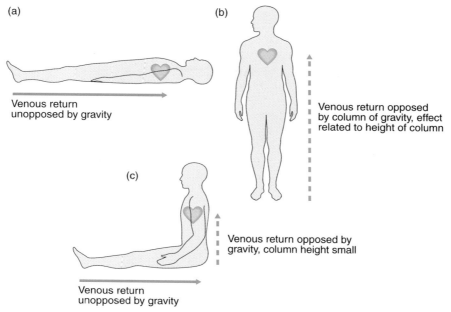

Fig. 8.8   *The effect of posture on venous return.*

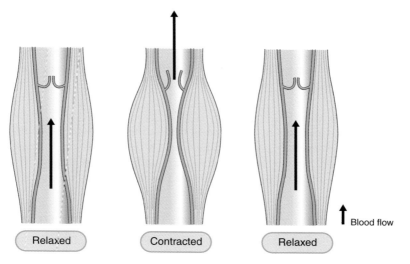

Fig. 8.9   *The muscle pump.*

pushes this blood further up the vessel. This step-by-step movement of blood up the veins happens most forcibly in physical activity, but the continuous rhythmic contractions of the posture muscles, as they keep the body upright, contribute to venous return.

Respiratory pump
This is the rhythmic pumping action produced by breathing in and out.

At inspiration, the thoracic cavity enlarges and consequently pressure here is

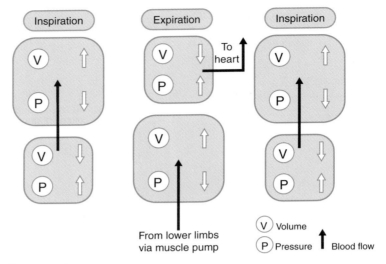

Fig. 8.10   *The respiratory pump.*

lowered. In the abdominal compartment, pressure is raised as the diaphragm is lowered and abdominal wall muscles are tightened. Because blood will move from higher to lower pressure, blood moves from the abdominal cavity to the lower-pressure thoracic compartment.

At expiration, the thoracic pressure is raised and blood in the thoracic veins moves to the area of nearest low pressure, which is the right atrium, thereby increasing venous return. The lower pressure now in the abdominal compartment allows blood to flow in from the lower limbs, ready for the next inspiratory stroke of the pump.

Venous tone

Veins are capable of constricting or dilating and therefore changing the pressure of the blood they contain. The effect is to increase or decrease the pressure of the blood flowing back to the heart and therefore change venous return (the mechanisms involved are considered in the next section).

REGULATION OF BLOOD PRESSURE BY VESSEL CAPACITY

Changes in vessel capacity can affect both the overall blood pressure and the pressure in local areas. Overall or systemic changes will affect diastolic pressure. Local changes can redirect blood from one area to another, increasing the supply to one tissue perhaps at the expense of another.

Vessel structure and function

The structure of a blood vessel determines its function. All blood vessels are lined with endothelium, which provides a smooth surface against which cells such as platelets are unlikely to stick and initiate clotting. Smooth muscle found in the walls allows the vessels to alter its diameter and therefore vary the pressure of the blood in the vessel (Ch. 12). The state of partial contraction allows the vessel to relax if the pressure rises and constrict if the pressure falls.

Elastic tissue is found in large arteries and allows the vessel to stretch and reduce the pressure but to then recoil and raise pressure. Vessels without elastin can stretch passively if subjected to high pressure. This is called *vessel compliance* and it is an important mechanism which avoids hypertension.

Large arteries

Large arteries, such as the aorta, have thick walls with smooth muscle and elastic tissue. They are sometimes called 'the pressure vessels' because, being nearest the heart, they are exposed to the highest and most pulsatile pressure. They must be able not only simply to withstand the pressure, but to stretch at systole and reduce pressure, then recoil and raise pressure in diastole. This moderates the peaks and troughs of pressure produced by the rhythmic pumping of the heart.

Smaller arteries

Smaller arteries have smooth muscle but less elastic tissue the further away they are from the pulsatile effect of the heart.

Arterioles

Arterioles are small arteries of narrow bore and relatively thick walls. Their structure gives them a particular role in the control of blood pressure and blood flow. They are 'the resistance vessels' and they contribute greatly to *peripheral resistance*, which in turn has a large overall effect on diastolic pressure.

Flow in a vessel is very strongly affected by the bore of the vessel. A small decrease in the diameter has a very large effect on the resistance to flow and, by changing the diameter using the smooth muscle in the thick walls, resistance can be increased in one part of a vascular bed and decreased in another. Blood will then take the path of least resistance, i.e. redirection of flow. There is never enough blood to fill every vessel and the arterioles have an important role in the control of blood distribution, moving blood from area to area and keeping the tissues perfused according to demand (see Fig. 8.11).

Capillaries

Capillaries are exchange vessels that do not constrict and dilate although they may be stretched. The walls have only occasional strands of smooth muscle. They are mainly composed of endothelium on a basement membrane and are therefore extremely thin. Permeability varies, depending on the gap between the cells; some capillaries are 'tight junction' and allow only restricted exchange. On the other hand, some capillaries have very large gaps allowing much larger molecules to pass through. Most capillaries will allow the passage of water, dissolved gases and small molecules in solution but not large molecules such as proteins or cells. In fact, the whole system of exchange between blood and tissue depends on the maintenance of the osmotic pressure provided by the plasma proteins and it is important that large amounts do not escape into the tissues.

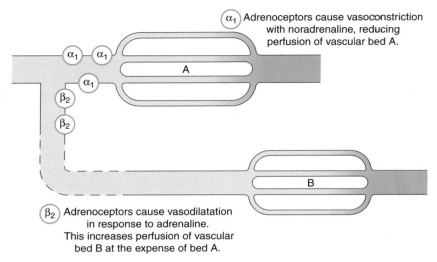

Fig. 8.11   *Redirection of blood flow by the catecholamines.*

Venules

Venules collect up the capillary blood at the end of the capillary beds. Although larger than capillaries and containing some smooth muscle, they are still small, thin-walled vessels. They are fewer in number than the capillaries that drain into them, therefore flow rate increases, but because they are larger, pressure is reduced.

Veins

Veins increase in diameter nearer the heart although the wall thickness remains much less than the arteries. The wall includes smooth muscle so they are capable of constricting and dilating; however, because of the relatively thin wall, they are able to stretch to accommodate extra blood volume (this is *venous compliance*). They are sometimes called 'the capacity vessels' and evidence of this compliance can be seen in the full veins in the legs of anyone standing for long periods.

> The blood circulates, from the ventricles and back to the atria, through the following system of vessels – the arteries, arterioles, capillaries, venules and veins – in that order.

Throughout the vascular system, the relative number of vessels affects both pressure and flow rate. Single arteries lead into a larger number of smaller arteries, which in turn supply many arterioles and even more capillaries. The effect is to progressively step down the pressure and slow the flow rate until the conditions are suitable for exchange at the capillary bed. The capillaries lead in to successively smaller numbers of larger venules and veins until the great veins are reached. Pressure continues to drop with increasing vessel size and distance from the pump, but, as the number of vessels coming after the capillaries decreases, flow rate increases so that the volume of venous return is large and fairly rapid even if the pressure is low.

Blood pressure and vessels

Vessels with smooth muscle can be stimulated to contract – *vasoconstrict*; this has the effect of reducing the capacity and increasing hydrostatic pressure. In smaller vessels particularly, it has the effect of increasing resistance to flow. The opposite effect is *vasodilatation*, brought about by relaxation of the vascular smooth muscle. This will reduce hydrostatic pressure and resistance.

Blood vessels in different circulations have different levels of contraction which would be considered as 'usual' for that site. This 'usual state' is called *basal tone* and it can vary from low tone, i.e. fairly relaxed vessel walls, to high 'basal tone', where vessels are much more contracted. Vessels with a low basal tone can be made to constrict to a much greater extent, but from their basal state they cannot dilate much more. Capacity vessels have a low basal tone compared with resistance vessels.

Regulation of vessel capacity

Vessel size can be altered overall (systemically) or locally and by numerous mechanisms.

The effects of the autonomic nervous system can be found systemically, but only where there are neural pathways going to the vessels or at sites where there are receptor sites for the neurohormones, noradrenaline and adrenaline. These are released into the circulation during sympathetic stimulation of the adrenal medulla.

The effects of the autonomic nervous system can be divided into those that are:

- caused by sympathetic activity arising from the brainstem; this may be reflex – the *vasomotor reflex* – or stimulated by the higher brain
- due to the neurohormones adrenaline/noradrenaline – the *sympathomedullary* response
- parasympathetic and arise from the higher brain but affect only a small number of tissues.

Centrally mediated sympathetic effects

This regulatory mechanism is part of an autonomic reflex called the *vasomotor reflex*. It is similar in function to the heart rate response and again uses baroreceptors. It is in operation continuously and therefore the vessels are in a sustained state of partial contraction or tone. The reflex works by raising and lowering the level of activity in the mechanism rather than switching it on and off and produces what is called a *tonic* state. A rise in blood pressure increases baroreceptor activity, which increases inhibition of the brainstem centre maintaining the level of vasoconstriction. The reduced vasoconstriction that follows reduces pressure, primarily diastolic pressure. The opposite effect happens if the blood pressure falls: baroreceptor activity is reduced, inhibition is reduced and the resulting vasoconstriction raises blood pressure. The sympathetic transmitter is noradrenaline and the receptor sites that bring about constriction are α_1.

This reflex, slightly slower than the heart rate reflex, continually monitors and adjusts blood pressure, and whereas the heart rate mechanism affects pump output and therefore systolic pressure; the vascular reflex directly affects diastolic pressure and systolic rises as a secondary response (see page 168). The effect produced by stimulation of the sympathetic system from the higher brain is not part of the reflex system. The cerebral cortex can directly affect the brainstem so that stimuli such as fear, excitement or embarrassment may affect the blood vessels. People might go red with embarrassment (vasodilatation) or white with fear (vasoconstriction).

Circulating noradrenaline/adrenaline

When the adrenal medulla is stimulated by sympathetic activity, noradrenaline and adrenaline are released into the circulation. Noradrenaline and adrenaline are called by the group name *catecholamines* and the response is the *sympathomedullary effect*. This mechanism, which can maintain blood pressure and at the same time redirect blood flow, depends on the ability of the catecholamines to use more than one type of receptor site. Noradrenaline has effects on blood vessels, acting mainly on α_1 sites and causing constriction. Adrenaline also acts on α_1 sites, causing constriction, but can also affect β_2 sites, which cause dilatation. The combined effects of constriction in some vessels and dilatation in others cause blood to move from the high-pressure, constricted area to the low-pressure, dilated area, i.e. there is redirection of flow (Fig. 8.11).

This effect is very obvious when there is a large drop in blood pressure and the catecholamine response redirects blood from the skin to vital organs. The resulting pale, cold skin is clear evidence that blood has been directed away from the skin by constricting the skin blood vessels almost to the point of closure.

> The diameter of blood vessels is influenced by the autonomic nervous system and by circulating hormones.

Parasympathetic effect on blood vessels

The parasympathetic system supplies only a few vascular sites. The effect is not tonic (i.e. it can be switched on and off), separate sites can be selected and it is controlled from the higher brain. The transmitter is acetylcholine and the receptors are cholinergic (muscarinic).

Examples of sites supplied are the blood vessels in the salivary glands, the tongue and the external sex organs. The effect at all these blood vessels is to cause vasodilatation.

Parasympathetic activity at these sites has little effect on overall blood pressure, but the local effects are important. For example, vasodilatation in the salivary glands provides the extra fluid required for the increased flow of saliva when eating and vasodilatation at the penis and clitoris allow engorgement and erection of the tissue.

The effects of temperature on blood vessels

Temperature affects blood vessels both at the level of central control in the brain and locally on the vessel itself.

The central effect is achieved by altering the sympathetic tone of the vessels. A reduction in blood temperature causes vasoconstriction and, conversely, a rise in blood temperature causes vasodilatation. The skin circulation is particularly affected by changes in body temperature and this is one of the mechanisms by which body temperature is maintained.

The local effect of temperature is also dilatation as the temperature rises and constriction as the temperature falls. The mechanism is not centrally mediated, however; it is a direct effect on vascular smooth muscle.

Substances that directly affect blood vessels

Many of the responses of blood vessels are mediated by substances that have direct effects on blood vessel walls, either on the smooth muscle by making it contract or relax, or on the capillaries by changing the permeability. These mediators may be released in response to neurotransmitters or hormones, or they may be released from cells that have been damaged, for example by injury.

There are many such mediators. One familiar example is histamine, which causes vasodilatation and increased capillary permeability seen as redness and swelling when the skin is injured. Histamine probably acts by releasing other mediators rather than directly. This highlights one of the difficulties of attributing physiological effects. As new information becomes available, there always seems to be another link in the chain.

One substance, for example, was named some time ago as 'endothelium-derived relaxing factor' (EDRF). As that name suggests, the substance is produced by endothelial cells and causes vasodilatation. It has now been found to be nitric oxide and is the mediator by which many vasodilator effects are achieved. Nitric oxide is the subject of much research interest and is now available for some therapeutic uses.

Metabolic regulation of local pressure and perfusion

Blood vessels must be able to respond to local conditions so that changes in demand can be exactly matched by changes in perfusion. Regulation by the metabolites produced by the tissue itself provides a means of doing this. Although all blood vessels respond to local conditions, metabolic regulation is particularly important in some areas: for example, in the coronary circulation that supplies the heart muscle itself. The blood vessels here must be sensitive to even very small changes in local conditions and be able to respond immediately.

When levels of carbon dioxide are elevated (hypercapnia) or when oxygen levels are low (hypoxia), the effect is to cause vessel dilatation. This reduces the pressure locally, and more blood flows in bringing more oxygen and washing out the carbon dioxide. Increasing levels of acid such as lactic acid also cause vasodilatation and, although it would be unusual for this to accumulate in a normal heart muscle, this would happen in skeletal muscle blood vessels.

The local effects of injury on blood vessels – the inflammatory response

The classical description of inflammation as 'hot, red, swollen and painful' indicates that at least some of the effects are on the local blood vessels. The inflammatory response involves vessels, surrounding tissue and cells recruited into the area. The term 'triple response', sometimes used instead, applies more strictly to the blood vessels. The triple response is described as a red line, followed by a spreading flare, then a raised weal.

At the site of a superficial injury, damaged cells release several mediators, which have a variety of effects.

Vasoconstrictors such as serotonin and the vasoconstrictor prostaglandins cause local constriction and the appearance of a white line or area over the site of the injury. Immediately following this, vasodilators such as histamine take effect and the area becomes locally reddened (in the case of a scratch, this would be the red line stage of the triple response). Vasodilator chemicals begin to spread into the surrounding area, the local nerve endings also induce vasodilatation and the redness spreads (the spreading flare). The increased volume of blood at the site causes some swelling and, as the concentration of mediators such as histamine increases, permeability of capillaries increases with the escape of fluid from the blood vessels into the surrounding tissue. This causes more swelling (the raised weal). If permeability is greatly increased, plasma proteins escape into the tissue spaces and fluid follows by osmosis, leading to more severe oedema in the injured area.

The increased perfusion and permeability are important features of the response to injury, because they allow access to the tissue of cells of the immune system and the blood-borne chemical factors involved in the repair of the damaged tissue.

'Special circulations'

Although it may have appeared that blood vessels behave in the same way wherever they are, some circulations have very particular conditions to meet and are adapted accordingly.

The coronary circulation, already mentioned, responds to local blood gases and metabolites in order that it dilates promptly on demand. In addition, the capillaries are very short and so numerous that almost every myocardial cell has its own capillary. Because the heart muscle acts as the driving force for the whole system, it is essential that this muscle, above all, is well supplied and records show that some hearts can stay fit and function well for a hundred years or more.

> The heart receives its own blood supply via the coronary circulation. The coronary arteries fill with blood when the heart is relaxed.

The skin circulation is adapted to allow the skin to act as part of the temperature regulatory system of the body. Its vessels are very sensitive to local changes in temperature and, in constricting and dilating, prevent the effects of changes in ambient temperature penetrating to the core body.

The cerebral blood vessels have a highly engineered 'sprinkler system' type of structure where pressure can be maintained equally around the many units that make up the brain. The carotid arteries have baroreceptors, which monitor the main cerebral supply of blood, but the brain vessels do not respond to the baroreceptor reflex and even when blood pressure is low in the rest of the system, cerebral vessels do not constrict.

The pulmonary vascular system is the most atypical of all the 'special circulations'. It depends on being a low-pressure system so that fluid can be reclaimed efficiently from lung tissue. If the pressure is too high, pulmonary oedema forms and the distance between air in the alveoli and the blood that will carry the gases increases to the point where the diffusion distance is too great and oxygen uptake is jeopardised (carbon dioxide is usually less affected because it is a more soluble gas and is less affected by diffusion distance). Pulmonary vessels also behave quite differently when exposed to hypoxia and hypercapnia. Where other circulations dilate, pulmonary vessels constrict. This is not as contrary as it might seem when the function of the pulmonary circuit is considered. The aim is to take up oxygen and unload carbon dioxide for the benefit of the body as a whole. There is little to be gained from increasing the perfusion in areas of lung that are poorly ventilated and therefore are poor sources of oxygen and already rich in carbon dioxide; it is better to direct the blood to more favourable areas of the lung. The giving of therapeutic oxygen to a hypoxic patient is important to maintain the patient's blood oxygen levels, but it may be even more important to reduce the pulmonary vessel constriction, which would limit the uptake of the oxygen provided.

REGULATION OF BLOOD PRESSURE BY CHANGES IN INTRAVASCULAR VOLUME

Regulation of intravascular volume (blood volume) is an important contributor to the regulation of blood pressure. Changes in volume take longer to achieve in normal circumstances than changes in either heart rate or vessel capacity but this slower rate of change tends to have a stabilising effect.

Hydrostatic pressure is regulated in parallel with osmotic pressure and mechanisms are stimulated not only by changes in blood pressure but some are also affected by changes in body water.

Fluid retention or excretion by the kidney (Ch. 11) is the most controlled process of regulation, although fluid regulation also takes place at the gut and skin. The mechanisms of adjustment use:

- antidiuretic hormone (ADH) (also called vasopressin)
- renin–angiotensin–aldosterone system
- atrial natriuretic peptide (ANP).

Antidiuretic hormone (ADH)

ADH is a hormone, produced in the hypothalamus and released from the posterior pituitary gland, which causes the reabsorption of water at the distal nephron. ADH also has another effect important in the regulation of blood pressure in that, as its alternative name suggests, it is a potent vasoconstrictor.

The release of ADH is stimulated by a drop in blood pressure signalled by baroreceptors located in low-pressure circulations such as the pulmonary circuit. Their activity inhibits the production and release of ADH. When their firing rate is decreased as pressure falls, the inhibitory effect is reduced and ADH is released. The retention of water by ADH plus its vasoconstrictor effect raises pressure, which in turn acts as a negative feedback on the reflex (Ch. 7).

If blood pressure is raised, inhibition of ADH will cause less water to be reabsorbed at the kidney, fluid output is increased and blood pressure reduced.

If pressure is adequate but body fluids are over-concentrated, ADH would again be released. This time the stimulus comes from cells in the hypothalamus sensitive to changes in concentration – osmoreceptors. The retention of water at the kidney by ADH has the effect of diluting body fluids and restoring osmotic pressure to normal. In physiological terms, hydrostatic pressure takes precedence over osmotic pressure, and where blood pressure is severely reduced, water will be reclaimed even if body fluids are already dilute.

Renin, angiotensin, aldosterone mechanism

This system takes longer to adjust the blood pressure than does ADH but it can be maintained over a longer period. It is initiated by a fall in blood pressure at the kidney and the release of the substance renin. This sets in train the series of reactions shown in Figure 8.12, the end result of which is the active reabsorption of sodium ions at the nephron and the passive reabsorption of water with the sodium.

The mechanism has the added advantage that angiotensin II acts as a vasoconstrictor of arteries and arterioles, reducing the overall capacity. It also promotes thirst and the intake of fluid. The whole mechanism, therefore, produces a rise in blood pressure by several regulatory routes.

Several drugs that inhibit the activity of angiotensin-converting enzyme (ACE) have been developed. These are the ACE inhibitors such as captopril and enalopril, which are used as antihypertensive agents.

Atrial natriuretic peptide

ANP is a chemical mediator released by the cells of the atria in response to excess filling of the atria. Its presence would indicate venous return at either high volume or high pressure.

It increases sodium (therefore water) output by the kidney, therefore reducing intravascular volume and systolic pressure. It also causes some vasodilatation, particularly at the arteries, thereby reducing peripheral resistance and diastolic pressure. ANP therefore reduces pressure by more than one regulatory route and reduces both systolic and diastolic pressures.

Fluid recovery from tissue

Tissues contain some fluid surrounding the cells, mainly in the form of a gel. If

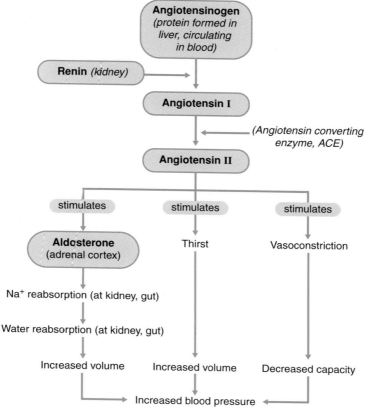

Fig. 8.12   *The renin, angiotensin, aldosterone mechanism.*

blood pressure drops to a value below that in the tissue, fluid will migrate into the vessels in response to the osmotic pressure of the plasma. In extreme hypotension, up to 500 ml can be retrieved in an adult. This is sometimes called internal fluid transfusion and evidence for its effectiveness can be seen in the low haematocrit of patients who have lost a large volume of blood.

PRELOAD AND AFTERLOAD

The heart as a pump obeys the laws of mechanics that apply to all pumps and as understanding of this aspect of heart performance has improved, the understanding and treatment of blood pressure abnormalities have also improved.

The principles of preload and afterload apply to the heart just as much as they would apply to a pump in a water supply, although the cardiovascular system has abilities to adapt to changes in pressure not available to pumps and water pipes. The mechanics can be simplified as follows.

Preload

Imagine the heart as a single chamber (Fig. 8.13). The chamber is filled from

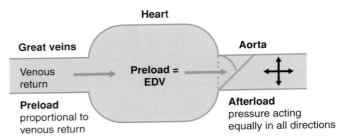

Fig. 8.13   *The principles of cardiac preload and afterload. EDV, end-diastolic volume.*

venous return until full at the end of diastole, i.e. at end-diastolic volume (EDV). EDV is the load that the heart will have to eject and it can be called *pre-load*. Preload = EDV, EDV is proportional to venous return, and therefore preload is proportional to venous return.

Some of the EDV will be ejected as stroke volume and some will remain behind in the ventricle as cardiac reserve. A large preload will normally produce a large stroke volume and cardiac output. A low preload underfills the heart and stroke volume and cardiac output are reduced. Preload is therefore related to systolic pressure.

Afterload

Stroke volume is ejected from the left ventricle into the aorta, where there is already blood at a pressure of perhaps 60–80 mmHg, i.e. diastolic pressure. The pressure generated by the ventricle at systole must be enough to overcome the pressure in the vessel outside so that the semilunar valve can be opened and the stroke volume can be expelled. The higher the pressure outside, the harder the heart must work to open the valve and eject the volume. The pressure outside keeping the valve closed can be called afterload:

1. The higher the diastolic pressure, the greater the afterload.
2. The ventricle must generate about half as much pressure again before afterload can be overcome; therefore, if diastolic pressure is 80 mmHg, systolic pressure must be about 120 mmHg.
3. High diastolic pressure, i.e. high afterload, increases the workload of the heart.

There are two rules:

1. The higher preload is, the greater systolic pressure is likely to be – see Starling's law of the heart.
2. The higher afterload is, the harder the heart must work to achieve ejection; therefore, a rise in diastolic pressure causes a rise in systolic pressure in a healthy heart.

'Preload' is the same as end diastolic volume and 'afterload' is the same as the peripheral resistance to blood flow.

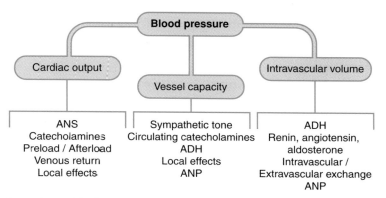

Fig. 8.14 *Mechanisms adjusting blood pressure.*

RESPONSE TO CHANGES IN BLOOD PRESSURE

Integrated response

Blood pressure, although variable, is maintained within a range of 'normal' values. The body has a complex array of mechanisms available to alter all the aspects of blood pressure. For example, systolic pressure and diastolic pressure can be adjusted independently. Blood can be moved from one circulation to another and adjustments can be made over a variety of time scales. Blood pressure must be able to respond to circumstances, to rise in activity and increase the supply to the capillary beds, and conversely to fall when the body is at rest. Figure 8.14 shows a brief outline of the main areas of adjustment.

Evidence of responses to an acute disturbance in blood pressure

The responses to pressure disturbance can most easily be seen when the disturbance is large. Smaller disturbances will be compensated by all the mechanisms above, but the effects may not be visible and may not even be measurable. A large haemorrhage, however, produces such an acute loss in pressure that signs of the compensatory mechanisms in action become obvious.

Table 8.1 lists the symptoms of acute haemorrhage that can be found in many textbooks and will be familiar to many practitioners. The cardiovascular symptoms are shown as either 'effect', i.e. attributed to the low pressure itself, or 'response', where they are due to physiological compensation for the fall in pressure.

SUMMARY

Appropriate blood pressure is central to healthy tissue function which requires efficient exchange of substances used or produced by cells. The complexity of the cardiovascular system arises largely from the continual need to adjust pressure.

TABLE 8.1	Symptoms of Acute Haemorrhage	
	Symptom	Effect or response
	Hypotension	Effect
	Blood pressure values	Low systolic pressure, low-volume venous return, low output – effect
		Elevated diastolic pressure, reflex vasoconstriction – response
		Narrow pulse pressure – result of the above
	Tachycardia	Baroreceptor reflex – response
		Circulating catecholamines – response
	Cold, pale skin	Baroreceptor reflex vasoconstriction – response
		Sympathomedullary response, redirection of flow – response
		Angiotensin II – response
		ADH (vasopressin) – response
	Oliguria	ADH – response
		Renin–angiotensin–aldosterone – response
		Low glomerular filtration rate – effect

The variable rate of exchange which allows tissues to function under different conditions, e.g. at rest and in exercise, is achieved by varying hydrostatic pressure at the capillaries. The many mechanisms which can be used by the body to achieve pressure changes are under the control of the hypothalamus which uses the autonomic and endocrine systems in an integrated and closely monitored association. These reflex adjustments to pressure are made in response to signals from receptors such as baroreceptors.

This chapter has considered the general principles of pressure regulation by changing cardiac output, vascular capacity and intravascular volume, with the changes modified by local chemical or temperature effects. Circulations such as the pulmonary and cerebral circuits show 'special' characteristics which fit them for their particular function.

Some evidence of reflex adjustments can be seen when there are small changes in pressure, for example, the tachycardia due to standing up. Dramatic evidence of acute changes in pressure, such as in haemorrhage, produce the syndrome described as 'shock'.

QUESTIONS

1. Describe the cardiac cycle.
2. What is cardiac output and how does it contribute towards blood pressure?
3. How is blood returned to the heart from the periphery of the body?
4. Describe the mechanisms which respond to a fall in blood pressure.

FURTHER READING

Herbert R, Alison J (1996) Cardiovascular function. In: Hinchliff S, Montague S, Watson R (eds) *Physiology for nursing practice, 2nd edn*. Baillière Tindall, London, pp 374–451

Watson R (1995) *Anatomy and physiology for nurses, 10th edn*. Baillière Tindall, London

9 Blood

Sheenan Kindlen and Jan Gill

After reading this chapter you should be able to:

- describe how blood flows in blood vessels
- list the components of the blood and their functions
- explain how blood is formed
- explain how gases are transported in blood
- understand ABO blood grouping
- describe the body's response to bleeding.

Blood is the transport system that supplies tissues with their requirements, such as water, oxygen and nutrients, and removes waste materials for excretion. Blood carries cell products exported to other tissues, and organs communicate with one another via blood-borne chemical messengers. As well as the transport and communication roles of whole blood, the many components of blood have their own independent roles.

Blood provides a means of achieving regulation of many aspects of the internal environment. The large volume and continual 'stirring' effect of the circulation allows the composition of the fluid bathing the cells to remain relatively constant, but at the same time, because the rate of exchange between blood and tissue fluid can be varied by altering the pressure gradient (Ch. 8), rapid changes can be achieved when required.

Regulation of the internal environment usually requires the cooperation of several body systems (Ch. 7) with circulating blood acting as a linking and interlocking mechanism. The management of body temperature by heat distribution is an example. During exercise, skeletal muscle produces a great deal of heat, which must be lost if the body is not to overheat, and it is transported by blood to the skin where it can be lost to the atmosphere. When the body is at rest, the heat produced by the liver from metabolic processes is transported to tissues that are much cooler, helping to maintain body temperature.

BLOOD FLOW CHARACTERISTICS

Blood must be able to flow along vessels, some of which may be smaller than the diameter of the red blood cell, which makes up the majority of the blood cell population. If the flow is impeded, blood becomes static, the tissue is deprived of oxygen, the metabolites are not removed and the tissue is damaged. If the lack of supply is prolonged, the tissue will die. This is the pattern of events in a 'heart attack', a myocardial infarct, where a piece of heart muscle dies because its blood supply has failed. This is a very dramatic event, but ischaemia (failure

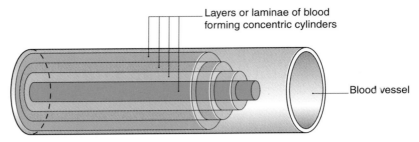

Fig. 9.1 *Laminar flow in large blood vessels.*

of the blood supply) would produce the same effects in any tissue affected in this way.

Blood has special properties that allow it to flow, regardless of the size of vessel, even in those vessels which are, at first sight, too narrow to allow red cells to pass. The physical structure of blood gives it special characteristics. Blood cells, which are suspended in plasma, are not rigid inflexible grains; they act more like microscopic droplets of one fluid suspended in another fluid. This unusual arrangement allows blood flow to adapt to different vessel sizes and remain unimpeded in the very narrow vessels.

Blood flow in larger blood vessels

In larger blood vessels, i.e. those larger than small arterioles, capillaries and small venules, the size of the cells is not a problem and flow is rapid and unhindered. Blood flows along as though it were made up of concentric cylinders (Fig. 9.1); this is called laminar flow or laminar streaming, each cylinder being a layer or 'lamina'. Each cylinder drags on the one next to it and the outer one drags on the vessel wall; the drag of the layers is called 'resistance' and the effect gives rise to the viscosity of blood. In this kind of flow, blood is behaving as a conventional fluid whose viscosity is constant at any one temperature and is not affected by the bore of the tube. This is sometimes called 'Newtonian flow'. The term 'resistance' has clinical significance. A reduction in the bore of the vessel – vasoconstriction – narrows the vessel, increases the drag between the layers and on the wall of the vessel and increases the resistance to blood flow. This is most likely to happen in arterioles (Ch. 8) and would be referred to as an increase in peripheral resistance.

Turbulent flow

If there is an obstruction to flow, an abrupt narrowing of the vessel or a sudden change in the direction of flow, the laminae may break and collide with one another (Fig. 9.2). The result is called turbulent flow.

Blood flow in small blood vessels

In smaller vessels, particularly capillaries, it is essential that blood flow is maintained, because this is the area in which exchange takes place between blood and tissue (Ch. 8). If the flow were to remain laminar in small-diameter vessels, the viscosity would reduce the rate of flow to an unacceptably low figure. The

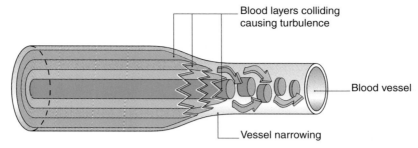

Fig. 9.2   *Turbulent flow in large blood vessels.*

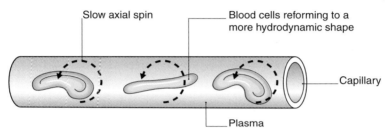

Fig. 9.3   *Axial flow in small blood vessels.*

blood cells, which may be larger than the bore of the vessel, would be at risk of becoming trapped in the vessel, forming an obstruction and causing ischaemia.

> The diameter of a capillary is smaller than the diameter of an erythrocyte, therefore erythrocytes have to be flexible in order to flow along capillaries.

The blood's 'emulsion' characteristic now causes a change in the dynamics. As the shear stress increases (this is the force exerted by one layer on another), the red cells begin to change shape. Their flexible or 'deformable' membrane allows them to elongate and twist and move into the centre of the stream. They also turn gently on their own axes, creating a small centrifugal force which keeps the plasma to the outside of the stream (Fig. 9.3). The wall of the vessel is therefore in contact with the component of blood that has the lowest viscosity (plasma), which reduces the drag and maintains the flow at an adequate rate. This is called axial flow or single line flow. This phenomenon was discovered in the 1930s and it was shown that blood viscosity in a capillary was effectively less than half that in a large arteriole. In a condition where the red cells are unable to change shape, for example in sickle cell anaemia, blood flow slows in these small vessels, tissues are inadequately supplied and one of the effects may be severe muscle pain during activity.

COMPOSITION OF BLOOD

Blood makes up about 7% of body weight in an adult, more in a young baby

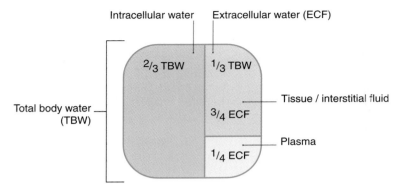

Fig. 9.4 *Body fluid compartments.*

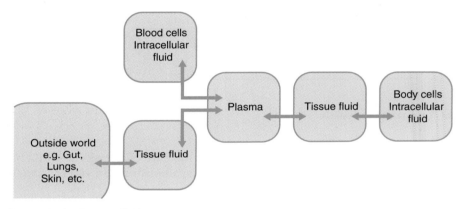

Fig. 9.5 *Communication between fluid compartments.*

and less in an elderly person. It is made up of plasma and cells. The fluid portion of blood is plasma, approximately nine-tenths of which is water. This is the source of the water used to hydrate all tissue cells.

Blood cells are sometimes referred to as 'formed elements', because one type, the platelet, is not a complete cell and lacks many of the typical cell structures. The expression is more often heard in classical physiology than in clinical situations, where 'blood cells' would be perfectly acceptable.

Plasma

Plasma is part of the total body fluid and is an important component in the distribution of water and solutes required by the body cells. The fluid compartments (Fig. 9.4) form a chain of communication between the outside environment and the inside of the cells (Fig. 9.5). The compartments can be described as follows:

1. Intracellular fluid is the fluid within the cell and bounded by the cell membrane.
2. Extracellular fluid is the environment outside the cells and, as such, it must

be carefully controlled to ensure the normal functioning of the cells. Plasma is extracellular fluid within the vascular system; interstitial fluid is extracellular fluid surrounding the tissue cells and outside the vessel walls.

> The fluid in the body can be described as being intracellular (that contained within cells) or extracellular (the plasma and interstitial fluid).

Plasma is a straw-coloured liquid and makes up about 55% of whole blood. It has many important functions:

1. It is able to distribute the heat produced in the body.
2. It acts as a transport system for a wide variety of substances, e.g. nutrients, gases, hormones, electrolytes such as Na^+, Cl^+, K^+, Ca^{2+}, etc. and waste products such as urea and creatinine.
3. It contains the plasma proteins, which constitute about 7% of the plasma weight and have an important role in maintaining the osmotic pressure of the blood (Ch. 1). Without the osmotic effect of plasma proteins it would be impossible to maintain blood volume inside the vascular system (Ch. 8). Plasma proteins also act as chemical buffers and help to regulate the acid/base balance (Ch. 1). The different plasma proteins have particular roles. Albumin, for example, because of its high concentration and small molecular size, makes a major contribution to plasma osmotic pressure, but also acts as a carrier for substances such as fatty acids and certain drugs. Plasma contains proteins required for the formation and later breakdown of blood clots, as described later in this chapter. Plasma also contains several classes of globulin proteins, e.g. the gamma globulins, which are immunoglobulins and essential to the body's defense mechanism (Ch. 14).

Blood cells

Bone marrow stem cells and haemopoiesis

Blood cells are formed, by the process of haemopoiesis, from the bone marrow stem cell or haemocytoblast, which is the common precursor cell for all blood cell lines (i.e. it is 'pluripotent').

> All the blood cells are formed in the bone marrow and are derived from a single type of pluripotent stem cell.

Only about one cell in a thousand in bone marrow is a stem cell and of those, at any one time, only 10% are active; the majority are 'resting' but capable of recruitment if required. The stem cells can self-replicate, each division increasing the number by a factor of 2, but the total number is regulated by a complex system of stimulatory and inhibitory factors. The huge resting reserve and the capacity for self-replication give an indication of the enormous potential capacity for haemopoiesis. In normal health, about 20 millilitres (ml) of red cells is produced every day, a growth rate matched only by skin epithelium and the gut mucosa. Production can be increased two to three times if blood is lost, and in extreme circumstances (provided iron and other nutrients are available) production can be increased six to eight times, amounting to perhaps 150 ml of red cells per day.

The uncommitted stem cell, because it is capable of giving rise to any one of a number of blood cell types, must be able to respond to signals that will decide its future development, i.e. its commitment, differentiation and maturation. The most primitive stem cells are most likely to self-replicate and, as they mature, they become increasingly sensitive to factors that will cause commitment. These factors are sometimes given the group name 'colony-stimulating factors', the most widely known of which is renal erythropoietin, which stimulates red cell production. Where bone marrow is to be damaged, e.g. by irradiation, stem cells can be harvested before treatment and allowed to multiply. After treatment, the stem cells are returned to the circulation and find their way back to their bone marrow 'niches' where they relocate using a mechanism rather like that at a receptor site (Ch. 5).

Following commitment and early differentiation, the cell begins the process of maturation towards the mature cell, which may be stored in bone marrow or released into the circulation. The cells of one type, at various stages, make up a cell line. The stages of haemopoieis in the cell lines are shown in Figure 9.6.

Packed cell volume or haematocrit

The volume occupied by the cells relative to plasma (expressed as a decimal fraction) is given by the 'packed cell volume' (PCV) or haematocrit (Hct) (Fig. 9.7). It is calculated by centrifuging a sample of peripheral venous blood in a calibrated tube, in which the blood separates into a layer of cells below the plasma. The red cells make up almost all the cell volume and the white blood cells and platelets form a small layer or 'buffy coat' on top of the red cells.

A normal range for males is approximately 0.4–0.54, and for females it is 0.37–0.47. The greater the value of the haematocrit, the greater the percentage of cells and the higher the viscosity of the blood. A greater pressure is required to force the blood through the capillaries as the viscosity rises.

Polycythaemia (excess red blood cells) and an elevated PCV is sometimes seen in dehydration caused, for example, by excessive sweating or where fluid has been lost as a result of diarrhoea. In this case, the total number of cells has not changed but the amount of plasma has been reduced. In cases of polycythaemia where there is excess production of red cells, the haematocrit may rise to 0.6 or 0.7; viscosity is greatly increased with the risk that blood flow, particularly axial flow, will cease and the deprived tissue will die.

A low PCV value would be indicative of overhydration, where the plasma volume had increased, or anaemia, where the red cell number was reduced.

After haemorrhage, there are characteristic changes in the PCV. Immediately after blood loss, the PCV remains normal, then falls as the lost plasma is replaced over 1–3 days; it then rises back to normal over 2–4 weeks as the red cells are replaced.

ERYTHROCYTES OR RED BLOOD CELLS

All body tissues need a constant supply of oxygen (O_2); however, not enough

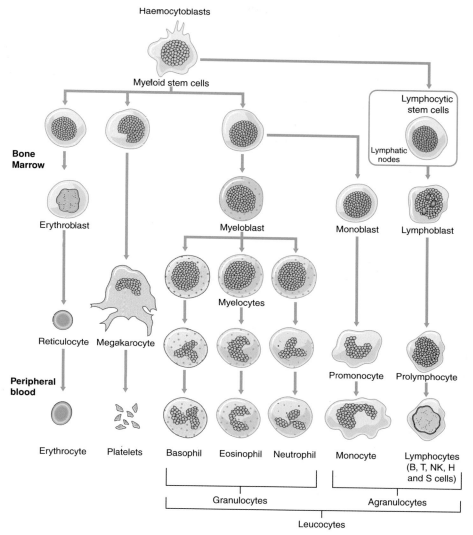

Fig. 9.6 *Haemopoiesis.*

oxygen can simply dissolve in the blood and most is transported bound to the carrier protein haemoglobin. This increases the oxygen-carrying capacity by about 70 times. Red cells have an equally important role in the carriage of carbon dioxide (CO_2), dissolved in the cytoplasm and attached to haemoglobin; the increased capacity here is about 17 times. Haemoglobin occupies about one-third of the volume of the red cell and gives it its characteristic colour.

The red cell shape and the characteristics of its membrane make it ideally suited to its role as a gas transporter. The familiar doughnut shape, a biconcave disc, increases the cell surface area allowing greater diffusion of gases across the cell membrane. The diameter of a red cell is approximately 7 micrometres (μm) while that of a capillary, where gas exchange actually takes place, may be as low as 3 μm; however, the flexible membrane of the red cell allows it to change shape and travel through the narrow capillaries by axial flow.

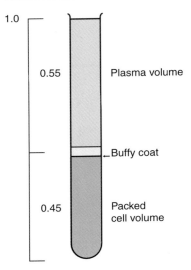

1.0

0.55   Plasma volume

Buffy coat

0.45   Packed
cell volume

Fig. 9.7   *Packed cell volume or haematocrit.*

The lifespan of a red blood cell is about 120 days. The components of old and damaged red blood cells are broken down and recycled by macrophage cells of the liver, spleen and lymphatic tissue. Very little is lost, and only the fragments of haem after the iron has been removed are excreted as bile pigments.

The red cell number is controlled by balancing loss against replacement. As red cells are destroyed, the oxygen-carrying capacity is reduced, the reduced oxygen level in blood stimulates production of the hormone erythropoietin by the kidney, and this in turn stimulates the production of red cells.

Functions of red blood cells

- Transport of oxygen
- Transport of carbon dioxide
- Haemoglobin and bicarbonate buffering of H^+.

General points about transport and exchange of gases

1. Gases such as oxygen and carbon dioxide must be in solution before they can be transported, exchanged or used by tissues.
2. Each gas is transported in several forms, each form in equilibrium with the others. If the amount of one form changes, this will have the effect of changing the others.
3. A gas will move from an area of higher concentration to an area where there is a lower concentration. An example of this is the carriage of oxygen, which is transported attached to haemoglobin in the red cell and in solution in red cells, plasma and tissue fluid. As the tissue cells use the oxygen and deplete their intracellular store, oxygen moves in from the tissue fluid along the concentration gradient. This reduces the oxygen level in the tissue fluid and oxygen moves into the tissue fluid from the plasma; the now lower level in plasma prompts the movement of dissolved oxygen from the cytoplasm of

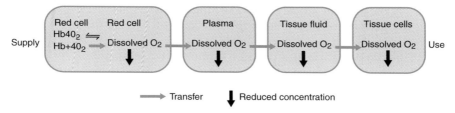

Fig. 9.8 *Disturbance of equilibrium and transfer of gas in solution.*

the red cell, where the lower level of dissolved oxygen in the cytoplasm causes dissociation of oxygen from haemoglobin (Fig. 9.8).

Transfer of carbon dioxide is the same in principle; however, the forms of carriage are more numerous (see under carbon dioxide). The direction of movement is opposite, with oxygen moving from lungs to tissue and carbon dioxide from tissue to lungs.

Haemoglobin

Some oxygen is transported in solution, but a much larger amount is carried combined with haemoglobin. Haemoglobin is a large protein molecule, consisting of four globin protein chains, each chain containing the chemical group haem, which has one bound atom of iron. It is this complex that gives haemoglobin its characteristic red colour. There are differences in the structures of the globin chains, which are named alpha, beta, gamma and delta. In adults, the most common form of haemoglobin (haemoglobin A), contains two alpha chains and two beta chains.

Fetal haemoglobin or haemoglobin F is the major form in the blood of the fetus and newborn and is made up of two alpha chains and two gamma chains. This form of haemoglobin has properties that allow it to compete successfully with the haemoglobin A of the maternal blood for available oxygen and to take up oxygen where the concentration is low. Oxygen is more tightly bound to haemoglobin F then to haemoglobin A, therefore it can carry as much as 20–30% more oxygen than can maternal haemoglobin.

Transport of oxygen

Each molecule of haemoglobin can bind four molecules of oxygen, one at each haem group, and in this form, haemoglobin is referred to as oxyhaemoglobin. Haemoglobin that contains no bound oxygen is called deoxyhaemoglobin or reduced haemoglobin, which is a much darker colour of red than oxyhaemoglobin. Venous blood, which has a lower level of oxygen, has a higher concentration of deoxyhaemoglobin and shows this darkening of colour. One important characteristic of the process of binding oxygen to haemoglobin is that it is reversible. In the lungs, where the amount of oxygen is high, oxygen binds to haemoglobin, but in the tissues, where the level of oxygen is low, oxygen is released by haemoglobin and diffuses to the cells.

The amount of oxygen taken up by haemoglobin is determined mainly by how much free oxygen is available and, similarly, the oxygen released is affected by the amount already free. The 'amount' of available oxygen can be related to its partial pressure. The partial pressure of a gas is the share of total pressure exerted by that gas when it is part of a mixture of gases. As sea level, in standard conditions, air is at a pressure (atmospheric pressure) of 760 mmHg and contains about 21% oxygen. In the mixture of gases that make up air, 21% of the pressure is exerted by oxygen, the partial pressure of oxygen in the air at sea level, or PO_2 = 21% of 760 mmHg = 160 mmHg.

When a gas is dissolved in liquid, e.g. in plasma water, the expression 'gas tension' is sometimes used, rather than 'partial pressure', which more correctly applies to gases in 'gas' form. The gas tension of oxygen would be shown as tO_2. Some clinical texts use the more correct expression of gas tension for blood gases, but it is still common to find 'P' and 'partial pressure' referring to a dissolved gas. Arterial blood has a PO_2 or tO_2 of about 95 mmHg, venous blood about 40 mmHg.

As the PO_2 of blood increases, it might be assumed that the amount of oxygen attached to haemoglobin would increase. This is only partly true: there is an increase but not a proportional increase; the expression used is that the increase is not linear. Instead, if a graph is constructed, the pattern would be a sigmoid or 'S'-shaped curve (Fig. 9.9). The amount of oxygen being carried by haemoglobin is expressed as 'the degree of saturation' of the haemoglobin molecules, e.g. if all the binding sites contained oxygen, haemoglobin would be 100% saturated. At lung level, haemoglobin is about 98% saturated and at venous level, where much of the oxygen has been given up to the tissues, the degree of saturation might be 70–75%.

The shape of the curve is important; if it were a straight line, life would not be possible. The most significant areas are the upper flat or plateau region and the middle region, which is very steep.

The plateau part of the curve relates to haemoglobin in blood which is nearest the air oxygen, i.e. in the lung capillaries. In these conditions, the haemoglobin molecule is almost fully saturated (about 98%) with bound oxygen. The flat section shows that, when haemoglobin is already saturated, an increase in PO_2

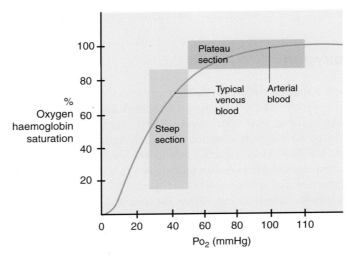

Fig. 9.9 *Oxygen/haemoglobin dissociation curve.*

cannot increase the saturation level any further. Breathing air at a lower P_{O_2} makes only a small decrease in the level of saturation, therefore a relatively wide variation in the lung P_{O_2} causes only a small change in the extent of the haemoglobin saturation and the oxygen uptake by blood.

The steep middle portion of the curve is important at tissue level. The structure of the haemoglobin molecule, with different globin chains enclosing the haem, allows it to respond differently to changes in oxygen levels in this section of the curve, and the difference is of great physiological and clinical significance. The blood that has arrived at the tissues from the lungs is around 98% saturated with oxygen with a P_{O_2} of about 95 mmHg. At the tissues, however, the P_{O_2} will be around 40 mmHg. The difference in P_{O_2} favours the movement of dissolved oxygen from plasma to tissue fluid and the release of oxygen from haemoglobin, which can then diffuse into the plasma (and from there into the tissue fluid).

> Oxygen is transported in erythrocytes by binding to haemoglobin. Conditions in which the body is physiologically stressed, such as exercise, decrease the affinity of haemoglobin for oxygen meaning that the oxygen is more readily given up to tissues that require it for greater metabolic activity.

The slope of the curve here is steep, small changes in P_{O_2} resulting in the unloading of large amounts of oxygen from the haemoglobin. Any change in tissue P_{O_2} as a result of extra tissue metabolic activity will be met by a rapid and large release of additional oxygen from the blood supply, automatically matched to demand. The evidence for unloading is the change in saturation from 98% at the lungs to about 70% in venous blood leaving the tissues.

In summary, at the plateau section, where oxygen is abundant, the P_{O_2} is high and the percentage saturation is high; large changes in P_{O_2} can take place with little effect on percentage saturation. At the steep slope, at tissue level, a small reduction in P_{O_2}, indicating tissue demand, results in the unloading of large amounts of oxygen from haemoglobin to meet the demand.

Factors that alter haemoglobin–oxygen dissociation

Several factors are able to vary the amount of oxygen released from haemoglobin. This is sometimes referred to as 'shifting the position of the curve to the right or left' (Fig. 9.10).

For example, in the case of a shift of the curve to the right, for a given blood P_{O_2}, the affinity of haemoglobin for oxygen is reduced and, at the steep slope, more oxygen can be unloaded.

Agents that cause a right shift in the position of the curve are increased concentrations of CO_2, acidity and a rise in temperature. Each of these factors might be associated with exercise; the effect of moving the curve would be an increase in the amount of oxygen available to the tissues and supply would be matched to demand. The compound 2,3-diphosphoglycerate (DPG) also moves the curve to the right. 2,3-DPG is found in red cells and its concentration is increased by several factors such as exercise and by hormones such as the thyroid hormones (Ch. 6). It is also increased where there is likely to be hypoxia, for example in people living at high altitude, or in people with anaemia or

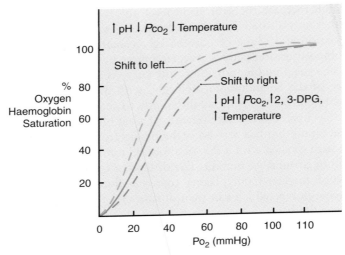

Fig. 9.10   *Shifting of the curve. 2, 3-DPG; 2,3-diphosphoglycerate.*

respiratory disease. The effect of increasing 2,3-DPG (and shifting the curve to the right) is to make more oxygen available to the tissue by unloading more from haemoglobin, again matching supply to demand.

A shift of the curve to the left is caused by a rise in pH, a fall in P_{CO_2} and a fall in temperature. The left shift causes less oxygen to be unloaded from haemoglobin, but, more importantly, another effect is to reduce the uptake of H^+ by haemoglobin, which helps to correct the pH.

Carbon monoxide (CO) also causes a shift of the curve to the left. Carbon monoxide is an extremely toxic substance found in cigarette smoke, car exhaust fumes and the fumes produced when household fuel is used incorrectly. It combines with haemoglobin at the same site on the molecule as oxygen, to form carboxyhaemoglobin (HbCO), which seriously affects the ability of the blood to transport oxygen. The affinity of haemoglobin for carbon monoxide is about 250 times its affinity for oxygen and many potential oxygen-carrying sites on haemoglobin become blocked by a compound that is very difficult to displace. In addition, because of the shift of the curve, any oxygen which is there becomes less available.

Transport of carbon dioxide

CO_2 is carried in several forms, in equilibrium and related to one another:

> Carbon dioxide is transported in erythrocytes mainly as bicarbonate ion.

1. It is transported to the lungs in three forms: about 90% as HCO_3^-, about 5% bound to haemoglobin as carbaminohaemoglobin, and about 5% in solution. The percentages differ in arterial and venous blood.
2. Haemoglobin transports CO_2 from the tissues to the lungs. CO_2 binds to the globin part of the haemoglobin molecule (unlike oxygen, which binds to the

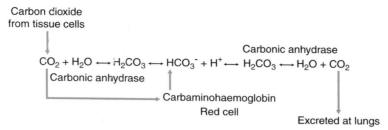

Carbon dioxide from tissue cells

Carbonic anhydrase

$$CO_2 + H_2O \longleftrightarrow H_2CO_3 \longleftrightarrow HCO_3^- + H^+ \longleftrightarrow H_2CO_3 \longleftrightarrow H_2O + CO_2$$

Carbonic anhydrase

Carbaminohaemoglobin

Red cell

Excreted at lungs

Fig. 9.11   *Carbonic anhydrase and the transfer of carbon dioxide.*

haem group) forming the complex carbaminohaemoglobin. CO_2 binds more easily to haemoglobin with less bound oxygen, therefore uptake of CO_2 at the tissues is encouraged by the offloading of oxygen from the haemoglobin molecule.

3. It is excreted at the lungs as CO_2. All the forms of transport are in equilibrium with one another (Ch. 1) and as loss of CO_2 from lungs reduces the concentration in plasma, bicarbonate dissociates to make up the concentration of dissolved CO_2 (Fig. 9.11). In turn, bicarbonate moves out of the red cell, encouraging the unloading of CO_2 from haemoglobin. (A bonus from this action is that haemoglobin is now in a state that makes it more likely to take up oxygen.) The deficit in CO_2 is made up by uptake of more at the tissues (Fig. 9.11).

4. The reversible reaction that combines CO_2 with water is too slow for biological purposes and one of the red cell enzymes, carbonic anhydrase, plays a vital role by speeding up the reaction. Because the reaction is reversible, the enzyme is important in the uptake of CO_2 from tissue cells and its eventual release at the lungs (Fig. 9.11).

The hydrogen ion, produced during the course of these reactions, is taken up by the bicarbonate buffer system, and by haemoglobin acting as a buffer inside the red cell, so that it does not significantly affect the acid/base balance (Ch. 1), although there is a small difference in pH between venous blood coming from the tissues and arterial blood which has recently passed through the lungs.

In summary, oxygen and carbon dioxide are carried in blood as shown in Table 9.1.

TABLE 9.1	*Transport of Oxygen and Carbon Dioxide in the Blood*	
Transport of O_2		*Transport of CO_2*
• From lungs to tissue		• From tissues to lungs
• Transported bound to haemoglobin		• ~5% is transported dissolved in blood
• The binding is loose and reversible: where the O_2 levels are high in the lungs, O_2 binds to haemoglobin, but where the O_2 level is low, as in the tissues, O_2 is released		• ~90% is transported as HCO_3^- ion
		• ~5% is transported bound to haemoglobin as carbaminohaemoglobin

Haemoglobin and bicarbonate buffering of H⁺

Haemoglobin is not only an important buffer in its own right, taking up and releasing H⁺ within the red cell, but is closely associated with the bicarbonate buffer, which acts both inside and outside the cell. The association of the two buffer systems allows the acid/base balance to be directly linked with respiration. The catalytic action of carbonic anhydrase rapidly converts CO_2 and water, yielding bicarbonate and H^+, bicarbonate moves out of the red cell into plasma and H^+ is taken up by haemoglobin. It is the continual removal of the products of the reaction that allows the continued uptake of CO_2 from the tissues. At the lungs, if CO_2 is to be continuously excreted, H^+ must be released from haemoglobin to combine with bicarbonate, eventually giving CO_2 and water (Fig. 9.11). Because CO_2 is always available from tissue cells, the bicarbonate buffer is rapidly renewable, and it is possible to control the pH of plasma by regulating the rate and depth of breathing (Ch. 10).

Red cells and blood groups

The red blood cell membrane contains many complex groups, 'inherited' antigens or agglutinogens, which have the ability to cause the production of antibodies. Antibodies are immunoglobulins produced by activated B lymphocyte cells (Ch. 14). The antibody combines with the antigen and promotes reactions which ensure that the antigen and the object carrying it (in this case, the red cell) are destroyed.

More than 30 blood groups have been identified, based on the various antigens found on the red blood cell membrane. Of these, those of the ABO system and the Rhesus (Rh) system are the most important.

When blood is to be transfused into a patient, it is vital that the donated blood and the patient's blood are compatible. If an individual receives blood of an incompatible type, antibodies against the 'foreign' antigens will be produced and the donated red cells attacked, causing agglutination (clumping of the cells) and haemolysis (rupture of the cells). Fatal transfusion reactions are possible, with death resulting from released haemoglobin damaging the kidney, agglutinated cells blocking small blood vessels and the systemic effects of a large inflammatory reaction (Ch. 14). The blood groups of both donor and recipient must therefore be carefully checked.

ABO system

Two antigens, A and B, occur on the surface of the red blood cell. A person may have:

- neither antigen – blood group O
- both antigens – blood group AB
- only A – blood group A
- only B – blood group B.

Very early in infancy, antibodies (or agglutinins) are formed to red cell antigens other than the individual's own and, thereafter, these are found in plasma:

In the ABO blood grouping, individuals with blood type A carry antibodies to blood type B and vice versa. Individuals with blood type O carry neither antibody.

- the plasma of group O contains antibodies to A and to B
- the plasma of group A contains antibodies to B
- the plasma of group B contains antibodies to A
- the plasma of group AB contains no antibodies to either A or B.

Within the UK population, approximately 46% of people are group O, 42% are group A, 9% are group B and 3% are group AB. Blood typing is done by adding sera containing either anti-A antibodies or anti-B antibodies to a sample of red cells and examining the cells for signs of agglutination. This is a rapid reaction and, for example, type A red cells put in anti-A serum will clump together and begin to haemolyse. Type B cells put in anti-A serum remain separate, freely moving and undamaged.

Normally the donation of whole blood with the same blood group type should be possible: for example, type A blood can be given to group A recipients; however, if blood of type B was given to group A, the recipient's plasma antibodies would react with the B antigens on the donor red cells and a transfusion reaction would occur. Type O whole blood may be given, in limited quantities, to either group A or group B recipients, because type O blood has neither antigen and would not be attacked by the recipient's plasma antibodies. The quantity is important, however, because the plasma of the O group donor will contain antibodies to both A and B cells and will cause a reaction with the recipient's red cells. Because the amount of antibody in the donated plasma will be relatively small and very much diluted by the recipient's plasma, the level of reaction, while not desirable, may be acceptable. The cardinal rule in blood transfusion is that 'the donor red cells must not antagonise the recipient's plasma antibodies', although the much increased use of blood products, where whole blood is separated into many different fractions, has resulted in whole blood being used less often.

Rhesus (Rh) blood group

The Rh antigen is also found on the surface of the red blood cell. People either have the antigen (Rh positive) or do not (Rh negative). About 85% of the UK population is Rh positive and 15% are Rh negative.

There is one important difference between this blood group system and the ABO system. Unlike the ABO system where the plasma antibodies develop spontaneously, the antibodies of the Rh system develop only after the person has been exposed to the Rh antigen. This exposure may be due to a blood transfusion with Rh-positive blood or may happen when a pregnant mother, who is Rh negative, has received some blood from her Rh-positive child either across the placenta or at its birth.

The reaction to the first exposure is short-lived and likely to pass without notice. The immune system, however, has been alerted to the Rh antigen and has formed the initial antibodies to it. A second exposure to the antigen will result in a rapid and large-scale 'memory response' in the immune system (Ch. 14). In the case of the Rh-negative woman now pregnant with a second Rh-positive baby, maternal antibodies are produced against the baby's blood. These can cross the placenta, damaging the fetal red cells and producing products likely to cause neural damage in the fetus. Identification of Rh-negative women and their subsequent treatment during and after delivery, by temporarily suppressing the immune response to the Rh antigen, has been so successful that few babies are now affected by haemolytic disease of the newborn.

LEUCOCYTES – WHITE BLOOD CELLS

Production of white cells (leucopoiesis) begins with commitment of the stem cells in the bone marrow. Lymphoid tissue is also important to the production of one type of white cell – the lymphocyte.

All of the white blood cells are involved in some way in protection of the body.

The roles of the leucocytes are to resist invasion by foreign material such as bacteria or viruses, to enclose and destroy cell debris and foreign material and to target and destroy cancer cells that can arise within the body.

The diagram of the haematocrit (Fig. 9.7) shows that white blood cells (WBCs), along with platelets, form the thin 'buffy coat' which lies above the main body of red blood cells, which outnumber the WBC by about 700 to 1. Although there are many fewer white cells in total (about $4–11 \times 10^9$/L), the number of each of the different types of white cells can be selectively increased in response to a specific threat. The substances that stimulate the manufacture of WBCs can be produced from tissue which has been attacked or produced by activated WBCs themselves.

There are five types of leucocyte. The classification is made on the basis of how they appear when stained and viewed with the microscope:

- neutrophils
- eosinophils
- basophils
- monocytes
- lymphocytes.

Neutrophils, eosinophils and basophils are classed as polymorphonuclear granulocytes, i.e. 'many-shaped nucleus, granule-containing cells'. Monocytes and lymphocytes are known as mononuclear agranulocytes, i.e. cells with a single nucleus and no granules in the cytoplasm.

Neutrophils

Neutrophils are the most common type of WBC, making up approximately 60% of the total white cell count. They form part of the first line of defence against invasion and have several important weapons in their 'armoury':

1. They can leave the bloodstream and enter tissue spaces by a process known as diapedesis, literally 'putting a foot through'. They have a rapid amoeboid movement and can travel several times their own cell length every minute.
2. They exhibit chemotaxis, i.e. they are attracted to 'signal' substances produced by damaged and inflamed tissues and move to the site of the signal.
3. They are very active and non-specific phagocytes and any particle of a

suitable size that is not living host material, i.e. cell debris, particulate material, bacteria, etc., is engulfed and destroyed.

The number of neutrophils increases in response to acute bacterial infections. Some young neutrophils are released from a 'holding pool' in the bone marrow and at the same time the bone marrow is stimulated to produce more of this cell line. The age of the neutrophil can be judged by the greater number of lobes on the nucleus as the cell ages and when shown on a chart, neutrophils are conventionally shown with the youngest cells on the left of the picture. A shift in distribution, i.e. a higher proportion of younger cells, and therefore a response to infection, would be referred to as 'a (neutrophilic) shift to the left'.

Eosinophils

Eosinophils make up about 2% of all WBCs. They have a specialist role in attacking parasites too large for phagocytosis and are also involved in allergic responses. They are found in increased numbers in people who are sensitive to allergens such as pollen, resulting in hay fever. Eosinophilia (an increased number of eosinophils) is also found in the blood and lung tissue of people who suffer from asthma.

Basophils

Basophils are the least numerous type of WBC, making up about 0.5% of the total WBC population. Their function is still not totally understood. They are able to store several chemicals, of which two are histamine and heparin. Histamine is a vasodilator and heparin is an anticoagulant. It is unlikely that the heparin acts as large-scale anticoagulant, but the combined effect of histamine and heparin may be important in keeping microcirculations open (Ch. 8) in the early stages of tissue damage. The histamine produced may also act as a chemotaxic signal to lymphocytes in some types of hypersensitivity reaction.

Monocytes

Monocytes are the largest WBC but make up only about 4% of the total number. They circulate in the blood for about 70 h, then migrate into tissue. There they mature and enlarge to form tissue macrophages (Ch. 14), which have an important phagocytic function and are essential to several stages in the wound healing process. They contain several chemicals that are important parts of the defence system, e.g. components of the complement system by which dead or infective material is disposed of. The pus sometimes evident at the sight of tissue damage is composed of dead tissue, neutrophils and both monocytes and tissue macrophages. Chronic infection is characterised by an increase in the number of circulating monocytes.

Lymphocytes

Lymphocytes vary in size from similar to red cells to two or three times larger. They account for about one-quarter to one-third of all WBCs. Although they, like all other blood cells, originate form the bone marrow stem cell, their development is dependent on the activity of lymphoid tissue (Ch. 14). Lymphocytes are found in many tissues other than blood, the majority in the lymphatic tissues. There are two major types, B and T lymphocytes, and a third, less numerous type, the non-B, non-T lymphocyte or natural killer (NK) cells.

B lymphocytes are concerned with the production of antibodies, which are 'tailor-made' to destroy foreign material. The chemical make-up of the invader is recognised by the cells as 'foreign' and this stimulates the production of antibody. The particular chemical group of the invader that invokes this response is the antigen.

T lymphocytes do not produce antibodies. Instead they directly destroy organised cellular tissue such as a graft, i.e. among other functions, they produce the 'host versus graft' response.

Non-B, non-T lymphocytes or NK cells make up about 15% of the lymphocyte population and differ from other lymphocytes in that they do not require to be sensitised to foreign cells. They form an important early line of defence, particularly against viruses, which they attack before the more specific B cell population is activated. They also attack cells that are becoming malignant and are therefore important in preventing these cells becoming established.

Abnormalties in white cell numbers

Leucopenia

This is a lower than normal WBC count. It is seen in cases of chronic stress and severe infections and also as a consequence of significant bone marrow disturbances due, for example, to exposure to radiation. The individual with leucopenia has reduced resistance to infections.

Leucocytosis

Leucocytosis is the term used to describe an abnormally high WBC count. It is usually due to an increase in the number of neutrophils and would be observed in many infectious diseases, where it is evidence of a response to an infective agent. Leucocytosis is a general term and gives no indication whether all types or only one type of white cell is affected; use of a term such as 'neutrophilic leucocytosis' would indicate which cell line was the main contributor to the increased number.

Two laboratory tests that give information on both leucopenia and leucocytosis are the total white cell count and the differential white cell count. The total white cell count estimates the total number of WBCs in the blood. Typical normal results would be 4000 to 11 000/mm^3 of blood. A result of 4000/mm^3 of blood may also be expressed as 4×10^6/ml or 4×10^9/L. A differential white count determines the percentage of each of the five types of WBC.

PLATELETS

Platelets are small cell fragments formed in the bone marrow from larger cells called megakaryocytes. The concentration of platelets in the blood is around

150 000 to 300 000 per mm^3 or 150–300 $\times$ 10^9/L. They survive in the circulation for about 15 days and are then removed by macrophage cells mainly in the spleen. Platelets have several properties of fundamental importance to the process of haemostasis and the prevention of blood loss:

1. On the outer surface of platelets is a glycoprotein that prevents platelets sticking to the walls of the blood vessel under normal conditions, so preventing inappropriate clotting. If the walls of vessels are ruptured or injured, however, platelets will stick to these sites and to each other, beginning the processes that will prevent further blood loss.
2. Platelets can contract and have cytoplasmic proteins that are very similar to those found in muscle. The contraction draws together the damaged edges of the vessel wall and shrinks the clot, once formed, making it structurally stronger.
3. Platelets also help to stabilise the blood clot itself by producing a compound, fibrin-stabilising factor, which acts to make cross-links between the long protein strands of the fibrin in the blood clot, making the long threads into a much stronger mesh structure.
4. Platelets can stimulate growth in other cells and therefore the healing process itself. Platelet-derived growth factors act on blood vessel cells to encourage multiplication and growth to repair damaged tissue.
5. Platelets manufacture several other important chemicals, e.g. adenosine diphosphate (ADP), prostaglandins and thromboxane A$_2$ (TXA$_2$), which control blood vessel diameter and affect platelet adhesion and chemical coagulation.

HAEMOSTASIS

Haemostasis is a complex process involving the vessel wall, platelets and chemical factors, some of which are in the blood itself. The response to damage to a blood vessel can be considered in three stages:

1. immediate response of the vessel
2. the formation of the platelet plug
3. the formation of a blood clot (coagulation).

Vessel response

The first response to damage, e.g. a cut, occurs within the blood vessel wall. The wall contracts as a result of neural reflexes around the cut, stemming the flow of blood. The amount of contraction that occurs increases with the amount of damage to the vessel wall. Where the blood vessel has been severed by a sharp cut, i.e. damage over a small area, more blood loss would be anticipated than from vessel wall damaged by crushing where the area of damage is much greater. The initial constriction is followed by dilatation due to histamine and other inflammatory agents released from the damaged cells. This also reduces blood loss, this time by reducing pressure (Ch. 8); in addition, the increased capillary permeability produced by the inflammatory agents allows white cell access to the surrounding damaged tissue.

The platelet plug

Contact of platelets with the damaged vessel walls causes several important changes. First, the platelets swell and become sticky so that they stick to the vessel wall and to each other. Chemicals, such as TXA_2 and ADP, are produced that act on other platelets causing these too to become sticky and attach to the platelets clumped together. The end product is a platelet plug, which, in cases of damage to very small-diameter blood vessels, may be enough to stem the flow of blood. Small vessels are constantly being damaged in the normal process of living and this method of preventing blood loss from small blood vessels is always at work. It is only where the number of platelets is low (thrombocytopenia), and bruising begins to appear, that small-scale blood loss becomes evident.

The formation of a blood clot – coagulation

If the platelet plug fails to stem the flow of blood, a blood clot will be necessary. A blood clot is composed of a network structure of the protein fibrin, enclosing 'trapped' platelets, blood cells and plasma.

Its formation requires a series of steps, one leading to the next in a cascade of reactions (Fig. 9.12). The principle in the clotting cascade is that each reaction produces a product, which in turn activates the next step; failure at any step of the process will stop the process. Cascade systems are common in biology and have useful features. Each step can bring about amplification of the previous one, giving a larger amount of product; a series of reactions, each with a smaller

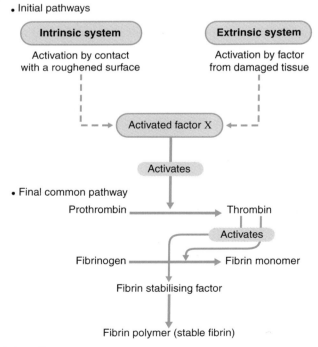

Fig. 9.12   *Clotting cascade in outline.*

energy requirement, is also more achievable than a single, huge reaction. Perhaps just as important, a series of steps is a safer strategy than a single reaction, which might go wrong; clotting is, after all, a potentially dangerous process.

Entry into the cascade

The cascade can be started when blood components come into contact with a roughened surface, such as a damaged blood vessel. No factor needs to be added from outside the blood, therefore this is the 'intrinsic pathway'. It is this pathway which is at work when blood is left in a container, e.g. a glass jar, and clotting is initiated by contact with the container's surface.

The other route into the cascade is via a factor added from damaged tissue; this is the 'extrinsic pathway'. The two pathways are usually active at the same time when there has been an injury.

The final common pathway

The two initial pathways come together in a final common pathway, with the activation of prothrombin and its conversion to thrombin. Prothrombin, like many of the clotting factors, is formed in the liver and circulates as a plasma protein. The conversion of prothrombin to thrombin is achieved by the action of prothrombin activator, produced as a result of completion of either the intrinsic or extrinsic pathways.

The next step is to use thrombin to activate fibrinogen. Fibrinogen is a plasma protein produced by the liver, the 'ogen' ending indicating that it is an inactive precursor. When fibrinogen is acted on by thrombin, it is converted to a long thread-like molecule, fibrin. At this stage, fibrin is a single unit, a monomer, but it rapidly joins with other fibrin molecules to form a polymer. The fibrin threads are only weakly held together, but fibrin-stabilising factor or factor XIII, present in plasma and platelets and trapped in the fibrin mesh, causes the formation of strong cross-links between the fibrin strands and also makes the fibrin stick to the vessel walls. Coagulation is now complete, the clot formed and the damage halted, if not yet permanently sealed.

Activation of the extrinsic pathway will cause blood clotting in as little as 15 s. The intrinsic pathway is generally slower (1–6 min). In practice, however, injury would normally result in the activation of both the intrinsic and extrinsic pathways because both tissue damage and blood trauma would occur simultaneously.

> Blood clotting takes place via two pathways. The extrinsic pathway works very rapidly to produce fibrin whereas the intrinsic pathway works more slowly. However, the intrinsic pathway produces greater amounts of fibrin than the extrinsic pathway.

Clot retraction

A few minutes after the clot is formed, clot retraction begins; the clot contracts and pushes out trapped fluid, which is serum (i.e. plasma without the clotting factors). Platelets have yet another important role to play in this process. They bind across different fibrin threads and, using their muscle-like proteins, are able to contract and pull the fibrin threads together. They also aid the clot retraction process by continuing to release the fibrin cross-linking agent factor XIII. The result is to thicken and strengthen the clot and to pull together the broken surfaces of the blood vessel encouraging vessel repair.

The importance of the platelet at this stage is seen clinically when a low circulating level of platelets is revealed by a failure of the clot retraction process and the continued presence of a soft spongy clot.

Physiological prevention of inappropriate clotting

Successful prevention of blood loss is an important factor in survival, but the formation of unwanted clots may be just as risky. The following are examples of some of the physiological mechanisms that help to avoid this:

1. The smooth surface of undamaged blood vessels prevents the binding of platelets and activation of clotting factors.
2. A protein within the blood capillary wall is able to bind any thrombin that has been activated and halt the coagulation process.
3. Within blood itself, antithrombin III binds thrombin and effectively inactivates it.
4. The fibrin threads of the clot itself also bind thrombin and so prevent its spread to other regions of the blood vessels.

Fibrinolysis

Once the vessel and surrounding tissue has been repaired, the clot has ceased to be of any use; in fact, it may become a hazard if allowed to remain in the vessel. It may impede flow in the vessel, causing ischaemia (Ch. 8) or attract platelets and become a focus for further clot formation, i.e. causing thrombosis. A clot may be detached from the site of its formation by the flow of blood and these clots, moving with the blood flow, are called emboli. If they are deposited in small vessels this can have serious consequences, e.g. blockage of brain blood vessels might result in a stroke.

The clot must be removed when it is no longer useful. It is broken down by the enzyme plasmin, normally present in plasma in the inactive plasminogen form. When it is trapped along with blood cells and plasma within the blood clot, it becomes activated (usually 1–2 days later) by several factors, including tissue plasminogen activator (TPA) released by the injured tissue (Fig. 9.13). TPA is now produced commercially and is used to break down clots formed, for example, in the coronary vessels at a myocardial infarct (Ch. 8). The process of fibrinolysis yields fibrin/fibrinogen degradation products (FDP), which can be measured to estimate the extent of fibrinolytic activity, particularly in immobile patients where the risks of thrombosis and embolism are increased. (Anticoagulant treatment may be given to minimise the risk of embolism formation, e.g. during and after an operation and in cases where the subject has been immobile for some time.)

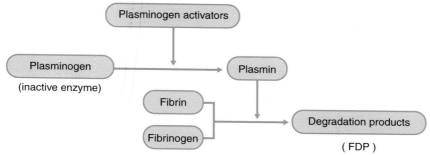

Fig. 9.13 *Fibrinolysis.*

Pharmacology

Therapeutic anticoagulants

Several drugs can be administered to reduce the extent of blood coagulation, one of which is heparin. This compound is found within the body and on its own it has very little anticoagulant action; however, its combination with antithrombin III greatly increases its effectiveness. Because heparin interferes with chemical reactions, its effect is immediate; it then decreases over a period of about 6 h and the dose is usually repeated every 4 h. Heparin is widely used clinically, but it cannot be used orally because it would be destroyed in the gut.

Another class of drug used as anticoagulants are the coumarins, of which warfarin is an example. Warfarin acts at the liver, at the site of formation of many of the blood coagulation factors. By competing directly with vitamin K, an important factor in the manufacturing process, warfarin is able to bring about decreased production of several important blood coagulation factors. This action of warfarin in preventing coagulation will not be immediately effective, because it takes time for the level of existing factors to be reduced and many hours may elapse before the coagulation process is sufficiently depressed. In practice, the two anticoagulants may be used together: heparin to produce an immediate effect and cover the time during which warfarin is taking effect. A coumarin-type drug, on its own, can then provide longer-term oral therapy.

Non-therapeutic anticoagulants

Other anticoagulants can be used to prevent the clotting of blood in a transfusion bag or in blood that has been removed to a test tube for subsequent analysis. Examples are citrate (non-toxic and can be used in a bag), oxalate and EDTA (toxic and used for sample analysis), all of which have the ability to chelate or bind Ca^{2+}, which is required at several stages in the clotting cascade.

Fibrinolytic drugs

Some drugs are used, not to prevent clotting, but to break down the clot once it has been formed. These are the fibrinolytic drugs (see fibrinolysis) such as streptokinase, urokinase and TPA, which all activate plasminogen. They promote the process of fibrinolysis, speed up the dissolving of the clot and limit the damage done by restoring the circulation and reducing the chances of forming other clots at the site of the first.

FAILURE OF BLOOD CLOTTING

Thrombocytopenia

This condition is characterised by low levels of circulating platelets. Failure to form the platelet plug results in excessive bruising even in very minor injuries. The clotting process itself is affected by low levels of platelet factors and even clot retraction is less efficient. Treatment is usually by transfusion of platelets.

Haemophilia is a group of conditions due to deficiency (usually inherited) of clotting factors and characterised by uncontrolled bleeding. The most common is due to a deficiency of factor VIII and occurs almost exclusively in males; other rarer forms of haemophilia are due to deficiency of other factors, e.g. Christmas disease. Treatment requires the replacement of the deficient factor.

Secondary clotting disorders

Any condition that affects adversely the functioning of the liver (where most of the blood clotting factors are formed) or the absorption or utilisation of vitamin K will have a detrimental effect on the process of blood coagulation. The synthesis of at least six of the factors requires vitamin K and a deficiency resulting in the lowering of their levels will slow the process of coagulation.

SUMMARY

Blood is a liquid tissue with numerous functions, some characteristic of blood itself, many attributable to its components. Its flow properties allow it to act as a carrier reaching the smallest vessels and its large volume and continuous stirring action allow rapid changes in composition to be moderated.

The plasma fraction, in addition to containing the proteins which provide the osmotic pressure which keeps the fluid within the vessels, also carries water, oxygen, substrates and regulatory factors required by tissue cells. Waste materials are removed for excretion.

The cell populations have functions which include non-specific to highly specific defence (white cells), gas carriage, acid/base regulation and blood type identification (red cells), and prevention of blood loss (platelets). The cells have a common precursor, the stem cell, which can be committed to any or all of the cell types. There is an extensive capacity for regeneration, giving blood the capability of huge replacement if required.

QUESTIONS

1. What is a pluripotent stem cell and what does it give rise to in the bone marrow?

2. Describe the features of the red blood cell which enable it to transport oxygen.

3. List which antibodies and antigens are present in the plasma and on the surface of the red blood cells in the ABO blood groups.

FURTHER READING

Montague S (1996) Blood. In: Hinchliff S, Montague S, Watson R (eds) *Physiology for nursing practice, 2nd edn.* Baillière Tindall, London, pp 323–373

Watson R (1995) *Anatomy and physiology for nurses, 10th edn.* Baillière Tindall, London

10 Respiration

Roger Watson

After reading this chapter you should be able to:
- list the components of the respiratory system
- describe the process of external respiration
- understand the lung volumes
- explain gas exchange in the lungs.

INTRODUCTION

Respiration is the process whereby oxygen in the atmosphere is exchanged for carbon dioxide in the tissues of the body and it takes place externally at the lungs and internally at individual cells that require oxygen in order to carry out their metabolic functions. This chapter is concerned with external respiration, which is necessary if internal respiration, and thereby the function of cells, is to continue. The material will be divided up into the mechanics of respiration whereby air is drawn into and expelled from the lungs, also known as breathing, and the process whereby oxygen and carbon dioxide are exchanged in the lungs. Before that, the structure of the lungs will be described.

THE LUNGS

The lungs lie in a pair on either side of the heart, as shown in Figure 10.1. The lungs are connected to the outside of the body through a system of tubes that starts at the mouth and nose and subdivides and extends down to the functional units of the lungs, which are called alveoli. If the structure of this tubular system is followed from the mouth to the alveoli, the first structure that is encountered is the pharynx. The pharynx is an area of soft tissue and is divided into three areas: the nasal pharynx, the oral pharynx and the laryngopharynx. These areas refer to the structures that lie in front of the pharynx, nose, mouth and larynx, respectively (Fig. 10.1).

The larynx is the 'voice box', which enables speech and contains the vocal cords, and at this point there is a division in the cavity into the oesophagus and trachea. The oesophagus, as discussed in Chapter 12, is the muscular tubular structure that delivers food from the mouth to the stomach. The trachea is the structure whereby air is delivered to the lungs and it is protected during swallowing by a flap of cartilage called the epiglottis, which covers it to prevent food from entering the lungs as it is swallowed. The larynx can be seen, especially in

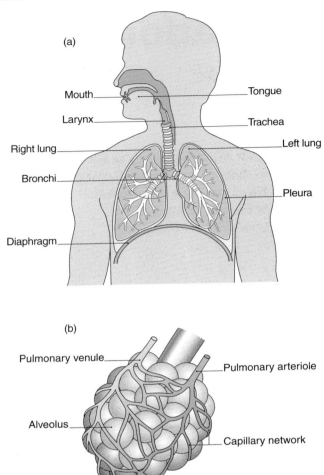

Fig. 10.1   *The respiratory tract. (a) Gross anatomy showing the main features. (b) Alveoli surrounded by the capillary network.*

males, in the front of the throat and is also known as the 'Adam's apple'; it is raised during swallowing and this can be observed or felt during swallowing.

The trachea and bronchi

From the larynx to the bronchi, the trachea – also known as the windpipe – is the route whereby air is drawn into the lungs during inspiration and passed out during expiration and, because of the pressure changes that take place here and to prevent it collapsing, it is lined with semicircles of cartilage, which can also be felt if the throat is rubbed below the Adam's apple. The trachea is lined with cilia, which are hair-like projections from single cells on the epithelium of the trachea. The epithelium of the trachea also secretes mucus and the purpose of this is to trap dust particles, which are then moved up and out of the trachea by the cilia, which move with a concerted wave-like motion.

At the base of the trachea the windpipe divides into the bronchi, which conduct air to either lung. Thereafter, the bronchi subdivide into primary bronchi (also lined with semicircles of cartilage), which successively subdivide into smaller tubular structures, the secondary and tertiary bronchi, leading to the bronchioles, which eventually supply individual alveoli. There are millions of alveoli, and therefore millions of bronchioles, in the lungs and the structure is also known as the respiratory tree (Fig. 10.1), which is an apt description if the whole structure is imagined upside down.

Air is transported to the lungs by a system of vessels that progressively decrease in size known as the respiratory tree.

The bronchioles

The bronchioles convey air from the trachea and bronchi to the alveoli and these exist as either respiratory bronchioles, conveying air to areas of the lung, or terminal bronchioles, which convey air to groups of alveoli. The structure of the alveoli differs from the trachea and the bronchi in that they are lined with circular smooth muscle, which enables them to change in diameter according to different conditions. Under conditions where more air is required, as in exercise, the smooth muscle relaxes, leading to bronchodilatation. In some pathological conditions such as asthma, the smooth muscle constricts abnormally leading to bronchoconstriction, which makes the inspiration, and particularly the expiration, of air from the lungs harder than normal.

The alveoli

The functional units of the lung are the alveoli and this is where the exchange of oxygen and carbon dioxide between the air in the lung and the bloodstream takes place. Essentially, the alveoli are small sacs and they are kept open by the presence of a detergent substance (Ch. 2) called surfactant, which reduces the forces in the alveoli that would tend to collapse them. The total area for gas exchange provided by the alveoli is estimated at being about the size of two tennis courts, one from each lung. There is a vast excess of alveoli and we do not normally use them all except in extreme exercise.

In order for oxygen and carbon dioxide to be exchanged freely between the air in the alveoli and the blood, the walls of the alveoli are very thin. This allows for diffusion, the movement of a substance from a region of high to a region of lower concentration, to take place easily and the distance is only one cell thick (Fig. 10.1). The alveoli are surrounded by networks of the smallest vessels in the cardiovascular system, the capillaries, and the combined structure of the alveoli and the capillaries (Fig. 10.1) can be imagined to be like a net bag full of oranges with the capillaries representing the net bag and the alveoli, which exist in clusters, as the oranges.

Clusters of alveoli are supplied with blood through capillaries from arterioles, which are branches of the pulmonary artery, and the blood is collected into venules, which return it to the pulmonary vein. Blood arriving at the alveoli is rich in carbon dioxide and depleted of oxygen and the blood leaving the alveoli is rich in oxygen and depleted of carbon dioxide. It should be noted, however, that the lung tissue does not receive its blood supply from the pulmonary circulation. Blood is supplied to the lung tissue via the bronchial artery, a branch of the aorta, and this allows it to carry out its normal metabolic functions.

EXTERNAL RESPIRATION

External respiration, commonly referred to as breathing, is the process whereby air is drawn into the lungs (inspiration) and forced out of the lungs (expiration). In order for this to take place, the volume of the lungs changes and this is directly in response to changes in the volume of the thorax, which are accomplished through the concerted action of the ribs, diaphragm and pleura. Each of these will be described below.

> External respiration refers to the exchange of oxygen and carbon dioxide between the blood and the atmosphere whereas internal respiration refers to the exchange of oxygen and carbon dioxide between the blood and the tissues. External respiration results from the action of the lungs and internal respiration results from metabolism.

The ribs

The ribs form part of the axial skeleton and are projections of the thoracic vertebrae of the spine. There are 12 pairs of ribs and 10 of these are connected via cartilage (costal cartilage) to the sternum or breast bone (Fig. 10.2) Collectively, this structure, formed between the ribs and the sternum, is called the rib cage and its primary function is respiratory. Between the ribs lie two layers of skeletal muscle, the internal and external intercostal muscles, respectively.

Contraction of the external intercostal muscles raises the ribs upwards and outwards and this increases the volume of the thorax. The movement of the ribs can be likened to the movement of a bucket handle when it is raised and the movement of the sternum can be likened to that of a pump handle. The internal intercostal muscles may be used to forcibly lower the rib cage.

The diaphragm

Lying below the lungs and separating the thorax from the abdomen is the diaphragm. The diaphragm is composed of skeletal muscle (Ch. 12) and, while it is possible to exert some control over its contraction and relaxation, it is mainly under involuntary control by a pacemaker region in the respiratory centre of the medulla at the base of the brain. However, this involuntary control cannot be completely overridden voluntarily, as can be demonstrated by attempting to hold your breath indefinitely.

Contraction of the diaphragm shortens it and, because of its upward convex structure when relaxed, this pulls it downwards and increases the volume of the thorax (Fig. 10.2). This takes places concomitantly with the contraction of the external intercostal muscles.

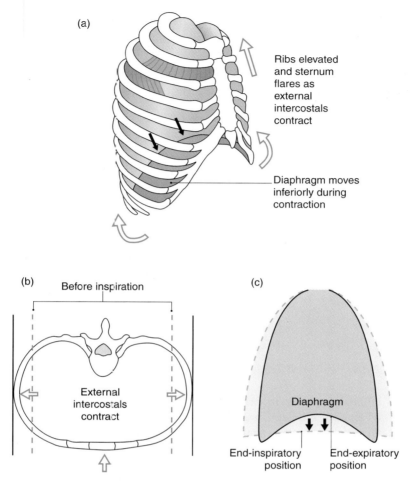

Fig. 10.2 *Changes in the thoracic volume upon inspiration. (a) Antero-posterior (pump handle); (b) lateral (bucket handle); (c) supero-inferior.*

The pleura

The lungs are surrounded by a double layer of tissue known as the pleura. The inner layer is the visceral pleura and the outer layer is the parietal pleura (Fig. 10.3). Between the pleura is a region, described as a potential space, known as the intrapleural space. There is actually no space. Instead, the two pleura lie in close proximity with a fluid, known as pleural fluid, lying between them. The pressure in the intrapleural space is negative relative to air pressure and this force holds the pleura together. The effect of this force can be visualised if you collapse an inflated balloon, knot the opening and then try to pull the surfaces of the balloon apart, which is very difficult.

The negative pressure in the intrapleural space is vital to the function of the lungs because there is no direct physical connection between the lung tissue and the diaphragm and rib cage. Instead, the 'connection' is made by the negative intrapleural pressure, which keeps the lungs inflated, even when the ribs are lowered and the diaphragm is relaxed. It is essential that the lungs are kept

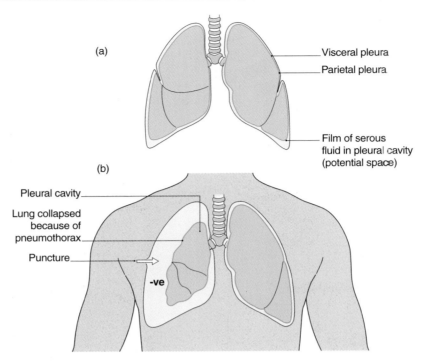

(a)

Visceral pleura

Parietal pleura

Film of serous
fluid in pleural cavity
(potential space)

(b)

Pleural cavity

Lung collapsed
because of
pneumothorax

Puncture

-ve

Fig. 10.3   *Expansion of the lungs. (a) Diagram of the pleura; (b) pneumothorax.*

inflated in order to prevent collapse of the alveoli, which can only function when they are kept open. Another consequence of the negative pressure in the intrapleural space is that changes in volume of the thorax, which take place during breathing, are followed by changes in the volume of the lungs and this effects respiration.

> The lungs are kept open and expanded by the negative pressure in the intrapleural space.

THE MECHANICS OF EXTERNAL RESPIRATION (BREATHING)

Breathing normally takes place involuntarily and is initiated by the respiratory centres of the medulla, which is situated in the brainstem. The involvement of the respiratory centres in the control of breathing will be considered below and this section is concerned with the events that follow the initiation of breathing.

Stimulation of the diaphragm and the external intercostal muscles leads to their contraction, which lowers the diaphragm and raises the rib cage upward and outward as described above. The consequence of these movements leads to an increase in the volume of the thorax by relatively small movements in three directions: from front to back (anteroposterior), from top to bottom (superoinferior) and from side to side (lateral) of the thorax (Fig. 10.2). The net effect of these movements, however, is large and the volume of the thorax increases by about 500 ml in normal breathing. The pressure within the thorax decreases and, due to the negative pressure in the intrapleural space, the volume of the lungs also increases and air is moved in from the atmosphere, through the respiratory tree, to the alveoli. This is the process known as inspiration.

Once inspiration is complete, the stimulus to breathe in stops and the lungs recoil, rather like a spring that is stretched. This is due to inherent elastic forces in the tissues of the thorax and the lungs, and air is forced out. This is the process of expiration.

The function of the intrapleural space in the process of inspiration can be demonstrated by the condition known as pneumothorax. A pneumothorax occurs when air is permitted to enter the intrapleural space and this may occur when either the visceral or the parietal pleura are punctured. The example of a puncture to the parietal pleura by a wound is shown in Figure 10.3. The consequence of a pneumothorax is that the affected lung collapses and no longer expands when the pressure in the thorax is decreased by the normal inspiratory movements of the diaphragm and rib cage. It is relevant to note that an understanding of the mechanics of respiration underlies the standard treatment of pneumothorax using sealed underwater chest drainage. In this procedure a drain is introduced into the enlarged intrapleural space through the wall of the thorax and the end of the drain is kept below the level of the lung and under water. With each inspiratory movement of the thorax the affected lung inflates slightly and air is forced out of the drain. Subsequent collapse of the lung is prevented by water which is drawn up the drainage tube and the process continues until the lung is fully inflated and water is no longer drawn up the tube. At this point it may be possible to remove the drain, ensuring that air does not enter the thorax again, and normal function of the affected lung resumes.

LUNG VOLUMES

In order to understand the functioning of the lungs as air is inspired and expired it is helpful, briefly, to consider the lung volumes, which demonstrate the extent to which the lungs are capable of filling with air under normal breathing and under physical stress such as exercise. Lung volumes are used in the diagnosis of disorders of the lungs and can be easily measured by asking a person to breathe into and out of an apparatus called a spirometer (Fig. 10.4); these measurements are known as lung function tests.

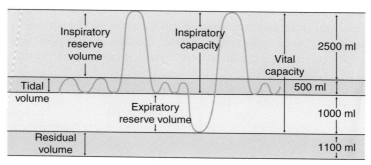

Fig. 10.4   *Lung volumes and capacities.*

The amount of air that is inspired and expired under normal breathing is called the tidal volume (Fig. 10.4) and is normally about 500 ml. Not all of the air that is inspired reaches the alveoli and is, thereby, available for gas exchange; this is due to a volume called the dead space. The dead space is a result of the tubular structures of the respiratory tree (the trachea, bronchi and bronchioles) as these are merely there to transfer air from the atmosphere to the alveoli. The volume of the dead space is about 150 ml, meaning that 350 ml (500 ml minus 150 ml) reaches the alveoli; this volume is known as the alveolar air.

> The volume of air in the lungs that is not available for gas exchange is known as the dead space.

Forced inspiration fills the lungs to their maximum capacity (about $5\frac{1}{2}$ L) and the volume of inspired air (about $2\frac{1}{2}$ L) is known as the inspiratory reserve volume. Conversely, forced expiration can expel about 1 L from the lungs and this is known as the expiratory reserve volume. The sum of the expiratory and inspiratory reserves and tidal volume (5 L) is known as the vital capacity and this can be achieved by forced expiration followed by forced inspiration. It should be noted that the lungs cannot be emptied completely; a residual volume of about 1 L always remains and this is due to the negative pressure in the intrapleural space, which prevents the lungs from collapsing completely.

An additional measure of lung function is the forced expiratory rate, which may be measured by forced expiration into a peak flow meter after normal inspiration. This test, which assesses the patency (openness) of the bronchioles, is used to diagnose asthma and to gauge the effectiveness of treatment.

OXYGEN AND CARBON DIOXIDE EXCHANGE

The exchange of oxygen and carbon dioxide in the lungs can be demonstrated by comparing inspired atmospheric air with expired air. The major component of atmospheric air is nitrogen (80%). In addition, atmospheric air contains 20% oxygen and a negligible amount of carbon dioxide. By contrast, expired air contains 16% oxygen and 4% carbon dioxide. The percentage of nitrogen remains unchanged because nitrogen is an inert gas; it does not react easily with other chemicals and is not taken up into the blood. These values are shown in Table 10.1. The observation is that the amount of oxygen in the expired air is lower than in the inspired air and the conclusion is that oxygen has been removed from the atmospheric air. Conversely, the amount of carbon dioxide increases, suggesting that carbon dioxide is released into the lungs. The exchange of oxygen and carbon dioxide is taking place at the alveoli.

TABLE 10.1	Composition of Inspired, Expired and Alveolar Air (%)		
	Oxygen	Carbon dioxide	Nitrogen
Inspired	20	<1	80
Expired	16	<4	80
Alveolar	14	<6	80

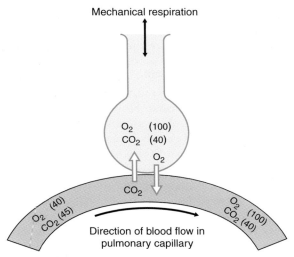

Fig. 10.5 *Gas exchange in the lungs. (All values in parentheses are in units of mmHg.)*

Gas exchange in the alveoli

The principle that governs gas exchange in the alveoli is diffusion, whereby the gases that are exchanged, oxygen and carbon dioxide, move from a region of high concentration to a region of low concentration. In the alveoli, oxygen moves from the lumen of the alveoli into the blood and carbon dioxide moves from the blood into the lumen of the alveoli.

In order to examine the exchange of gases in the alveoli it is convenient to consider the levels of oxygen and carbon dioxide in terms of their partial pressures. The partial pressure of a gas is the contribution that it makes to the overall pressure of gases in a fluid (a gas or a liquid) and it may be expressed in millimetres of mercury (mmHg). The partial pressure of oxygen in the inspired air is 100 mmHg. Alveolar air contains a higher partial pressure of oxygen than the blood entering the capillaries that surround the alveoli (Fig. 10.5). Because there is only a very thin physical barrier between the alveolar air and the pulmonary capillary blood, the oxygen diffuses into the pulmonary blood and raises the partial pressure of oxygen in the blood to 100 mmHg.

> The exchange of gases between the blood and the alveoli takes place by diffusion and is driven by the relative partial pressures of oxygen and carbon dioxide in each.

The converse situation takes place with respect to carbon dioxide, which has a partial pressure of 46 mmHg in the pulmonary blood approaching the alveoli. The partial pressure of carbon dioxide in the alveoli is 40 mmHg and carbon dioxide diffuses into the alveoli thereby lowering the partial pressure of carbon dioxide in the pulmonary blood leaving the alveoli.

The transport of oxygen and carbon dioxide by the blood

Oxygen is delivered from the alveoli to the blood and carbon dioxide is delivered to the alveoli by the blood. However, these gases are not simply dissolved in the blood; they are transported by the erythrocytes and it is the transport of these gases from the alveoli to the peripheral tissues, in the case of oxygen, and vice versa in the case of carbon dioxide, which is the link between external and internal respiration.

Oxygen is sparingly soluble in water and, indeed, a very small amount of oxygen is dissolved in the plasma. However, the amount of oxygen transported in the blood is far in excess of the amount that could be dissolved and this is due to the unique properties of the erythrocyte. The erythrocyte is a highly specialised cell in the sense that it has dispensed with many of the functions of other body cells in order to fulfil its function of oxygen transport. It does not reproduce and only breaks down glucose by glycolysis, and towards these ends it has no nucleus and no mitochondria. It also has a unique biconcave shape and its diameter is almost exactly the diameter of the smallest capillaries where stacks of erythrocytes pass through, thereby maximising the number in a capillary at any one time. The shape of the erythrocyte produces a minimal distance for the diffusion of oxygen and carbon dioxide into and out of the cell.

The principal feature of the erythrocyte is that it is packed full of haemoglobin in structures called cristae. Haemoglobin is a protein with a quaternary structure (Ch. 2): it has four similar subunits of globin protein and each subunit contains a haem group with iron attached. The iron in the haem group is capable of changing valency and can bind and release oxygen. Each haem group can bind one molecule of oxygen; therefore, each haemoglobin molecule can bind four molecules of oxygen in a reversible reaction. Haemoglobin in solution rapidly and strongly binds oxygen and the binding of oxygen as its partial pressure is increased is represented graphically by a hyperbolic curve, as shown in Figure 10.6. This should be contrasted with the binding of oxygen to haemoglobin under physiological conditions, when the haemoglobin is contained in erythrocytes, where the binding of oxygen to haemoglobin is represented by a sigmoidal curve (Fig. 10.6) (see also Ch. 9).

The sigmoidal curve is physiologically advantageous because it permits the

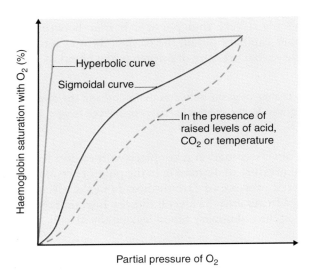

Fig. 10.6   *Oxygen/haemoglobin dissociation curve.*

binding of oxygen to haemoglobin at high partial pressures of oxygen, which occur in the lungs, and also the release of oxygen at low partial pressures, as occur in the peripheral tissues. If the binding of oxygen to haemoglobin under physiological conditions was represented by a hyperbolic curve then the partial pressure of oxygen in the peripheral tissues would have to be extremely low before oxygen was released and this would not allow cells to function. Clearly, the sigmoidal binding of oxygen to haemoglobin is more responsive to changing partial pressures of oxygen throughout the body. Furthermore, the sigmoidal binding of oxygen to haemoglobin is also physiologically beneficial in that the curve is also sensitive to other factors such as increasing levels of carbon dioxide, increasing temperature and lowered pH, all of which indicate that more oxygen is required. The response of the sigmoidal curve to these changes is to move to the right, as shown in Figure 10.6, and this means that oxygen is more readily released by the haemoglobin.

Carbon dioxide

Some carbon dioxide is dissolved in blood and some attaches to haemoglobin in the erythrocyte. However, the vast majority (approximately 90%) is transported in the erythrocyte as bicarbonate ions (Ch. 9). Carbon dioxide enters the erythrocytes and a reaction catalysed by the enzyme carbonic anhydrase ($CO_2+H_2O \rightarrow H_2CO_3$) results in the formation of carbonic acid. Carbonic acid, which is a weak acid, further dissociates into bicarbonate ions and hydrogen ions ($H_2CO_3 \rightarrow HCO_3^-+H^+$). All of these reactions are reversible and under conditions where carbon dioxide is being produced, such as in the peripheral tissues (e.g. muscle), there will be a tendency for the reactions to move in the direction of carbonic acid production. Conversely, in conditions where carbon dioxide levels are low, such as in the lung, the reactions will move in the direction of carbon dioxide production and the carbon dioxide will be blown off as a gas during expiration. As described below, this system is sensitive to changes in levels of carbon dioxide in the body.

> The exchange of carbon dioxide between the atmosphere and the blood and between the blood and the peripheral tissues is made possible by the reversible reaction catalysed by carbonic anhydrase.

NORMAL RESPIRATION

Respiration is controlled by the respiratory centres in the medulla oblongata of which there are two: an inspiratory centre and an expiratory centre. Signals are sent from the inspiratory centre via the nervous system (the phrenic and intercostal nerves) to the respiratory muscles in the diaphragm and external intercostal muscles, respectively, to stimulate inspiration: the rib cage is raised and the diaphragm flattens. Inspiration lasts for about 2 s, after which time the expansion of the lungs is sensed by stretch receptors, which send inhibitory signals to the inspiratory centre thereby causing it to stop sending signals to the respiratory muscles. Owing to the elastic forces in the thorax, it automatically recoils and expiration, which lasts for about 3 s, takes place.

During normal expiration the expiratory centre in the medulla oblongata does not send any signals to the respiratory muscles. However, in exercise or in certain lung diseases where forced expiration is necessary, the expiratory centre does play a role. Examples of such lung diseases are emphysema, where the elasticity of the lungs is decreased, and asthma, where there is difficulty in expiring due to constriction of the bronchioles.

Control of respiration

Respiration is a dynamic process in that it changes in response to changing bodily conditions. For example, we are familiar with what happens to our breathing when we take exercise: it increases in depth and, to some extent, in rate. The reason for this change in respiration during exercise is to increase the delivery of oxygen to the blood, and to the skeletal muscles, and to increase the removal of carbon dioxide from the blood. Without this responsiveness of respiration our skeletal muscles would become deprived of oxygen and carbon dioxide would increase in the blood thereby increasing the hydrogen ion concentration and making the blood more acidic. The cells of the body cannot function outside of a narrow range of pH and this would be detrimental. Respiration, therefore, serves a homeostatic function (Ch. 7) in maintaining a constant internal environment with respect to oxygen delivery to peripheral tissues and the pH of the blood.

As control of respiration is a homeostatic process it is possible to identify the three key elements of a homeostatic mechanism – a sensor, a control centre and effector – and these are, respectively, the chemoreceptors, the respiratory centres of the medulla oblongata and the respiratory muscles.

The chemoreceptors are located in the aortic arch and in the carotid sinus (co-located with the baroreceptors which respond to changes in blood pressure). The medulla also acts as an indirect sensor for control of respiration. The chemoreceptors are responsive to increases in carbon dioxide in the blood by sensing the decrease in pH that results from the carbonic anhydrase catalysed reaction, referred to previously in this chapter. Carbon dioxide and water react to produce carbonic acid, which dissociates to produce bicarbonate ion and hydrogen ions. The higher the carbon dioxide levels in the blood, the more the equilibrium of these reactions is pushed towards the production of hydrogen ion, thereby lowering the pH, and vice versa.

When the chemoreceptors sense a drop in pH they send signals to the medulla whereby the rate and depth (mainly the latter) of respiration are increased. Increasing the rate and depth of respiration allows more oxygen to diffuse into the blood from the alveoli and excess carbon dioxide to diffuse into the alveoli from the blood. As a result of this process, carbon dioxide is literally 'blown off' at the lungs and the lowered levels in the blood lead to an increase in pH, which prevents signals being sent from the chemoreceptors, thereby turning off their stimulation of the medullary inspiratory centre. This is a classic negative feedback loop, which restores respiratory rate and depth to normal. It should be noted that control of respiration does not primarily respond to changes in the level of oxygen in the blood, except when this level is extremely low.

SUMMARY

The function of the lungs, in terms of the mechanics of breathing and exchange of gases which are collectively called external respiration, have been considered in this chapter. Ventilation of the lungs is achieved by the coordinated action of the diaphragm and the intercostal muscles and air is drawn into the lungs via a system of tubular structures that ultimately supply individual functional units of the lungs, called alveoli. Exchange of oxygen and carbon dioxide is facilitated at the alveoli by virtue of the fact that they present a very small distance for the diffusion of these two gases. The erythrocytes are responsible for the transport of both oxygen and carbon dioxide in the lungs. External respiration is a homeostatic mechanism, which responds primarily to changes in the level of carbon dioxide in the blood ensuring an adequate supply of oxygen to peripheral tissues and removal of carbon dioxide from the peripheral tissues under changing physiological circumstances.

QUESTIONS

1. Starting at the mouth, list the components of the respiratory tree down to the alveoli.

2. What part does the intrapleural space play in respiration?

3. What part does carbon dioxide play in regulating respiration?

FURTHER READING

Stocks J (1996) Respiration. In: Hinchliff S, Montague S, Watson R (eds) *Physiology for nursing practice, 2nd edn.* Baillière Tindall, London, pp 530–581

Watson R (1995) *Anatomy and physiology for nurses, 10th edn.* Baillière Tindall, London

11 Kidneys

Roger Watson

After reading this chapter you should be able to:
- describe the position and structure of the kidneys
- list the functions of the kidney
- explain how urine is produced
- explain the part the kidneys play in acid-base balance in the body.

INTRODUCTION

In terms of homeostasis, the kidneys play several crucial roles. They regulate the amount of body water, filter the blood in order to excrete unwanted substances, principally nitrogenous waste in the form of urea, and retain valuable substances. They also help to regulate the pH of the blood (Ch. 1). This chapter will consider the structure of the kidneys in relation to the above functions and explain how they are able to fulfil these multiple homeostatic functions. The kidney is also involved in the production of erythrocytes by the secretion of a hormone called erythropoietin, but this function will not be covered in the present chapter (Ch. 9). Control of blood pressure via the renin–angiotensin system was described in Chapter 8.

The importance of the kidneys is reflected in the fact that they receive almost 25% of the cardiac output, meaning that the entire blood volume passes through the kidneys more than 300 times per day. The product of the kidneys is urine, of which we excrete approximately 1500 ml daily. The composition and amount of urine excreted can be regulated in response to the needs of the body. How this is achieved will be described below.

ANATOMICAL FEATURES OF THE KIDNEYS

There are two kidneys, which are located at the rear of the abdomen on either side of the vertebral column, as shown in Figure 11.1. The kidneys receive their blood supply from branches of the aorta via the right and left renal arteries and blood leaves the kidneys via the right and left renal veins. There is another output from the kidneys via vessels called the ureters, which collect urine and transport it to the urinary bladder where urine is stored and ultimately released from the body in the process of micturition. These anatomical relationships are shown in Figure 11.1 and a key to understanding the structure of the kidneys is that branches of all these vessels can be found inside the kidneys in an intimate relationship whereby the function of the kidneys may also be understood.

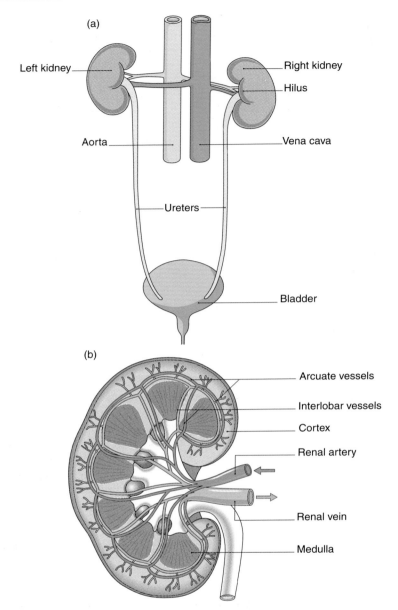

Fig. 11.1 *The kidneys. (a) Rear view; (b) cross-section.*

The blood vessels entering the kidney, the renal arteries, successively subdivide into smaller vessels which supply blood to regions of the kidney called lobes and, thereafter, into lobules. Ultimately, these vessels become capillary-like structures that end at the glomeruli (singular, glomerulus). The vessels that collect blood from the kidneys are initially capillary-like structures know as the vasa recta and these collect blood into successively larger vessels which, ultimately, emerge as the renal veins. This relationship between the vessels is summarised in Figure 11.1.

Each glomerulus is a network of capillaries surrounded by a structure called

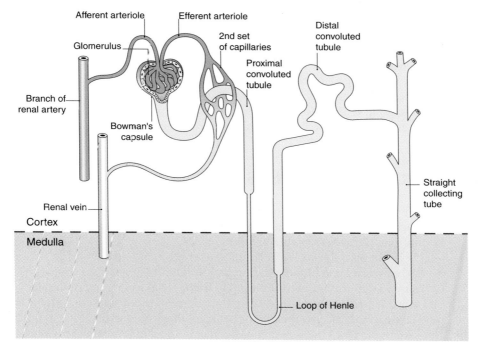

Fig. 11.2   *A nephron and the blood vessels associated with it.*

the Bowman's capsule and this, in turn, is part of a structure known as the nephron. The nephron is the functional unit of the kidney where all of the homeostatic functions referred to above take place and the nephron is surrounded by another network of capillaries formed by the vasa recta, as shown in Figure 11.2. Arterial blood arrives at the nephron via the afferent arteriole of the glomerulus, leaves via an efferent arteriole and passes to the vasa recta. From the vasa recta it is collected into venules and these transport the blood to the renal veins.

> The functional unit of the kidney is the nephron, which is surrounded by a system of capillaries called the vasa recta.

The anatomical features of the nephrons, of which there are many millions in each kidney, are shown in Figure 11.2. The kidney is a compact organ with a cortex and a medulla and the glomeruli are located in the cortex with the descending and ascending limbs of the nephron – known as kidney tubules – located in the medulla. Some nephrons extend deeper into the medulla than others and this anatomical orientation is essential to their function.

Kidney tubules

The kidney tubules begin at the Bowman's capsule. The first part of the tubule is convoluted and is called the proximal convoluted tubule and this leads to the descending limb. Linking the descending limb to the ascending limb is a loop known as the loop of Henlé. Another convoluted tubule (the distal convoluted tubule) lies at the end of the ascending limb and this leads to the collecting duct. These structures are shown in Figure 11.2.

The product of the nephrons is urine and this is gathered in the collecting ducts in the renal medulla and taken to the ureters, which leave the kidney near the point where the renal artery and renal veins enter. This area is known as the renal pelvis. Urine flows down the ureters to the urinary bladder.

FUNCTION OF THE KIDNEYS

The function of the kidneys can be summarised as filtration, reabsorption and secretion. These functions will be considered below after the mechanisms maintaining filtration pressure are described.

If the blood pressure is compared in the renal artery and the renal vein (in other words, the blood entering and leaving the kidneys, respectively, it is measured at approximately 100 mmHg in the renal artery and 5 mmHg in the renal vein. It can be seen, therefore, that there is a considerable pressure gradient across the kidneys and this pressure gradient is used to filter blood from the glomerulus into the Bowman's capsule. In the glomerulus the pressure that tends to push fluid out into the Bowman's capsule, called hydrostatic pressure, is approximately 60 mmHg. There is hydrostatic pressure inside the Bowman's capsule, which tends to push fluid back into the glomerulus, of approximately 15 mmHg. The osmotic pressure in the blood, of 27 mmHg, also tends to prevent fluid from moving out of the glomerulus. If all these pressures are accounted for, as shown in Figure 11.3, then there is a net filtration pressure of approximately 18 mmHg at the glomerulus.

> The movement of fluid from the blood into the kidney tubules is influenced by hydrostatic pressure and osmotic pressure. Normally, the combination of hydrostatic pressure in the blood exceeds the combined hydrostatic pressure in the tubules and the osmotic pressure of the blood.

There are mechanisms acting on the kidney which ensure that the net filtration pressure is maintained within a reasonably narrow range. This ensures, on the one hand, that filtration does not stop and, on the other hand, that damage to the glomerulus and kidney tubules does not occur through a very high filtration pressure. These mechanisms are shown in Figure 11.3. If the filtration pressure is going to rise, it can be lowered by constricting the afferent arteriole through sympathetic nervous stimulation. Alternatively, if the filtration pressure is going to fall, it can be raised by constricting the efferent arteriole and this is effected by the release into the blood of a potent vasoconstrictor called angiotensin. An isolated kidney is also capable of autoregulating filtration pressure by the release of local hormones called prostaglandins. The above mechanisms are only capable of regulating the filtration pressure within a limited range and, ultimately, if the renal arterial blood pressure falls suddenly or to a very low level as in shock, then filtration will stop and this is called renal failure.

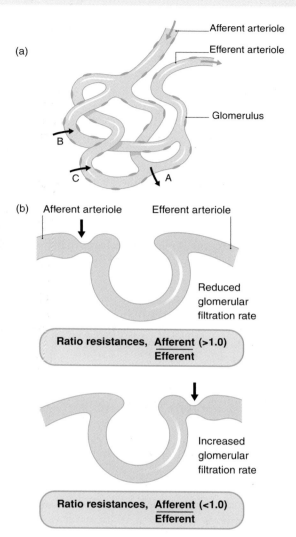

Fig. 11.3   *Glomerular filtration. (a) Pressures at the Bowman's capsule A = 60 mmHg, B = 15 mmHg, C = 27 mmHg; net filtration pressure = A − (B + C) = 18 mmHg. (b) Control of filtration.*

Filtration

Filtration is achieved at the glomerulus by a series of filters formed by the inner lining of the capillary (the endothelium), which contains pores called fenestrations, the basement membrane of the glomerulus and the filtration slits, which are formed around the glomerular vessels by the podocyte cells. The above structures restrict the passage out of the glomerulus of different sizes of particles. The fenestrations restrict the passage of erythrocytes, the basement membrane restricts the passage of large proteins and the filtration slits restrict the passage of small proteins.

As a result of the action of filtration pressure at the glomerulus and the system of filters, the resulting filtrate that is formed in the proximal tubule contains water, electrolytes (such as sodium and potassium; Ch. 1), urea, polypeptides, sugars (such as glucose) and amino acids (Ch. 2). Large proteins and erythrocytes normally remain in the blood. However, blood or protein in the urine may indicate that the function of the glomerulus has broken down and kidney damage has occurred.

Reabsorption

The amount of several substances filtered per day at the glomerulus is given in the first two columns of Table 11.1. The ease with which certain substances cross into the proximal tubule, e.g. water and sodium, and the restriction of others to the blood, e.g. protein, is demonstrated by the data. However, the third column shows that most of these substances are not excreted in the urine. It is clear, therefore, that there is a mechanism whereby most of the substances are removed from the tubules and this is called reabsorption.

TABLE 11.1	Daily Filtration by the Kidneys		
Chemical (unit)	Plasma	Filtrate	Urine
Water (L)	180	179	1.5
Protein (g)	9000	10	0
Sodium (g)	540	540	3
Glucose (g)	180	180	0
Urea (g)	53	53	25
Creatinine (g)	1.5	1.5	1.5

Reabsorption is essential if the body is not to lose essential nutrients such as glucose and amino acids and electrolytes such as sodium. Moreover, without reabsorption the body would lose all its water very quickly via the kidneys and dehydration would take place.

Reabsorption takes place throughout the kidney tubules. However, different substances are reabsorbed at different points and this is summarised in Table 11.2. Reabsorption takes place by several mechanisms, including pinocytosis, osmosis, active transport and passive transport (Ch. 4). Most filtered substances are reabsorbed at the proximal tubule, including sodium, glucose, amino acids and other cations (positively charged electrolytes), and these are reabsorbed by active transport. Water is reabsorbed by osmosis following the reabsorption of the above solutes. Reabsorption of the solutes raises the concentration of water in the tubule and it moves out of the tubules into the surrounding tissue of the kidney. Active transport of sodium continues in the ascending limb of the loop of Henlé in the distal tubule and chloride follows by passive transport in the ascending limb. Water is reabsorbed by osmosis in the descending limb of the loop of Henlé and the collecting duct is normally impervious to water, except in the presence of antidiuretic hormone (ADH), and the significance of this in the production of urine will be explained below.

TABLE 11.2	Reabsorption in the Kidney		
	Region of kidney	Substance	Process
	Proximal convoluted tubule	Sodium	Active transport
		Glucose	Active transport
		Amino acids	Active transport
		Water	Osmosis
		Small proteins	Pinocytosis
	Descending loop of Henlé	Water	Osmosis
	Ascending loop of Henlé	Sodium	Active and passive transport
		Chloride	Active and passive transport
	Distal convoluted tubule	Sodium	Active transport (aldosterone controlled)
		Anions	Passive transport
	Collecting tubule	Water	Osmosis (ADH dependent)
		Urea	Passive

Secretion

Some substances are secreted into the proximal and distal convoluted tubules and this helps the kidneys to regulate more efficiently the levels of certain substances in the body. This is particularly the case with substances that influence the acid/base balance of the blood. Substances secreted into the kidney tubules include potassium ions, hydrogen ions, ammonia and phosphate. Some drugs, e.g. penicillin, are also secreted into the tubules.

> Three processes take place in the tubules: filtration, reabsorption and secretion.

URINE PRODUCTION

Under conditions where the body is adequately hydrated, all of the above processes take place and filtrate, in the form of urine, passes from the kidney tubules to the collecting duct. The collecting duct is impervious to water and a dilute urine is produced that flows down the ureters to the urinary bladder.

However, under conditions where water needs to be preserved by the body, when it is dehydrated, the kidneys are also capable of forming a concentrated urine. All of the processes described above take place but, under the influence of ADH, the collecting ducts become permeable to water and water is reabsorbed into the blood. The mechanism whereby this takes place is thought to be enabled by countercurrents established between the descending and the ascending tubules of the kidney, and the outcome, as shown in Figure 11.4, is that a concentration gradient of sodium chloride is established in the medulla of the kidney. As the collecting duct descends through this concentration gradient, water is drawn out by osmosis and returned to the blood by the blood vessels of the vasa recta.

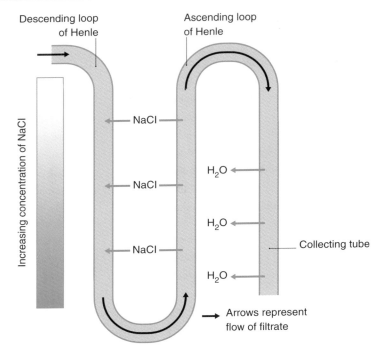

Fig. 11.4   *The mechanism of countercurrent exchange.*

Depending upon the needs of the body the kidneys are capable of producing either a concentrated or a dilute urine in order to either conserve water or get rid of water from the body, respectively.

Countercurrent

The countercurrent mechanism (Fig. 11.4) depends on the differing permeabilities of the ascending and descending limbs of the kidney tubules and the fact that filtrate flows in different directions in each limb. The ascending limb of the kidney tubule actively transports sodium and chloride out into the medulla but is impermeable to water. On the other hand, the descending limb of the kidney tubule is permeable to sodium, which may enter from the surrounding medulla, and it is also permeable to water, which will move out to regions of high osmolarity in the surrounding medulla.

Effectively, therefore, a countercurrent mechanism is established whereby sodium is actively transported out of the ascending limb and taken up by the descending limb. This has the effect, due to the loop connecting the two limbs, of maintaining a higher concentration of sodium chloride at the loop than at the top of either the descending or ascending limbs. The descending limb is permeable to water and this moves out into the medulla by osmosis.

Clearly, if the water that is transported out of the ascending limb and the collecting duct by osmosis is not removed then the process would eventually reach an equilibrium and the concentration gradient would be destroyed. Excess water in the medulla is removed by the vasa recta, which also descends into and ascends out of the medulla. As the vasa recta descends into the medulla, sodium chloride is taken into the blood by diffusion and water moves out into the medulla by osmosis as the blood in the vasa recta reaches areas of very high osmolarity. As the vasa recta ascends out of the medulla, sodium chloride diffuses out in response to the decreasing concentration of sodium chloride and water moves into the blood as a result of the decreasing osmolarity. The net effect is that water is removed from the medulla and returned to the blood, thereby maintaining the concentration gradient. These processes are summarised in Figure 11.4.

The production of a concentrated urine is made possible by the action of ADH on the collecting duct. As the collecting duct descends through the medulla of the kidney, water moves by osmosis into the medulla in response to the concentration gradient and this water is removed by the vasa recta as described above.

ACID/BASE BALANCE

An important function of the kidneys is to participate, along with the lungs and the blood buffering systems, in maintaining the acid/base balance of the blood within physiological limits. The normal pH of the blood is 7.35–7.45. There are three buffering systems in the kidney involving bicarbonate ions, ammonia and phosphate, and these will be considered in turn.

Bicarbonate ions are secreted into the lumen of the kidney tubules and combine with secreted hydrogen ions to form carbonic acid. The carbonic acid is, in turn, broken down into carbon dioxide and water by carbonic anhydrase, which is found in the lining of the tubule. The water is excreted and the carbon dioxide is taken up again by the cells of the kidney tubule where it is combined with water to form carbonic acid, by carbonic anhydrase in the tubule cells. The bicarbonate formed by the dissociation of the carbonic acid into bicarbonate and hydrogen ions is reabsorbed into the blood, the hydrogen ion being secreted into the lumen. These processes are summarised in Figure 11.5. Under conditions where excess hydrogen ions are present in the body, and the pH of the blood falls (acidosis), the uptake of bicarbonate ions by the kidney into the blood is increased and this returns the blood pH to normal. Alternatively, where the pH of the blood rises (alkalosis) as a result of excess production of carbon dioxide, the uptake of bicarbonate by the kidneys into the blood is reduced in order to return the pH of the blood to normal.

Under conditions where excess hydrogen ions are produced and secreted into the lumen of the kidney, they cannot be allowed to accumulate because this would result in a very acidic urine being produced. There are two ways in which excess hydrogen ions in the kidney tubules are, effectively, 'mopped up' involving ammonia and phosphate, both of which are present, as a result of metabolic activities, in the kidney tubules. In the case of ammonia the hydrogen ions combine with it to form ammonium ions and these may combine with other ions, such as chloride or sulphate, to form soluble salts, which are excreted in the urine. Similarly, phosphate ions may combine with hydrogen ions and sodium to form soluble sodium phosphate, which is likewise excreted in the urine. These processes are summarised in Figure 11.5.

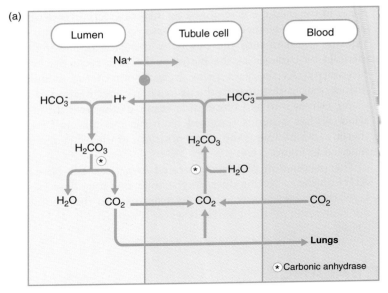

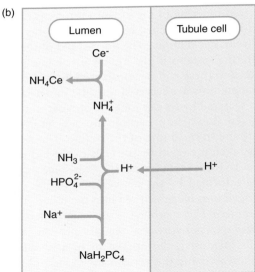

Fig. 11.5   *Renal buffering systems. (a) Bicarbonate buffering system; (b) ammonia/ammonium and phosphate buffering.*

MICTURITION

The process whereby urine is expelled from the body is called micturition and this takes place when the urinary bladder fills up, beyond a certain level, with urine. Urine is constantly produced by the kidneys and trickles down the ureters, assisted by gravity and peristaltic waves in the ureters, into the urinary bladder. The urinary bladder is composed of smooth muscle (Ch. 12), which is known as the detrusor muscle. Smooth muscle is extensible beyond its resting state and the fibres run in many directions in the detrusor, meaning that it can be stretched to accommodate a large volume of urine. Normally urine is voided when there is about 200 ml in the bladder but where there is obstruction to outflow via the urethra, it can hold over 1 L of urine.

The outflow of urine is prevented by two sphincters, an internal and an external sphincter, formed by smooth and skeletal muscle, respectively. The skeletal muscle sphincter is controlled voluntarily while the smooth muscle sphincter is under autonomic control.

The detrusor muscle contains stretch receptors which send signals to the brain and, by this means, there is an awareness that the bladder is filling. In very young children, up to about 2 years of age, the bladder empties by a reflex action once it fills. However, in adults, it is possible to suppress the reflex desire to void urine until it is personally and socially acceptable to do so.

> The skeletal muscles that control the outflow of urine from the bladder are formed from the pelvic floor muscle and these become stretched in childbirth in women, which can lead to stress incontinence of urine.

Micturition takes place when suppression of the reflex to void is voluntarily lifted and the external sphincter is relaxed. The internal sphincter also relaxes and the detrusor muscle contracts, thereby expelling urine from the bladder via the urethra.

SUMMARY

In this chapter the gross anatomy of the kidney and the microstructure have been outlined. The functions of the kidney in terms of filtration, reabsorption and secretion have been described and the process of urine production has been explained. Particular attention was paid to the countercurrent mechanism whereby a concentrated urine may be produced under conditions where the body needs to conserve water. Finally, the process of micturition was briefly described.

QUESTIONS

1. Describe the system of blood vessels in the kidney from the renal artery to the renal vein.

2. What is the functional unit of the kidney and what are its main features?

3. Explain the countercurrent mechanism in the kidney.

FURTHER READING

McLaren S (1996) Renal function. In: Hinchliff S, Montague S, Watson R (eds) *Physiology for nursing practice*, 2nd edn. Baillière Tindall, London, pp 582–617

Watson R (1995) *Anatomy and physiology for nurses*, 10th edn. Baillière Tindall, London

12 Muscles and Movement

Roger Watson

After reading this chapter you should be able to:
- describe the different types of muscles
- describe the composition and structure of muscle tissue
- state where these different muscles may be found
- explain how the different types of muscles are activated
- explain how movement is possible in the skeleto-muscular system.

INTRODUCTION

This chapter is concerned, in the first instance, with muscle in the different forms in which it is present in the human body. The secondary aim of this chapter is to consider movement and, in this respect, the focus is on the cooperative action of skeletal muscle and the bony skeleton of the body in producing movement at joints and, thereby, movement of the body. Neither the skeleton nor the anatomical skeletal musculature of the body will be considered in any detail and the student should refer to a more comprehensive anatomy and physiology textbook in order to fill in these details. The main concern in this chapter is to describe the different types of muscle and to explain how the skeleto-muscular system works.

Muscle is a tissue that is concerned with movement and it has the ability to change in length and thickness by a process of contraction. There are three different types of muscle: skeletal, cardiac and smooth. Skeletal muscle, together with nervous tissue and cartilage (which is specialised as tendons), is the major component of the muscles which are organs of the skeleto-muscular system, which serves to maintain posture and enable movement of the body. The muscles of the skeleto-muscular system also generate heat in the body. Cardiac muscle is unique to the heart, which is, essentially, an organ composed of muscle which acts as a pump in the cardiovascular system. Smooth muscle forms part of organs in the cardiovascular system, respiratory system, digestive system and in some other organs such as the eye where it is mainly concerned with changes in the diameter of hollow organs.

The purpose of this chapter is to explain how muscle tissue works and, thereby, to demonstrate how it serves its function within the various systems in which it is located. The essential similarities and differences between the three types of muscle referred to above will also be explained.

Muscle is an excitable tissue: in other words, its cells are capable of transmitting electrical activity across their surface. Nervous tissue has already been described in Ch. 5 and the principles that operate there largely apply to muscle tissue. The origin for the electrical activity in muscle tissue differs between the three types of muscle.

SKELETAL MUSCLE ACTIVATION

In skeletal muscle the origin is nervous stimulation by motor nerves which originate in the motor cortex and which synapse in the spinal cord. A motor nerve running between the brain and the spinal cord is called an upper motor neurone and a corresponding motor nerve running from the spinal cord to a skeletal muscle is called a lower motor neurone. The structure of skeletal muscle will be described below but it should be understood at this point that the structure formed by a lower motor neurone and the muscle cell that it supplies is known as a motor unit. The lower motor neurones do not physically connect with the muscle cells. Instead, they form a structure known as the neuromuscular junction, which is very similar to a synapse between two nerves (Ch. 5). The electrical activity in the lower motor neurone is transmitted chemically to the muscle in precisely the same way as electrical activity is transmitted chemically between two neurones at a synapse. The arrival of electrical activity, through stimulation of a nerve, at a neuromuscular junction leads to the release of acetylcholine. The acetylcholine crosses the gap between the neurone and the muscle cell at the neuromuscular junction and binds to receptors on the muscle cell. The binding of the acetylcholine to the muscle cell leads to depolarisation through an influx of sodium ions and this sets up an action potential, which spreads along the muscle cell. The events that follow the spread of the action potential will be continued below in describing the function of skeletal muscle.

> Skeletal muscle is an excitable tissue which is stimulated by electrical activity in motor neurones. The electrical activity in the motor neurones is transmitted chemically to the skeletal muscle where electrical activity is generated and spreads across the skeletal muscle.

CARDIAC MUSCLE ACTIVATION

Electrical activity arises spontaneously in cardiac muscle and the nervous supply to cardiac muscle serves the function of modulating this spontaneous electrical activity. All of the cardiac muscle, of which the heart is mainly composed, is capable of spontaneous electrical activity. However, a specific area in the heart, near the sino-atrial node, is responsible in health for regulating the electrical activity over the whole of the heart. This area is known as the pacemaker and the events that take place here are an influx of sodium ions into the cardiac cells in this area, leading to depolarisation (Ch. 5), which then spreads across the heart following a distinct path in the healthy heart. The heart has two nervous supplies: a sympathetic and a parasympathetic supply. The sympathetic supply goes to all regions of the heart, where it releases noradrenaline onto the cardiac muscle leading to acceleration and strengthening of the heart. The parasympathetic supply is mainly to the sino-atrial node, via the vagus nerve, where it releases acetylcholine, which slows down the heart and reduces the strength of contraction. Effects on the speed of the heart are known as chronotropic effects and effects on the strength of contraction are known as inotropic effects. Noradrenaline, therefore, is positively chronotropic and positively inotropic whereas acetylcholine is negatively chronotropic and negatively inotropic. The specific electrical events and the events that follow will be described below when the function of cardiac muscle is considered. Cardiac muscle also displays changes in its activity in response to circulating hormones, principally the catecholamines, in the blood.

> Cardiac and smooth muscle are both capable of spontaneous electrical activity but this is controlled by nervous and chemical factors.

SMOOTH MUSCLE ACTIVATION

Smooth muscle plays a wide variety of roles in the human body and the different types of smooth muscle, apart from differing in their structure, as will be described below, also differ in their electrical activity. Some smooth muscle displays spontaneous electrical activity and some only responds to external stimuli. In smooth muscle with spontaneous electrical activity the nervous supply plays a modulating role and this smooth muscle also responds to circulating hormones. The external stimuli, therefore, that influence smooth muscle include nervous stimulation and circulating hormones.

An example of smooth muscle which displays spontaneous electrical activity, coordinated by a pacemaker, is the smooth muscle of the stomach. The smooth muscle of the stomach constantly displays waves of contraction and these increase in size when, for example, the presence of food is sensed by sight and smell. The size of the contractions in the stomach is increased by several hormones released into the blood and also by the parasympathetic nervous system. The nerve supplying the stomach with parasympathetic stimulation is the vagus nerve, which releases acetylcholine onto the smooth muscle. (Note how nervous stimulation from the parasympathetic nervous system has opposite effects on the cardiac muscle and on the smooth muscle of the stomach.) Conversely, sympathetic stimulation decreases the activity of the smooth muscle of the stomach when noradrenaline is released onto the smooth muscle of the stomach and also when noradrenaline and adrenaline are released into the blood, e.g. in the 'fight or flight' reaction experienced by humans if they are frightened.

The smooth muscle lining the vessels of the cardiovascular system does not undergo spontaneous depolarisation but its activity is modulated by a nerve supply, mainly sympathetic, and by circulating hormones. Most of the sympathetic nerve supply to the blood vessels releases noradrenaline, which leads to contraction and thereby constriction of the blood vessels. However, in the blood vessels to skeletal muscle, there are sympathetic nerves that release acetylcholine leading to relaxation and thereby an increase in the diameter of these blood vessels. Circulating noradrenaline and adrenaline generally lead to constriction of the blood vessels.

A final example is the smooth muscle in the radial muscle in the iris of the eye. This smooth muscle is responsible for changing the diameter of the pupil of the eye under different intensities of light. The radial muscle is supplied by the sympathetic and parasympathetic nervous system and is also sensitive to circulating hormones. The sympathetic nerves release noradrenaline onto the radial muscle and this leads to relaxation of the muscle and dilatation of the pupil. The parasympathetic nerves, which release acetylcholine, have the effect of contracting the radial muscle and constricting the pupil. Circulating adrenaline and noradrenaline lead to dilatation of the pupil. (Note that the effects of noradrenaline and acetylcholine on the radial muscle are opposite to their effects on the smooth muscle of the cardiovascular system.)

Electrical activity in nerve fibres is transmitted to smooth muscle cells by means of chemical transmission and this is analogous to the system in skeletal muscle at the neuromuscular junction. However, the junction between autonomic nerves and smooth muscle is called the neuroeffector junction and the substance released from the autonomic nerve is noradrenaline. The exception is some neuroeffector junctions that release acetylcholine onto the smooth muscle of blood vessels in the skeletal muscles.

SKELETAL MUSCLE

Skeletal muscle conforms to several shapes in the human body and the shape of the muscle indicates something about its properties and function. Some muscles are relatively short, others are flat and others are thick. Generally speaking, the longer a skeletal muscle is the more able it is to contract and the thicker a skeletal muscle the stronger it is. A typical skeletal muscle that displays both length and thickness is the biceps muscle, which is used to reduce the angle between the arm and the forearm, as shown in Figure 12.1. The function of skeletal muscle can be described adequately by considering the structure and properties of a typical muscle such as the biceps.

A skeletal muscle such as the biceps clearly has an orientation, its length is greater than its breadth and the muscle contracts along its long axis. If the structure of the muscle is examined in more detail, from those features visible with

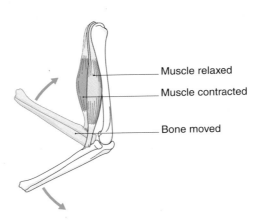

Muscle relaxed

Muscle contracted

Bone moved

Fig. 12.1   *Bone movement as muscle contracts.*

the naked eye to those that require microscopic magnification, then a gross arrangement of longitudinal structure called fascicles can be seen. Fascicles, in turn, are composed of muscle fibres and these fibres are the functional units of skeletal muscle.

Skeletal muscle fibres are, in fact, single muscle cells. However, unlike other cells, muscle cells are multinucleate; in other words, they have many nuclei and such cells are called syncytia (singular, syncytium). During the process of their development the walls between the cells break down and the result is long muscle cells, with several nuclei along their length, which are packed full of muscle proteins. It is the shortening of these cells that is responsible for the contraction of skeletal muscles.

> Skeletal muscle cells, also known as fibres, are long cells with many nuclei known as syncytia.

Muscle proteins

If a skeletal muscle cell is viewed under high magnification it has a particular striated or striped appearance and a typical microscopic picture is shown in Figure 12.2. The observed pattern results from the arrangement of muscle proteins (Ch. 2) in the muscle fibres and this is shown diagrammatically in Figure 12.2. There are two major proteins in skeletal muscle, actin and myosin, and these are arranged in long structures called myofibrils such that strands of myosin lie between strands of actin with a movable head on the myosin strands connecting the myosin to the actin.

Actin strands are arranged such that they project in two directions away from an anchoring region called the I band. The distance contained between two I bands is known as a sarcomere and this is the functional unit of skeletal muscle. When skeletal muscle contracts, the sarcomeres shorten and this can be observed under a microscope by a shortening of the distance between striations in contracted compared with relaxed skeletal muscle.

Contraction of skeletal muscle takes place when the heads of the myosin molecules move such that they pull the actin strands and move the I bands towards one another. The heads of the moving molecules can bend in order to pull the actin strand and then detach, return to their original position and repeat the movement. In this way considerable tension can be generated in a muscle and it all results from these small microscopic movements of proteins. This movement is know as the sliding filament theory and one way in which it is convenient to visualise the movement of the myosin heads is like the oars on a long boat. The 'oars' pull the myosin along the actin rather as synchronised oars pull a long boat through the water.

> Contraction of muscle takes place due to the action of specific contractile muscle proteins.

The process of muscle contraction is energy dependent and the energy is provided by ATP. The myosin head is capable of binding to a specific site on the

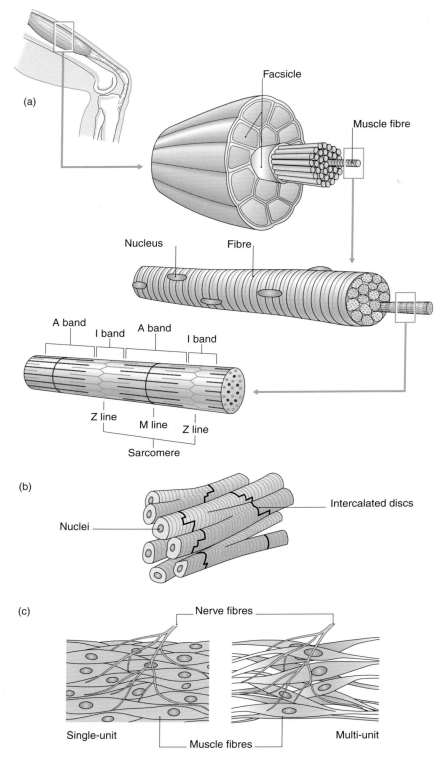

Fig. 12.2   *Types of muscle. (a) Skeletal muscle; (b) cardiac muscle; (c) smooth muscle.*

actin molecule and moving and, during this process, it splits the ATP molecule to form ADP and inorganic phosphate, which releases the energy required for the movement to take place. The process is stimulated by the presence of calcium ions, which initiate a change in the shape of the actin to allow formation of a link (a cross-bridge) between actin and the myosin head. The myosin head acts as an enzyme to catalyse the breakdown of ATP. After contraction has taken place, calcium ions are removed from the muscle cell and the actin returns to its original shape whereby the cross-bridge with the myosin head cannot be formed.

Calcium

Calcium is essential for the contraction of muscle and it is stored in skeletal muscle in a structure know as the sarcoplasmic reticulum. It is necessary to store the calcium in such a structure in order to control its release and, thereby, to control the process of muscle contraction. Calcium is released into the muscle fibres, from the sarcoplasmic reticulum, when an electrical impulse passes through the muscle cell and over the sarcoplasmic reticulum. The source of this electrical impulse, the action potential, is stimulation of the muscle by a motor nerve and the mechanism whereby the impulse spreads across the muscle is depolarisation (Ch. 5). Calcium acts by removing a protein complex (composed of three protein molecules) from the actin thereby allowing the myosin head to bind to the actin and pull it, causing muscle contraction. In the process of this movement the ATP (Ch. 1) is split into ADP and inorganic phosphate, thereby providing the chemical energy for the movement.

CARDIAC MUSCLE

Cardiac muscle is found uniquely in the heart and the muscle proteins are similar to those found in skeletal muscle. The contraction mechanism is also broadly similar and the storage and release of calcium from the sarcoplasmic reticulum is also similar. However, the cellular structure of cardiac muscle is quite different from that of skeletal muscle (Fig. 12.2). In contrast to the long syncytial cells of skeletal muscle, the cells of cardiac muscle are mononucleate, short and branched and interconnected by intercalated discs. These latter features have mechanical components that hold the cells tightly together called desmosomes and also gap junctions, which permit the passage of electrical activity easily between the cells. In fact, the ease of transmission of electrical activity between cardiac muscle cells leads to its description as a functional syncytium; in other words, many cells behave as if they were one.

When an action potential arises at the pacemaker it spreads across the atria of the heart and arrives at a structure known as the atrio-ventricular node where the electrical activity is slowed down and channelled along a specific pathway comprised of the bundles of His and the Purkinje fibres, which take the electrical activity to the bottom of the ventricles of the heart. The electrical activity that spreads across the heart causes an influx of calcium ions from the sarcoplasmic reticulum leading to contraction of the cardiac muscle. However, the function of the atrio-ventricular node serves to ensure that the atria, which are responsible for the final filling of the ventricles, contract before the ventricles, which propel blood out of the heart and into the systemic circulation.

SMOOTH MUSCLE

Smooth muscle is similar to skeletal and cardiac muscle inasmuch as it contains many of the same muscle proteins. It differs from skeletal muscle in that its cells, also called fibres, are single mononucleate cells but, unlike cardiac muscle, these are not interconnected (Fig. 12.2). The contractile proteins are found in bands on the surface of smooth muscle cells and smooth muscle exists as single unit, with fewer nerve fibres than muscle fibres, or as multiunit with one nerve fibre per muscle fibre. Single-unit smooth muscle is found in the hollow organs of the body such as the bladder and stomach and tends to undergo waves of contraction with the nervous supply playing a modulating role on the contractions. Multiunit smooth muscle, in contrast, is capable of rapid contraction such as those required in the iris of the eye and the nervous supply initiates contraction and relaxation.

Cardiac and smooth muscles are not syncytia; however, cardiac cells are arranged such that they work together and this is called a functional syncytium.

THE HUMAN SKELETON

The human skeleton consists of 206 bones arranged in two parts: the axial and the appendicular skeleton. The axial skeleton forms the long axis of the body and is mainly concerned with the protection of delicate organs, such as the brain and the spinal cord in the case of the skull and the vertebral column, respectively. The thorax, which also plays a protective function, is responsible for changing the volume of the thorax during breathing (Ch. 10). The axial skeleton is mostly only capable of limited movement and these movements are mainly concerned with the posture of the body. The appendicular skeleton, with which the axial skeleton articulates, is comprised of the upper and lower limbs and the pelvis and is capable of greater movement whereby the body may move, as in the case of the legs, or perform very fine movements such as the grasping of the hands. Generally speaking, the further away from the axial skeleton the bones of the appendicular skeleton are, the greater the range of possible movement.

There are 206 bones in the adult human skeleton.

Bones come in a variety of shapes and the greatest contrast is between the flat bones and the long bones. Flat bones are flat, as described, and are mostly concerned with protection of, for example, the skull. Long bones have greater length than breadth and these bones are mostly involved in movement; the most obvious examples are the long bones of the limbs but the bones of the fingers and toes are also examples of long bones. Series of long bones are interconnected by muscles and it is via this system of attachment of muscles to long bones that the major movements of the body are enabled.

MOVEMENT

Wherever two bones in the skeleton are next to one another it is possible that they will move relevant to one another, however limited that movement may be. The points in the skeleton where such movement may take place are called joints or articulations and to illustrate the variety of joints the point at which a tooth enters the jaw bone is a joint, but the movement here is extremely limited – except in children who lose their milk teeth and in adults where there is dental disease. In contrast, there is a joint at the shoulder between the shoulder blade (scapula) and the bone of the upper arm (humerus) whereby the arm may be moved through a very wide range of movement.

The bones of the skeletal musculature are attached to the bones of the skeleton by tendons and some bones are attached to one another by ligaments. Tendons allow the movement of articulated bones (joints), and ligaments, while holding some bones together, also allow a range of movement at some joints. The remainder of this chapter will be concerned with the different ways in which movement may take place at joints and, while examples will be given, the anatomical details should be obtained from a more comprehensive textbook.

Levers

In order to understand movement at the articulations between long bones it is necessary to understand the principles of levers and this also provides insight into the different types of movement that are capable at the various joints in the body. There are three classes of levers – first, second and third class – and these will be described, using simple diagrams and giving examples, in turn. The common components of all lever systems are the fulcrum, around which movement takes place, and the effort and load which are applied and moved, respectively, in order to provide movement. In the skeleto-muscular system the effort is provided by a muscle or muscles and the load is the part of the body that is moved. The efficiency of a lever system describes the extent to which the applied effort is transformed into moving the load.

> Movement in the body takes place as a result of the physical arrangement of skeletal muscles and the bones of the skeleton through a system of levers.

First-class levers

The first-class lever is the most efficient class of lever in which the fulcrum occupies a position between the effort and the load, as shown in Figure 12.3. A good example of a first-class lever is provided in the movement whereby the head is raised. The fulcrum in this movement is the atlanto-occipital joint between the top of the vertebrae and the base of the skull, and the effort is provided by the muscle that pulls the back of the head down, raising the load, which is the front of the skull (Fig. 12.3).

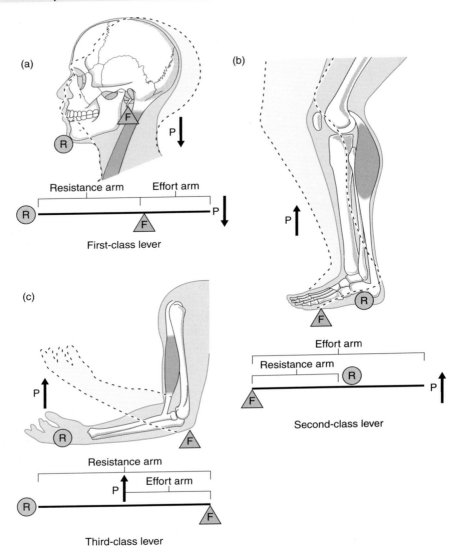

Fig. 12.3　*Levers. (a) First-class lever; (b) second-class lever; (c) third-class lever. F, fulcrum; P, force; R, resistance.*

Second-class levers

In a second-class lever the load occupies a position between the effort and the fulcrum (Fig. 12.3) and an example of such a lever is the movement whereby the heel is elevated when the body is raised on tiptoes. The fulcrum is provided by the ball of the foot, the effort is provided by muscles at the back of the leg and the load is the body (Fig. 12.3).

Third-class levers

Third-class levers are the least efficient class of levers, where the effort occupies a position between the fulcrum and the load (Fig. 12.3). Raising the hand towards the shoulder is an example of a third-class lever system where the fulcrum is the elbow, the effort is provided by a muscle running from the arm to the forearm and the load is the hand and forearm (Fig. 12.3). Third-class levers are the most common class of levers in the body.

Range of movements

The range of movements of which the body is capable is wide and varied and depends on several factors including the size and shape of the bones involved and the nature of the articulation between the bones. As described above, the widest range of movement is possible at synovial joints and the least movement at the joints between the jaw and the teeth. However, with this variety of joints the following movements of the body can be performed: reaching, handling, standing, walking, lifting, running, jumping, throwing, eating, breathing and speaking. In addition, the body is capable of complex movements such as cycling and swimming.

Movement involving non-skeletal muscle

In addition to the obvious movements of the body, i.e. those that can be observed by watching the body, there is also movement taking place within the body as a result of the functioning of cardiac and smooth muscle. It is possible to sense the movement of the cardiac muscle, which may be felt as a pulse where an artery, carrying blood away from the heart, passes close to the surface of the body and over an underlying bone, e.g. at the wrist. What is being sensed when a pulse is felt is a pressure wave passing through the cardiovascular system which is being generated by the movement of the cardiac muscle, which expels blood from the ventricles of the heart as the cardiac muscle contracts, and which is maintained by the smooth muscle tone (slightly contracted state) in the circular muscles of the blood vessels. This was considered in more detail in Chapter 8.

Smooth muscle is responsible for the movement of ingested food from the oesophagus, through the gastrointestinal tract, to the rectum. Waste residue from digestion is then expelled from the rectum, through the anus, by the cooperation of smooth and skeletal muscle. Swallowing food is accomplished by the coordination of the skeletal muscle of the tongue and the skeletal and smooth muscle of the oesophagus. Some rapid movements, such as the dilatation and constriction of the iris of the eye in response to changing light intensity, are achieved by the smooth muscle of the eye but, perhaps, the most characteristic movement achieved by smooth muscle is that of peristalsis in the gastrointestinal tract and this will be described below.

Peristalsis

Peristalsis is an involuntary action of the smooth muscle of the digestive tract, the function of which is to move food in one direction, from the oesophagus to the rectum. Peristalsis takes place in the oesophagus, stomach and intestine. Peristalsis only takes place in the oesophagus as a reflex action upon swallowing a bolus of food. The top third of the oesophagus is comprised of skeletal muscle and the lower two-thirds of smooth muscle. Thereafter, with the exception of the external anal sphincter, the remaining musculature of the gastrointestinal tract is comprised of smooth muscle and peristalsis, while changing in intensity, takes place constantly.

To understand peristalsis it is necessary to consider the structure of the gastrointestinal tract. While each region of the tract has a unique structure and specific secretory or absorptive properties, each region also has an arrangement of smooth muscle that allows movement. The inner and outer layers of the tract are epithelial, with a mucus-secreting layer (mucosa) on the inner surface. From the perspective of peristalsis the middle muscular layer is of interest and this is comprised of longitudinal muscle, running the length of the region of the tract, and circular muscle, which encircles regions of the tract. Clearly, contraction of the longitudinal muscle shortens the tract and contraction of the circular muscle reduces the diameter of a region of the tract.

Peristalsis can be visualised as rhythmic waves of alternate contraction and relaxation of the circular and longitudinal smooth muscle of the gastrointestinal tract, as shown in Figure 12.4. The effect of a peristaltic wave is to move food and partly digested food down the oesophagus to the stomach, from the stomach to the small intestine and through the small intestine to the large intestine and down to the rectum. In addition to the gastrointestinal tract, peristalsis also takes place in the ureters, which run from the kidney to the urinary bladder and assist in the movement of urine from the kidneys to the bladder.

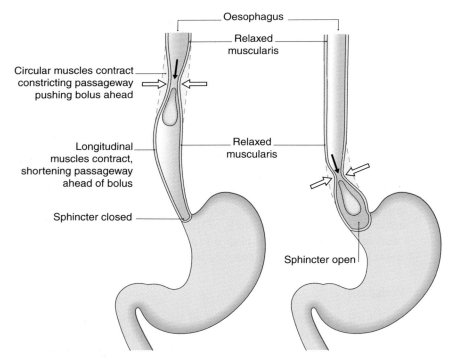

Fig. 12.4   *The oesophageal stage of swallowing showing peristalsis.*

Movement of food through the smooth muscle of the gastrointestinal tract takes place as a result of peristalsis.

Other movement in the gastrointestinal tract

While peristalsis is taking place in the gastrointestinal tract there are other movements taking place in the stomach, small intestine and large intestine. In the stomach, in addition to the longitudinal and smooth muscle, there is also a layer of oblique muscle with an axis approximately 45° to the longitudinal and circular muscle. The combined actions of contraction and relaxation of the three muscle layers of the stomach ensure thorough mixing and mechanical breakdown of the contents of the stomach and this ensures that the food comes into contact with the chemical agents, hydrochloric acid and the enzyme pepsin, in the stomach and this begins chemical breakdown or digestion producing chyme.

In the small intestine there are sharp pinching movements of alternate adjacent section of this region, which are called segmentations. This process ensures further mixing and mechanical breakdown of the contents of the small intestine and serves the same function as the movements of the stomach, i.e. mixing of contents with enzymes that complete the digestion of the food.

Peristalsis and segmentation continue in the large intestine. In this region, however, the contents are mainly moved onwards by mass movement, which involves contraction of the longitudinal muscles, shortening of the colon and movement of the contents down to the rectum in preparation for expulsion through defecation. The contents are prevented from moving backwards into the small intestine by a valve (the ileo-caecal valve), formed by a sphincter, and these valves will be described next.

Sphincters

Sphincters are rings of smooth or skeletal muscle which are essential in the control of movement of the contents of the gastrointestinal tract both in terms of the rate and direction of movement. There is a sphincter at the base of the stomach, where it connects to the small intestine, and this controls the emptying of the stomach. It is necessary to keep food in the stomach for long enough to achieve partial digestion and the sphincter, known as the pyloric sphincter, only allows a few millilitres of chyme into the small intestine. The ileo-caecal valve plays a similar role and, because it is closed when mass movement takes place, it prevents movement of the large intestine contents into the small intestine.

Sphincters are rings of muscle that control the movement of substances from one region of the body to another.

Two important sets of sphincters, controlling expulsion of contents from the body, are the anal sphincters and the sphincters of the urinary bladder. In both cases they are comprised of both smooth and skeletal muscle with the smooth muscle being under involuntary control and the skeletal muscle being under voluntary control. The relaxation of both smooth and skeletal muscle sphincters is necessary for defecation and micturition (passing urine) (Ch. 11), respectively, and it is only after about 2 years of age that children learn to control the skeletal muscle elements of each.

SUMMARY

The consideration of aspects of movement in the body has not been comprehensive. Nevertheless, a sufficient range of movements and a description of the ways in which skeletal, cardiac and smooth muscle function should provide general principles that may be applied to any organ or system of the body that includes muscle tissue.

QUESTIONS

1. Compare and contrast the structure and function of the different types of muscle.

2. Describe the different systems of levers operating in the skeleto-muscular system and provide one example of each.

3. Where is peristalsis found and how does it work?

FURTHER READING

McLaren S (1996) Skeletal muscles. In: Hinchliff S, Montague S, Watson R (eds) *Physiology for nursing practice, 2nd edn*. Baillière Tindall, London, pp 261–283

McLaren S (1996) Bones. In: Hinchliff S, Montague S, Watson R (eds) *Physiology for nursing practice, 2nd edn*. Baillière Tindall, London, pp 284–301

McLaren S (1996) Joints. In: Hinchliff S, Montague S, Watson R (eds) *Physiology for nursing practice, 2nd edn*. Baillière Tindall, London, pp 302–319

Watson R (1995) *Anatomy and physiology for nurses, 10th edn*. Baillière Tindall, London

APPLICATIONS

13 Microbiology

Jennie Wilson

After reading this chapter you should be able to:

- understand what microorganisms are including bacteria, fungi, protozoa and viruses
- describe how bacterial cells differ from animal cells
- know what microorganisms require for growth
- state how bacteria reproduce.

INTRODUCTION

In Chapter 4 we looked at the structure and function of animal cells. Now we shall turn to microbes – organisms that are so small that they cannot be seen without the aid of a microscope (Box 13.1). Microorganisms are an incredibly diverse form of life, inhabiting almost every type of environment, even the most hostile. The majority are very useful; they provide an important first link in the food chain, they fix atmospheric nitrogen in soil enabling it to be used by plants and they release nutrients by decomposing dead matter. Microbes are involved in the production of many types of food such as cheese, bread, yoghurt and wine and are increasingly used to manufacture drugs such as insulin and hepatitis B vaccine.

A few microorganisms cause disease and in the past these were responsible for considerable mortality. However, the application of microbiological discoveries during the past 300 years has had a major effect on the way that we live and on our life expectancy. We can now effectively treat most infectious diseases, we can vaccinate to prevent many others, we have better methods of preserving our food and we live in cleaner, more sanitary conditions.

The classification of microbes is somewhat problematic because they may be eucaryotic cells such as the protozoa, algae and fungi, prokaryotic cells such as bacteria and blue-green algae or neither, such as viruses. Box 13.2 lists the main groups of microorganisms and Figure 13.1 demonstrates their relative size.

BACTERIA

Structure of prokaryotic cells

Prokaryotic cells are much smaller, about the size of a mitochondrion, and far less complex than eucaryotic cells. They have no internal skeletal structure;

BOX 13.1	*The Microscope*

Individual cells are far too small for the detailed structure to be seen with the eye. Microscopes are used to magnify objects and are an essential tool for the study of both the cells of higher animals and plants and of micro-organisms.

The standard type of microscope is called a *compound light microscope*. It consists of two sets of lenses, one next to the object to be viewed (the objective lens) and one next to the eye of the viewer (the ocular lens). Light travels from a lamp in the base of the microscope, through the sample into the objective lens where the image of the sample is magnified. The image will be magnified again in the ocular lens. Modern microscopes contain several objective lenses of differing strengths enabling magnification of ×10, ×44 and ×100. The ocular lens then magnifies by a further ×10 so that the final image can be between 100 and 1000 times larger than the actual sample. Even at this level of magnification, ordinary light microscopes cannot be used to distinguish the internal structure of small cells. This is because the limit of their resolving power (the ability to distinguish between two adjacent objects) is dependent on the wavelength of the visible light used as the light source. The smallest object discernible in a light microscope will be at least 0.2 micro-metres (μm); bacteria range in size between 0.3 μm and 1 μm. The main value of the light microscope is to establish the shape and staining properties of the cells.

The *electron microscope* uses a stream of electrons instead of visible light to magnify an image. The wavelength of these electron beams is much shorter and enables adjacent objects only 0.001 μm apart to be distinguished by projecting the image onto a photographic plate. These microscopes can magnify ×100 000 and are therefore used to study the internal structure of even the smallest cells. To detect fine details of cell structure the samples have to be sliced very thinly and examined in series. Scanning electron microscopes focus a fine beam of electrons over the specimen to obtain three-dimensional images.

instead, the shape of the cell is determined by a rigid cell wall. There are also two main shapes of bacterial cell: spherical (cocci) and rod-shaped (bacilli). A few species are shaped like curved rods, e.g. vibrios, or spirals, e.g. treponema. The way in which cocci congregate together tends to be characteristic of particular species and can be a useful clue in determining the identity of a pathogen (Fig. 13.2).

Bacteria can be seen under a light microscope, but not easily, because the cells appear colourless. Stains are therefore used to enable cells to be seen more clearly and to distinguish their size, shape and arrangement. Most stains are made of basic dyes; the colour is carried by charged ions, which bind to other charged molecules in the cell wall.

The internal structures present within prokaryotic cells do not have their own membranes like the organelles of eucaryotic cells, but are simply extensions of the cytoplasmic membrane. This membrane has to carry out most of the functions that in eucaryotic cells are performed by the organelles (Fig. 13.3).

BOX 13.2	*A Classification of Microorganisms*

A. Eucaryotes – microscopic animals
   1. Protozoa (unicellular), e.g. amoeba, malarial parasites
   2. Helminths (multicellular), e.g. tapeworms, flukes, roundworms
B. Eucaryotes – microscopic plants
   1. Fungi, e.g. yeasts, moulds
   2. Algae (all non-pathogenic), e.g. green, brown and red algae
C. Prokaryotes
   1. Bacteria (true bacteria), e.g. staphylococci
   2. Actinomycetes (filamentous bacteria), e.g. *Streptomyces, Nocardia* sp.
   3. Rickettsias (parasitic intracellular bacteria)
     (a) Rickettsias, e.g. typhus fever
     (b) Chlamydias, e.g. psittacosis
   4. Mycoplasma (bacteria without cell walls), e.g. *Mycobacterium pneumoniae,*
     M. hominis
   5. Phototrophic bacteria (produce oxygen in sunlight)
     (a) Cyanobacteria, e.g. blue-green algae
     (b) Photosynthetic, e.g. purple and purple sulphur bacteria
D. Viruses – non-cellular micro-organisms, e.g. influenza, poliomyelitis

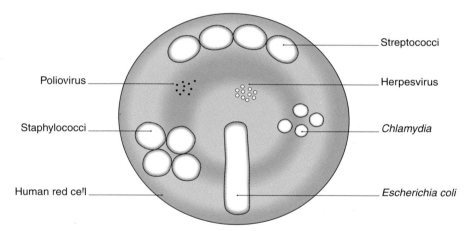

Fig. 13.1   *Relative sizes of microbes. The human red cell is 7–8 μm in diameter. Staphylococci and streptococci are about 1 μm in diameter. A Gram-negative rod such as* Escherichia coli *is about 1 μm in diameter and 3–5 μm long. The cells of* Chlamydia *are smaller (0.2–0.5 μm in diameter) and viruses are smaller again. Seven hundred of these red cells side-by-side would cover the full stop at the end of this sentence.*

Cytoplasmic membrane

Like eucaryotes, the cytoplasm of prokaryotic cells is contained by a thin membrane called the cytoplasmic membrane, which acts as an interface between the cell and the external environment. In prokaryotic cells, the cytoplasmic membrane is particularly important because it carries out many functions of the cell, such as:

• transport of electrons for respiration (ATP formation)

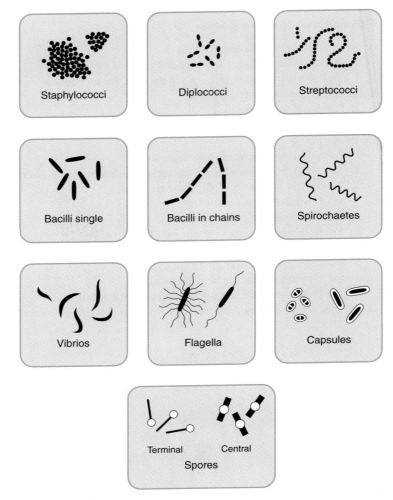

Fig. 13.2   *Some common bacterial shapes and arrangements.*

- nutrient transport systems to take the substances required for the cell to grow from the environment
- synthesis of cell wall components
- secretion of enzymes and toxins
- segregation of DNA during cell division.

Many bacteria have involutions in their cytoplasmic membranes called mesosomes and these are thought to increase its surface area and facilitate the action of enzymes involved in transport systems. Some mesosomes may also be involved in the separation of chromosomes during cell division and the secretion of proteins out of the cell.

Cell wall

A major component of bacterial cell walls is a unique substance called peptidoglycan. This network of carbohydrates and amino acids gives the cell its basic

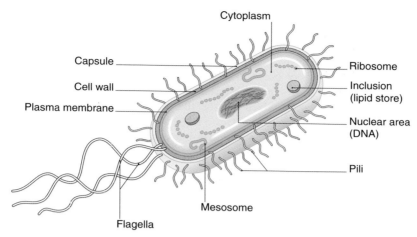

Fig. 13.3   *Structure of a bacterial cell.*

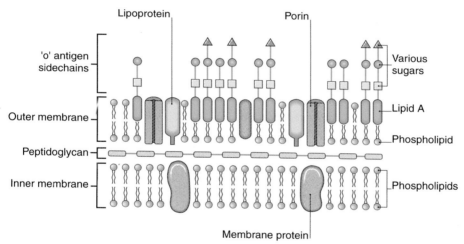

Fig. 13.4   *Structure of the cell wall of bacteria. Both inner and outer membranes are made of phospholipid. The porins in the outer membrane enable substances to pass into the cell. The sugars and side-chains attached to the outer membrane are antigenic. The layer of peptidoglycan between the membranes is thicker in Gram-positive cells.*

rigidity and helps it to withstand the high osmotic pressure exerted by the strong concentration of solutes in the cytoplasm (Fig. 13.4). Whilst the basic structure of peptidoglycan is the same in all bacteria, the arrangement of the wall varies considerably between the two major types of cell: Gram positive and Gram negative (see Box 13.3 for more information about Gram staining).

Gram-positive bacteria

These have a very thick mesh of peptidoglycan interspersed with polysaccharides and proteins. Small molecules are able to penetrate this mesh relatively easily. Whilst this allows nutrients into the cell, several harmful substances such as dyes, detergents and antibiotics can also reach the cytoplasmic membrane

BOX 13.3	*The Gram Stain*

One of the most important staining methods is the Gram stain, named after the physician who developed it in 1884, Christian Gram. It distinguishes between the two main types of bacteria, Gram-negative and Gram-positive, by exposing the cells to two dyes – gentian violet and safranin. Gram-positive cells have thick, mesh-like cell walls, which take up the gentian violet and they therefore appear blue under the microscope. Gram-negative bacteria have much thinner cell walls, which do not absorb the blue dye but appear red under the microscope after counterstaining with safranin.

easily and Gram-positive organisms are therefore relatively sensitive to these agents. Proteins can also pass out of the cell through the peptidoglycan and some Gram-positive bacteria are able to secrete enzymes, called exotoxins, which cause damage to the tissues of the host. Gram-positive bacteria are also susceptible to enzymes that attack the cell wall, such as the lysozyme secreted in tears. This enzyme weakens areas of the cell wall, causing the cell membrane to bulge through and the cell to break open. The thick layer of peptidoglycan has advantages for resisting the immune system of the host because it prevents the complement complex of the immune system from reaching the cytoplasmic membrane (Chs 2 and 4).

Gram-negative bacteria
These have more complicated cell walls. The layer of peptidoglycan is quite thin, is not attached to the cytoplasmic membrane and is surrounded by an outer membrane made up of proteins, phospholipids and lipopolysaccharide (LPS). The LPS of all Gram-negative bacteria is toxic to mammals and it is responsible for many of the symptoms associated with infection by these bacteria. In particular, it is pyrogenic (stimulates the hypothalamus to cause a fever), it decreases the number of white cells in the blood, causes local tissue damage by activating the complement system and causes widespread coagulation of the blood by activating the clotting system. Patients with serious infection caused by Gram-negative bacteria can develop serious abnormalities in the circulatory system including vasoconstriction (chills) followed by vasodilatation, impaired blood circulation, shock, organ damage and acidosis. Because the LPS is not secreted by the cell but is part of its structure, it is known as an endotoxin. The basic structure of LPS is similar in all Gram-negative bacteria but variation occurs in the polysaccharide side chains. The differences can be detected by serological techniques and are an important part of the identification and classification of Gram-negative bacteria.

Nutrients travel through channels formed by the porin proteins whilst other proteins are involved in actively transporting larger nutrient molecules into the cell. The lipids in the outer membrane are not easily penetrated by hydrophobic (water-hating) molecules and Gram-negative bacteria are therefore often able to grow in solutions of detergents that would rapidly destroy Gram-positive bacteria. They are also more resistant to penetration by a variety of other harmful substances such as antibiotics, phenols and dyes, but with a much thinner layer of peptidoglycan are less able to withstand a dry environment.

Capsules

Many bacteria secrete a layer of gelatinous material around the cell. This can be either loosely associated with the cell, in which case it is referred to as slime, or adhere strongly to the cell surface, when it is called a capsule. The structure and composition of the capsule can vary widely, even between different members of the same species. Capsules are an important determinant of the virulence of the bacteria, protecting the cell from phagocytosis and enabling it to adhere to hard surfaces such as teeth and intravascular devices.

Endospores

These are highly resistant casings that form around the cell and allow it to remain in a dormant state for prolonged periods. The casing is made of a thick layer of peptidoglycan surrounded by a very tough protein similar to keratin. These layers are extremely resistant to chemicals or physical disruption and will even survive in boiling water for a long time. They cannot be destroyed by most disinfectants, but will be killed by exposure to high-pressure steam in an autoclave. Spores are formed by some bacteria in response to a poor nutrient supply or other adverse conditions. Most bacteria that are able to form spores live in soil and the only ones that are significant pathogens in humans are from the genera *Bacillus* (e.g. *Bacillus cereus*, which is a cause of food poisoning) and *Clostridium* (e.g. *Clostridium perfringens*, the cause of gas gangrene). Spores will germinate in response to an improvement in environmental conditions such as a supply of nutrients or the presence of moisture.

> Bacteria can secrete protective capsules or form spores which make them very resistant to the normal defensive mechanisms of the body.

Flagella

These are hollow filaments, usually several times longer than the cell. They move the cell by acting like a rotating propeller. Bacteria use flagella to swim towards concentrations of nutrients or away from repellent chemicals in a process called chemotaxis. Different species of bacteria have a different number and arrangement of flagella around the cell. For example, *Pseudomonas* has a single flagellum, whilst *Proteus* has over 100. Flagella are found on both Gram-positive and Gram-negative cells, on half of the bacilli and nearly all spirilla, but rarely on cocci.

Fimbriae or pili

These are filaments on the surface of the cell but are thinner and shorter than flagella. Their purpose is to enable the cell to adhere to other cells. They are only found on Gram-negative bacteria and are an important factor determining the ability of an organism to cause disease. Different strains of the same organisms can carry fimbriae that are able to adhere to different types of tissue and therefore determine the type of infection caused by the bacteria. Special fimbriae called sex pili are used to join two cells for the exchange of genetic information in a process called conjugation.

Chromosome

As with eucaryotic cells, this is composed of DNA (Ch. 2) and provides the blueprint of the cell, determining both its activity and ability to replicate itself. Unlike eucaryotic cells, the chromosome in bacterial cells is not contained in a nucleus surrounded by a nuclear membrane, but simply lies within a nuclear region. Some bacteria, such as *Escherichia coli*, only have one chromosome whereas others have more than one. When the cell divides, chromosomes are attached to the cytoplasmic membrane and as the membrane grows they are segregated into each daughter cell. In bacteria, the genes coding for a particular set of proteins are all arranged together along the chromosome. This is necessary because, unlike in eucaryotes, the mRNA copied from the DNA is not rearranged before being translated into protein. The clusters of genes coding for a particular function are called operons and their transcription is regulated by a single control region on the chromosome which coordinates the production of different proteins as they are required by the cell.

> Bacteria only have one chromosome but can also carry other pieces of genetic information called plasmids which can be passed to other bacteria.

Plasmids

Many bacteria carry additional genetic information which is not part of the chromosome and not necessary for the cell to grow. These occur as small, circular pieces of double-stranded DNA of varying size and gene content called plasmids and most bacteria have between one and six. Often they contain genetic information that enables the cell to inactivate antimicrobial agents but can also carry factors that increase the virulence of the cell, facilitate adhesion (e.g. fimbriae) or damage tissues (e.g. enterotoxins, a cause of gastroenteritis, or exotoxins such as those that cause the symptoms associated with tetanus and botulism).

Plasmids can be transferred between cells of the same, or different, species and genetic information can also be exchanged between different plasmids. Some plasmids are 'self-transmissible', which means that part of their genetic information codes for sex pili and DNA transfer enzymes.

Ribosomes

Proteins are synthesised on the ribosomes (Ch. 4). These are smaller than those in eucaryotic cells and are liberally distributed throughout the cytoplasm.

Growth and cell division

Unlike higher eucaryotic cells, which can take between 8 and 24 h to divide, the simpler cell structure of bacteria enables them to divide in less than 30 min.

Bacteria, supplied with all the nutrients they need, will grow and divide at this rate until the supply of nutrients is exhausted or the environmental conditions become unfavourable. The ability of bacteria to multiply rapidly enables them to respond easily to changes in their environment.

To grow and divide, bacterial cells must be able to obtain all the molecules necessary to make up the cell. Many bacteria can synthesise a large proportion of their cell constituents and can therefore grow in very simple media containing only carbon sources and inorganic ions. Other bacteria cannot synthesise all their cell components and require a source of specific amino acids or vitamins. There are a few substances that are essential to support the growth of all microorganisms, in particular carbon, nitrogen and inorganic ions.

Carbon source

Carbon is necessary both as a source of energy and to make compounds that from the structure of the cell. Energy is captured by breaking down organic carbon containing compounds such as carbohydrates (Box 13.4). However, almost any source of carbon can be used by bacteria, including substances as diverse as wood, phenols and hydrocarbons. Some bacteria are able to obtain carbon from carbon dioxide in the atmosphere and use chlorophyll to capture the energy of the sun in the same way as plants.

BOX 13.4   *Respiration and Fermentation*

Catabolism is the breakdown of organic substances such as carbohydrates to release energy. Electrons generated as part of this process are passed along a transport chain, the energy released as a result of the reactions is stored in the form of adenosine triphosphate (ATP) and the electrons are ultimately passed to an electron-accepting compound. Where catabolism of the organic energy source occurs by respiration, the final electron acceptor is an inorganic compound, usually oxygen. A few strict anaerobes use another inorganic compound, such as nitrogen or sulphur, as the final electron acceptor.

Catabolism can also occur by fermentation, although it is a far less efficient method of producing energy than respiration. In fermentation, organic compounds are used as the source of energy as well as the final electron acceptor. The end product of the process can be lactic acid, acetic acid, ethanol, acetone, glycerol and a wide variety of other compounds. Fermentation is used as a method of generating ATP by many strict anaerobes. Most facultative anaerobes switch from respiration to fermentation in the absence of air, although some, notably lactobacilli, always use fermentation regardless of the presence of air.

The byproducts of fermentation have important uses in industry, such as brewing beer, production of vinegar, yoghurt and cheese and antibiotics, e.g. penicillin.

Nitrogen source

Nitrogen is needed to make proteins, nucleic acids and other components of the cell. A few bacteria can convert atmospheric nitrogen into ammonia and incorporate this into the cell. Others use inorganic sources such as nitrates or ammonia. Most pathogenic species are less versatile and need a source of organic nitrogen such as the amino acids glutamine, asparganine or arginine.

Inorganic ions

All organisms require phosphate, which is both a component of lipids and nucleic acids and is also used to store energy in the form of ATP. Many other ions are required to make amino acids, e.g. sulphur, or to act as co-factors for enzymes, e.g. magnesium, sodium and calcium. Iron is a growth requirement of all organisms as it is an important consistent of many enzymes and other proteins. In eucaryotes, iron is bound to proteins such as lactoferrin in milk or ferritin in liver. In solution, iron usually forms large complexes which cannot be absorbed into the cell and bacteria and fungi excrete iron chelators which can extract iron from these complexes.

The cytoplasmic membrane controls which substances pass into the cell; smaller molecules such as sugars and amino acids can pass through easily by simple diffusion, provided that their concentration is higher outside the cell than inside. Where this is not the case, carrier proteins or active transport mechanisms are used to carry the required molecules into the cell. Larger molecules may be present in the tissues or body fluids of their host but are too big to pass through the membrane. To facilitate this process, microorganisms frequently secrete enzymes into their environment to digest proteins, polysaccharides and lipids into smaller compounds, which can then be absorbed and used by the cell. These extracellular enzymes can be an important feature of the ability of an organism to invade a host.

Environmental conditions

The rate at which bacteria grow is also affected by environmental conditions, particularly temperature, oxygen supply and pH (Ch. 1). Clean, dry surfaces are unlikely to support the growth of microorganisms but they will survive and multiply happily in old solutions of disinfectants, poorly cleaned equipment and buckets of dirty mop water.

Temperature

Pathogenic bacteria are all mesophiles, i.e. they grow at temperatures between 10°C and 45°C and grow best when the temperature is between 20°C and 40°C. They are therefore ideally suited for growth and multiplication at body temperature. This range of temperatures is important when it comes to managing food safely. Thorough cooking will destroy pathogenic bacteria and provided the food is then kept at temperatures either above 60°C or below 10°C, any mesophilic bacteria left in it cannot multiply. Bacteria are very adaptable and can grow in environments where no other organism could survive. Thermophilic bacteria are adapted to temperatures of between 25°C and 100°C and can be isolated from compost heaps, hot springs and volcanic thermal vents.

Some bacteria can survive at a much wider range of temperature and pH than cells of the body.

pH

Microorganisms can be found in environments with almost any pH but each species will have an optimum pH for growth. Most grow best at neutral or slightly alkaline pH (7.0–7.4), although many fungi will grow at a pH of 4. The cell cannot maintain the internal pH in its cytoplasm when the gradient between the inside and outside of the cell is more than 2 or 3 units.

In the body, pH can provide a means of protecting against invasion by harmful microorganisms. In the stomach the normally acidic pH will kill many pathogens that might be ingested, whilst in the vagina a pH of between 4 and 5 is maintained as a result of the lactic acid produced by the normal flora of lactobacilli, discouraging the growth of other organisms.

Osmolarity

Microorganisms need moisture to grow but the concentration of solutes in the medium affects their rate of growth. In solutions with a high osmolarity the cell has to accumulate a large number of ions to maintain its internal osmolarity and above a certain osmolarity the cells will be destroyed. Concentrated solutions of salt and sugar have been used as a means of food preservation for centuries.

Oxygen

Bacteria can be classified according to their ability to grow in the presence of oxygen. Those that can make enzymes such as catalase, which can deal with the highly reactive and toxic byproducts of the respiration process, can grow in the presence of oxygen and are called aerobes. Obligate aerobes use respiration in their metabolism and therefore require oxygen to grow, e.g. pseudomonads and mycobacteria. Obligate anaerobes do not possess catalase and use fermentation, rather than respiration, as a means of energy production, e.g. *Clostridium* species. Many are extremely sensitive to oxygen and will die rapidly if exposed to air and special methods are therefore needed to isolate them from clinical specimens. Clostridia are normally found in human faeces and soil. They may contaminate up to 40% of septic wounds but are only able to cause severe infections, such as gas gangrene, in large necrotic wounds with a poor blood supply and heavily contaminated with dirt. For this reason such infections are usually only seen in serious injuries associated with road traffic accidents or in extensive war wounds. *Bacteroides fragilis* is another anaerobe that thrives in human intestines and can cause intra-abdominal abscesses where trauma or surgery has resulted in the contents of the intestine contaminating the peritoneal cavity.

Facultative anaerobes such as enteric bacteria and staphylococci can grow either with or without oxygen and can change their metabolic pathways in response to the conditions. Some species, e.g. streptococci and lactobacilli, use fermentation rather than respiration to derive energy but can survive in the presence of oxygen, although they will grow best where it is present in low levels.

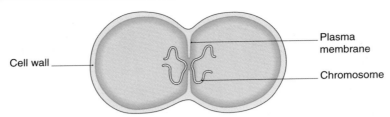

Fig. 13.5 *Binary fission in prokaryotic cells. The chromosome replicates and the daughter copy is separated into a new cell by the growth of plasma membrane between them.*

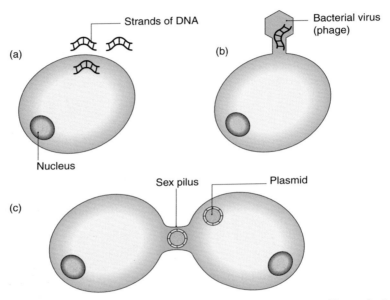

Fig. 13.6 *Methods used by bacteria to exchange genetic information. (a) Transformation; (b) transduction; (c) conjugation.*

Cell division

Prokaryotic cells multiply by simply dividing into two in a process called binary fission (Fig. 13.5). The chromosome is replicated and the cell wall and cytoplasmic membrane grow inwards to form a new cell wall across the inside of the cell.

Exchange of genetic information

In bacteria, exchange of genetic information does not occur by the fusion of two haploid cells as occurs in eucaryotic organisms. Instead, small fragments of the genome can be exchanged between bacteria of the same or different species in three ways (Fig. 13.6).

Transformation
Fragments of DNA released from bacterial cells, which have lysed and released

their contents into the medium, are absorbed into the cell. DNA can only be absorbed by cells with appropriate structures on their surface to enable the DNA to bind to and then enter the cell. Generally only DNA obtained from closely related species will be expressed.

Conjugation

DNA is transferred from one cell to another via a special tube called a sex pili which forms between them. The plasmid DNA in the donor cell replicates and one copy is sent into the recipient cell. The genetic information necessary to make the sex pili and DNA transfer proteins are carried on some plasmids and conjugation can therefore only occur where a cell carries one of these plasmids.

Transduction

DNA can be introduced into the cell by a bacterial virus (bacteriophage). Sometimes, part of the DNA of the host cell is copied by mistake during the replication of the virus genes. This host cell DNA is then taken out of the cell with the new viruses and the bacterial DNA incorporated into the genome of the next cell invaded by the bacteriophage.

Recombinant DNA techniques

A knowledge of how genetic information can be transferred between different bacteria has given rise to several specialised techniques which can be used for many purposes both in research and industry. A range of special enzymes called restriction endonucleases recognise specific sequences of bases in a strand of DNA. Using these enzymes it is possible to separate specific genes from a length of DNA, incorporate them into a plasmid and introduce the plasmid into a bacterial cell by conjugation or into a eucaryotic cell by other specialised techniques. The modern vaccine against hepatitis B has been made by introducing a plasmid carrying fragments of DNA from the virus into a yeast. The yeast produces viral proteins as it multiplies and these are purified to make the vaccine. Recombinant DNA techniques are also used to study the genes from all forms of life and to provide very rapid and specific tests for infectious agents based on the presence of specific DNA sequences found in particular species of microorganisms.

FUNGI

Fungi are eucaryotic organisms, similar to plants but without the green pigment chlorophyll. They range from large forms such as mushrooms and toadstools to microscopic moulds and yeasts. Of the 100 000 different species of fungi, only a few cause disease in humans. Most are found in soil and water where they play an important role in decomposing and recycling plant material. Like bacteria, they can use a wide variety of organic compounds as an energy source, using either respiration or fermentation for catabolism. Some produce toxins which have, rarely, been associated with food poisoning, e.g. aflatoxin.

Most fungi are harmless and some are even useful.

Structure of fungi

Most comprise a mass of cytoplasm with many nuclei, enclosed within a rigid branched system of tubes. This structure is called the mycelium; it cannot move but the cytoplasm can stream within the tubes.

Fungi reproduce asexually by forming and releasing spores from the tips of the branched tubes and each spore contains one or more nuclei. When the spore germinates, growth starts as a long thread called a hypha, which then branches to become the mycelium. Growth will continue indefinitely as long as a supply of nutrients is available; consequently, a large mass of mycelium can become visible. Many fungi have specialised spore-bearing structures above the surface (e.g. mushrooms), whilst the mycelium remains obscured under the ground or other structure.

Fungi are classified into several groups according to their structure and method of sexual reproduction. Some species have lost the mycelial form of growing and instead have become small, unicellular organisms. The generic term for these forms is yeasts and they are not confined to a single group of fungi; unicellular forms can be found across all the main groups of fungi. Yeasts multiply by forming buds on the side of the cell which gradually enlarge until the nucleus divides and a cross-wall forms between the two cells. They can also reproduce sexually by dividing by meiosis and forming two haploid daughter cells. Most yeasts do not live in soil but are adapted to living in a high concentration of sugar, which they ferment. They are therefore commonly found on the surface of fruits and flowers and are widely exploited for fermentation processes.

Diseases caused by fungi include superficial infections of the skin, hair and nails (e.g. *Tinea pedia* (athlete's foot) and *Tinea corporis* (ringworm)), a range of infections caused by yeasts (e.g. oral and vaginal candidiasis), cryptococcus and serious, systemic infections often associated with an immunocompromised host, e.g. aspergillosis.

THE PROTOZOA

Protozoa are eucaryotic cells but are neither plants nor animals; instead, they are now thought to belong to a separate sub-kingdom. They are microscopic, single cells that can carry out most of the activities of other forms of higher life. Most are aquatic but some are obligate parasites of animals and they occur in a wide variety of shapes and sizes.

Protozoan cell structure is very similar to that of other eucaryotes; they have a cytoplasmic membrane, one or two nuclei, mitochondria and structures to support their mobility, and they obtain nutrients by ingesting solid particles of food through a mouth-like opening. The food is then enclosed in a vacuole and digested by enzymes into soluble substances, which can then be transported into the cytoplasm of the cell. Undigested material is expelled from the cell when the vacuole breaks open on the surface. Under adverse conditions some protozoa can form cysts by secreting a protective coat around them. This often helps parasitic forms to survive outside the host until they are able to gain entry to a new host.

Protozoa generally reproduce asexually by dividing into two. Some can reproduce sexually and some have complex reproductive cycles involving several stages in the life cycle lived out in different hosts, such as plasmodium, the cause of malaria.

Protozoan cells are neither animal nor plant but they are eucaryotes and some, such as the malarial plasmodium, are harmful to humans.

VIRUSES

Viruses are quite different from any other type of microorganisms. They are not plants, animals or bacteria. In fact, they are not even a cell, but are a piece of genetic information wrapped in a coat of protein. With no organelles and no metabolism, they are intracellular parasites, entirely dependent on the host cell for their replication.

Viruses vary considerably in size but all are too small to be seen under a light microscope. Instead an electron microscope is used to identify them and study their structure (see Box 13.1). The outer protein coat or capsid is made from many identical subunits of polypeptide, formed into symmetrical shapes such as icosohedrals or spheres. The capsid protects the genetic information inside and provides a binding site to enable the virus to attach to specific receptors on the surface of the host cell. Some viruses have an outer lipid membrane or envelope, acquired from the host cell as the virus leaves by budding through the cell membrane. These envelopes have virus-specified glycoproteins on their surface, which the virus uses to attach to and enter a new host cell.

Viruses usually have only one molecule of nucleic acid, although some viruses have several fragments, and it can be either DNA or RNA, single or double stranded and linear or circular. Depending on the size of the virus the genetic information can code for between three to several hundred proteins (Fig. 13.7).

Not all cells carry receptors for all viruses and the presence of a particular receptor determines which cells are targeted by the virus. The human immuno-deficiency virus (HIV), for example, infects cells that carry the CD4 molecule on their surface. This molecule is mostly found on cells in the immune system such as the CD4+ helper T lymphocyte and macrophages. Cells without the receptor are resistant to invasion by the virus. When a virus infects a cell the whole virus enters through the cell membrane, the capsid is removed and the viral nucleic acid is released. The nucleic acid is transcribed and replicated in either the cyto-plasm or the nucleus of the host cell depending on the virus.

Viral replication

Although a few of the larger viruses carry genes coding for some of the proteins required for their replication, most viruses depend entirely on the mechanisms in the host cell for the transcription and translation of their genetic material. In DNA viruses, the genome is usually transcribed in sections. The early mRNAs make enzymes or other factors required for the regulation of the process and the transcription of the remaining viral genes. Some RNA viruses can be translated directly as mRNAs; others carry an enzyme to convert their RNA into mRNA

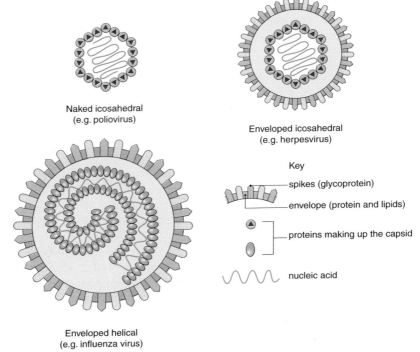

Naked icosahedral
(e.g. poliovirus)

Enveloped icosahedral
(e.g. herpesvirus)

Key

— spikes (glycoprotein)

— envelope (protein and lipids)

— proteins making up the capsid

nucleic acid

Enveloped helical
(e.g. influenza virus)

Fig. 13.7   *The shapes of viruses. The viruses of animals are naked or enveloped, icosahedral or helical. Poliovirus is a naked icosahedral virus, influenza an enveloped helical virus and herpes an enveloped icosahedral virus.*

once it has been released from the protein coat. Retroviruses have a genome made of RNA, which must first be transcribed into DNA before the corresponding mRNA can be made. This is catalysed by a polymerase enzyme called reverse transcriptase, which is carried by the virus and activated once the protein coat has been removed.

> Viruses cannot survive and replicate on their own. Viruses contain protein and either an RNA or DNA genome. The RNA has to be transcribed into host DNA before it can be replicated.

Once the viral proteins have been synthesised, they are assembled in either the cytoplasm or the nucleus and the nucleic acid is then inserted. Enveloped viruses are released by budding through the cell membrane; other viruses are released by lysis of the cell (Fig. 13.8).

Growth requirements

Because viruses depend on living cells for their replication, it is not possible to culture them in conventional nutrient media in the same way as bacteria. Eucaryotic cells can be grown artificially in culture by immersing them in a

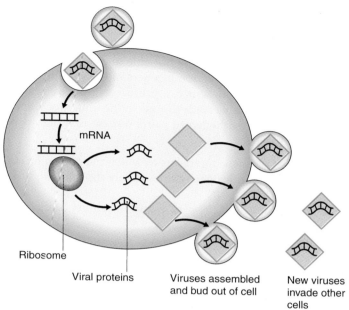

Fig. 13.8   *Replication of a virus within a host cell. The virus enters the host cell and its genome moves to a ribosome where it is transcribed, to make many copies of viral proteins and nucleic acids. The protein coats and genomes are assembled and then bud out of the cell, collecting part of the cell membrane of the host cell on the way out.*

Ribosome

Viral proteins

mRNA

Viruses assembled and bud out of cell

New viruses invade other cells

medium containing essential amino acids, vitamins, salts, sugars and serum and these cell cultures can then be used to support the replication of most viruses.

RELATIONSHIPS BETWEEN MICROBES AND MAN

Of the hundreds of different species of microorganisms, only a small proportion cause disease in humans. The surfaces of the body are populated by a variety of microorganisms, with the number and type of species varying according to the local conditions of nutrient supply, oxygen level and temperature. These microbes are described as commensals because they do not harm their host. Indeed, they can be of considerable benefit, for example by preventing the surface being occupied by other more harmful species.

Infection occurs when microorganisms invade the body, multiply and cause damage to the tissues. The infection can be recognised by the presence of both localised and systemic symptoms such as inflammation, pain and fever. Microorganisms that cause disease are called pathogens. Recognition of these clinical signs of infection is important because even pathogens can live on the body without invading the tissues to cause infection, and their presence in a microbiological specimen is not necessarily indicative of infection in the absence of any symptoms. Some commensals can become pathogenic if they are transferred from their normal location on the body to another vulnerable site. For example, *Escherichia coli* is part of the normal flora of the intestine but it will cause a urinary tract infection should it gain access to the bladder from the perineum. Hospital patients are particularly vulnerable to infection by commensal organisms on the skin, e.g. *Staphylococcus aureus*, because the normal defences against infection are commonly breached by invasive procedures such as surgery or devices such as intravascular catheters. Some pathogens are described as opportunistic because they are not able to cause disease in normal, healthy people, but can establish infection in a person with an impaired immune system: for example, *Pneumocystis carinii*, a protozoan that is commonly found in the respiratory tract but only causes disease in the immunocompromised.

The ability of a pathogen to cause disease in a host depends on several factors, in particular:

- the number of microorganisms to which the person has been exposed (the greater the infectious dose the less likely the immune system will be able to repel the attack)
- the general health of the person and the ability of their immune system to respond to the invaders
- the ability of the organism to cause disease, referred to as its virulence.

Virulence

Many factors contribute to the virulence of an organism and in the case of bacteria this may vary between strains of the same species according to which plasmids the cells contain. The ability of bacteria to cause infection in a particular host or particular type of tissue depends on their adherence to the surface of cells. In Gram-negative bacteria, adhesion is mediated by fimbriae. Adhesion prevents the bacteria from being washed away, for example by urine in the urinary tract or peristalsis in the gastrointestinal tract. Adhesion is extremely specific; a particular species of bacteria will only be able to recognise and bind to types of tissue that carry specific carbohydrate markers on their surface. They may only be able to bind with that tissue in a limited number of animals and this will dictate the host range of a particular infection. Bacteria that can adhere to cells in the urinary tract, e.g. *Escherichia coli*, can cause infection there but on other tissue of the body, such as the respiratory tract, cannot adhere easily and are therefore unlikely to cause infection. Often pathogens are species specific, i.e. they can adhere to tissue in one animal but not others: for example, *Neisseria gonorrhoeae* can only adhere to cells of the human genital tract but not to cells in other types of tissue or the genital tract of other animals. This explains why gonorrhoea can only be transmitted by sexual contact between humans.

SUMMARY

Microbes are organisms so small that they can only be seen under a microscope, they inhabit a wide variety of environments and many have very important ecological functions. Some are able to cause disease by invading and adhering to tissue cells. Hospital patients are particularly vulnerable to infection because their normal host defences are commonly breached by invasive procedures or devices.

Bacteria are prokaryotic cells; they have a very simple structure with the cytoplasmic membrane performing many of the functions of the cell. Their cell walls contain a unique substance called peptidoglycan and some can form a highly resistant wall called a spore, which enables them to survive in adverse conditions. Bacteria reproduce by simply dividing in two. In conditions where there is an ample supply of nutrients, a bacterial cell can divide in less than 30 min. They can exchange their genetic material between cells and this is commonly associated with the acquisition of resistance to antimicrobial agents. Fungi are also microscopic cells but are more similar to plants. They form branched tubes called mycelium and reproduce by forming spores. Protozoa are single eucaryotic cells and occur in a variety of forms. They obtain nutrients by ingesting solid particles of food and can survive in adverse conditions by forming cysts. Viruses are not like plants, animals or bacteria but are simply DNA or RNA wrapped in a coat of protein. They are entirely dependent on host cells for their replication.

QUESTIONS

1. What are the main features of prokaryotic cells which differ from eukaryotic cells?

2. How are some microorganisms able to withstand extremes of environment such as cold, dehydration and heat?

3. How are RNA viruses able to reproduce?

FURTHER READING

Wilson J (1995) *Infection control in clinical practice.* Baillière Tindall, London

14 Protection

Jennie Wilson

After reading this chapter you should be able to:
- understand how the body is protected and what it needs protection from
- know how specific and non-specific protection differ
- explain how immunisation works.

INTRODUCTION

The body has a range of mechanisms that enable it to protect itself against harmful microorganisms or foreign substances (antigens) and these are also an important part of the process of repair that follows tissue injury. Antigens are molecules recognised as non-self by the cells of the immune system. They can be small or large molecules, complex proteins or carbohydrates, or entire microorganisms. Some of the defences are non-specific, i.e. they do not recognise a particular microorganism but have the same general effect against any antigen. These include the physical barriers that protect the portals of entry to the body, and the internal cellular responses of phagocytic cells and the complement proteins. The immune system is also able to make a specific response to particular microorganisms or antigens it has encountered before. This is achieved through the production of two types of white blood cell or lymphocyte: the B lymphocytes, which recognise a particular antigen and produce specific immunoglobulins (antibodies) that bind to it; and the T lymphocytes, which both coordinate the activity of the different components of the response and deal with host cells that have been invaded by microorganisms. Microorganisms and other antigens are removed by phagocytic cells, which ingest and digest them. Different components of the immune response act in concert, facilitating and promoting the actions of each other.

The defences of the body can be divided into those which are non-specific and those which are specific. The non-specific defences act each time the body is invaded by a foreign body and the specific defences, which are triggered by specific foreign bodies, act on subsequent invasions by foreign bodies encountered previously.

NON-SPECIFIC DEFENCES AGAINST INFECTION

External defences

The first line of defence against invasion by harmful microorganisms is the

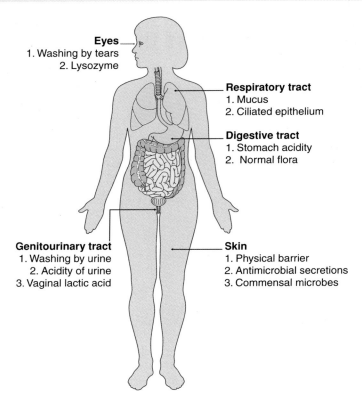

Fig. 14.1 *External defences to invasion by microorganisms.*

body's mechanisms for preventing their access in the first place (Fig. 14.1). The most important of these is skin, which, when intact, cannot be penetrated by microorganisms, but if sections are destroyed, for example following burns, this can give rise to serious infection. In addition to providing a physical barrier, the skin presents a hostile environment for many potential pathogens. Lactic acid and fatty acids in secretions from sebaceous glands generate a low pH on its surface, which will prevent the survival of many species. Harmless bacteria, which normally live on the skin, e.g. diphtheroids and staphylococci, thrive in these conditions and discourage colonisation by other species.

The normal microbial flora of the intestinal tract and vagina protect these surfaces against invasion. These microorganisms prevent the growth of many potential pathogens by competing for the available nutrients or by producing inhibitory substances. The lactobacilli in the vagina produce lactic acid as a byproduct of their metabolism; this gives rise to a local pH of between 4 and 5, which is sufficiently low to prevent the growth of many other species. Antimicrobial therapy can disrupt these defences by killing the normal flora and allowing it to be replaced by other pathogenic species, such as *Candida* in the vagina and *Clostridium difficile* in the gut.

Many of the secretions that bathe mucous membranes contain antibacterial substances. Tears, nasal secretions and saliva contain lysozyme, an enzyme that breaks down bacterial cells. Gastric juices are highly acidic and the resulting pH of between 2 and 3 destroys most ingested microorganisms; bile in the small intestine also inhibits bacterial growth.

Microorganisms cannot invade the body unless they are able to adhere to the host's cells. Mucus secreted by the membranes lining the inner surfaces of the body provides a barrier against adherence. In the respiratory tract, microorganisms trapped in this mucus are gradually expelled from the tract by the action of cilia, which move them back towards the mouth where they can be swallowed. Hairs in the nose that filter out larger particles, together with the cough reflex, prevent most microorganisms from entering into the bronchial tree. Adherence to other mucosal surfaces is prevented by washing with fluids such as urine, saliva or tears.

Internal defences

If microorganisms do penetrate the external defences, the body has several non-specific responses that are intended to confine the invaders and to destroy as many of them as possible.

Phagocytic cells

Phagocytosis is a process by which invading antigens are ingested by white blood cells (Fig. 14.2). It occurs when a microbe adheres to the surface of the phagocytic cell, triggering pseudopodia to form around it and rapidly enclose it in a vacuole. Enzymes are then discharged into the vacuole to kill and digest the microbe. There are two basic types of phagocytic cell: the polymorphonuclear neutrophil (PMN) and the macrophage.

PMNs are leucocytes derived from stem cells in the bone marrow (Fig. 14.3). They are the main white cells in the bloodstream, they do not divide and only circulate in the blood for 6–8 h. They have a nucleus divided into several segments and contain large numbers of granules, which store the range of enzymes used to attack and destroy the microorganisms that they ingest. They have high-affinity receptors for both complement proteins (C3b) and antibodies (immunoglobulins) and are able to attach to microorganisms that have been coated by these molecules.

Macrophages are concentrated in the lung, connective tissues and around small blood vessels. They are also present in the linings of the spleen and lymph

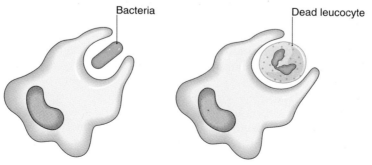

Fig. 14.2 *The process of phagocytosis.*

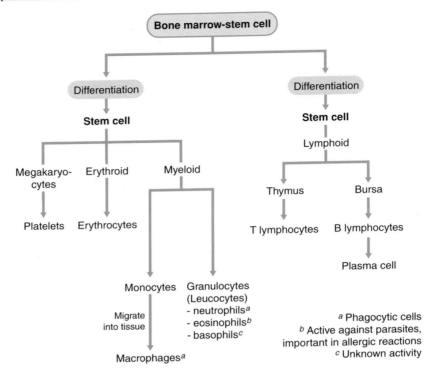

Fig. 14.3   *Differentiation of blood cells.*

nodes where they can filter out foreign material as it circulates through the lymph system. Macrophages are derived from stem cells in the bone marrow (Fig. 14.3) but unlike the neutrophils, they are long-lived. They are particularly important for attacking chronic infections and microorganisms that are capable of living inside the cells of their host. They secrete enzymes that increase the permeability of blood vessels, enabling them to pass through into the tissues, and contain lysozyme and peroxidases to digest ingested microorganisms. Some microorganisms, e.g. tubercle bacilli, are phagocytosed but can prevent these enzymes being released and continue to multiply within the macrophage. In tuberculosis, infected macrophages congregate into a nodule, called a tubercle, which becomes surrounded by connective tissue.

Macrophages ingest and process the microorganisms and then present them to the T and B lymphocytes, which are involved in the specific immune response. Phagocytic cells are attracted to the site of infection by a variety of chemotactic factors, including products from bacterial cells, damaged tissue cells, antigen–antibody complexes and complement proteins. Their activity is stimulated by the T lymphocytes.

Complement

The process of phagocytosis is dependent on microorganisms adhering to the phagocytic cell; this is facilitated by a complex set of about 20 proteins called complement. These proteins are involved in a series of reactions, with the product of one reaction catalysing the next (Fig. 14.4). The outcome of these reac-

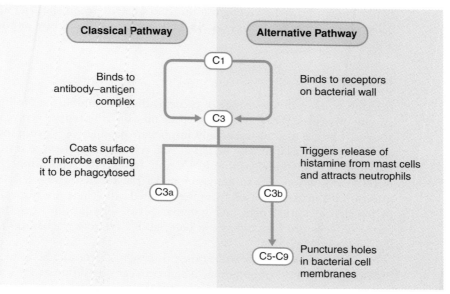

Fig. 14.4   *The complement cascade. The first complement protein (C1) can be activated in two ways to form an enzyme which splits the C3 protein into C3a and C3b. A series of catalytic reactions then convert C3b from C5 through to C9 to form a membrane attack complex.*

tions is to produce a large number of protein molecules known as C3b, which coat the surface of the invading microorganism. Phagocytic cells have receptors for these molecules and can bind to and ingest the coated microorganisms. In addition, other proteins in the series form a complex that attacks the membrane of the microbe, puncturing a hole in it and causing fluid and enzymes to flood in and lyse the cell. Complement can be triggered by encountering an antibody–antigen complex but an alternative pathway of reactions can also be triggered by a complement protein binding directly to the surface of some microorganisms.

Eosinophils

Large microorganisms such as parasitic protozoa and helminths cannot be phagocytosed and, instead, are attacked by granular polymorphonuclear cells, similar to neutrophils, called eosinophils. These cells recognise the C3b complement molecules deposited on the surface of the parasite and are triggered to release enzymes that attack its membrane.

Natural killer cells

These are large granular lymphocytes, which, although similar to the B and T lymphocytes, do not react to specific antigens. They monitor the body for malignant cells and parasites, which they bind to and destroy by releasing the contents of their granules into the space between them and the target cell. The granules contain lysosomal enzymes and proteins such as perforin, which, like complement, can punch holes in cell membranes. The activity of natural killer cells (NK cells) seems to be enhanced by lymphokines, such as interferon, but it is not known how they recognise target cells. Other non-specific killer cells (K cells) work in the same way as NK cells but are activated by antibody-coated antigens.

Interferon

Interferons are a diverse range of proteins that can inhibit the proliferation of a variety of viruses. They are produced by all cells when they become infected by a virus, but are also an especially important product of T lymphocytes. They bind to specific receptors on neighbouring cells, causing them to start producing enzymes that degrade viral mRNA and inhibit its replication by reducing mRNA translation. These activities make the neighbouring cells resistant to infection by viruses released from the infected cell. There are three main classes of interferon: alpha, beta and gamma. Most cells produce interferon alpha, epithelial cells produce interferon beta, and T lymphocytes and NK cells produce interferon gamma.

Interferons also have a wide range of other effects on the immune system, providing a method of communication between the different cells and coordinating their response. They help to switch on the cell-mediated part of the immune response operated by T lymphocytes, when intracellular pathogens invade the body or malignant or foreign cells are encountered. At the same time, they appear to switch off antibody production by B lymphocytes, which are more effective against pathogens that multiply outside cells. They are particularly important for macrophage activity, stimulating them to degrade microorganisms they have ingested and display their antigens on their surface ready for recognition by T lymphocytes.

In recent years the ability of interferons to mobilise an immune response against tumour cells has been recognised and they are being used to treat hairy cell leukaemia and Kaposi's sarcoma, with clinical trials being conducted for many other types of cancer. They are also used to treat some chronic viral infections, e.g. hepatitis B and C, and autoimmune disease, e.g. certain forms of multiple sclerosis. Unfortunately, interferon therapy is associated with severe, flu-like side-effects and bone marrow suppression but potentiating their effect by using them in combination with other drugs may overcome some of these problems.

SPECIFIC IMMUNE RESPONSE

The complement system and phagocytic cells are not able to deal with all invaders. Complement proteins cannot attach to the surface of many bacteria and some microorganisms have developed mechanisms to avoid phagocytosis. To overcome these problems the body has another component in its array of defences – the antibody. Antibodies are molecules that can stick to any microorganism by recognising specific structures on their surface. Antibodies are made by B lymphocytes; these circulate in the bloodstream and tissue fluids and are called the humoral (meaning 'of body fluids') immune system. A second type of lymphocyte, the T lymphocytes, are also able to recognise specific antigens and play a crucial role in destroying infected host cells and abnormal tumour cells

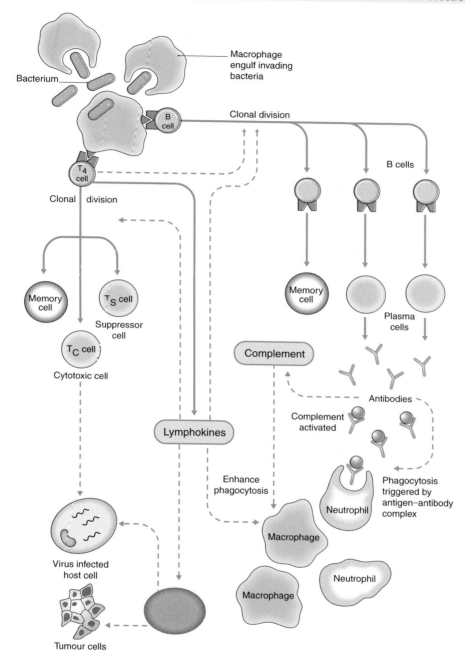

Fig. 14.5 *The specific immune response. The B cells, T cells and macrophages all interact to fend off the attack from invading microorganisms.*

and in coordinating the activity of other parts of the immune response. They are called the cell-mediated immune system. The interactions between the various parts of the immune system are illustrated in Figure 14.5.

The specific defences of the body work through cellular systems and through antibodies but both are specific to foreign bodies and both involve the lymphocytes.

Antibodies

Antibodies are Y-shaped proteins called immunoglobulins. They have three distinct regions as part of their structure: one region attaches to complement, activating the cascade of reactions, another region is recognised by phagocytes and a third region sticks to an antigen. The first two regions are in the stem of the Y and are the same in every type of antibody; the third region is on the two arms of the Y and varies from antibody to antibody, enabling each to attach to different antigens.

A specific antibody is needed for each of the many thousands of antigens that might be encountered. Antibodies are able to attach to a specific antigen because they have complementary shapes, and are able to fit together rather like a lock and key. Once close enough, the antigen is held to the antibody by a range of electrostatic forces such as hydrogen bonds (Ch. 1), van der Waals forces and hydrophobic bonds. These are relatively weak bonds so that the attachment can be readily reversed.

Antibodies are made by B lymphocytes. Each B lymphocyte is programmed at the time they are made to make a unique antibody; this is displayed on the outer surface of the lymphocyte, acting as a receptor for passing antigens. Antigens may be bacteria or viruses that are circulating in the blood or tissue fluids, toxins or other foreign substances. An antigen will bind to the antibody that fits its shape most effectively. If an antigen does bind with the receptor, this triggers the lymphocyte to convert into an antibody-forming plasma cell, which can secrete large quantities of antibody identical to the one that acted as the receptor on the original lymphocyte. The plasma cells then divide rapidly to accumulate a supply of identical plasma cells, called clones, all producing the same antibody. This means that large amounts of antibody can be produced to combat a specific infection without the need to store large numbers of each type of plasma cell in the blood.

When an antibody binds to the surface of a microorganism it activates the first protein in the complement system; when a second antibody attaches, it triggers phagocytic cells to ingest the microorganism. B lymphocytes need to be able to coordinate their activity with T lymphocytes. They do this by having surface receptors for lymphokines, which are proteins released by T lymphocytes.

Classes of immunoglobulin

There are five main classes of immunoglobulin and these can be distinguished by their structure: IgG, IgM, IgA, IgD and IgE. Each type can be produced by the same B lymphocyte and recognise the same antigen, but they have slightly different roles in the immune response (Table 14.1). IgM is the first immunoglobulin to be produced by a plasma cell; after a few days the same plasma cell starts to produce IgG instead. This switch is triggered by the activity of T lymphocytes.

TABLE 14.1	Types of Immunoglobulin	
	Immunoglobulin	Activity
	IgG	The most abundant type of immunoglobulin, it is able to diffuse from blood vessels into tissue fluids and cross the placenta in the last 3 months of pregnancy. It coats bacteria, facilitating phagocytosis and neutralising toxins
	IgM	This large immunoglobulin molecule is the first to appear in the immune response, but is confined to the blood. It assists phagocytosis by coating the antigen and binds with complement very efficiently
	IgA	This immunoglobulin is found in the secretions of the respiratory, reproductive and gastrointestinal tracts where it coats microorganisms and prevents them adhering to the epithelial cells
	IgE	This is mainly found attached to mast cells. If it encounters an antigen it triggers the release of histamine from the mast cell. It is associated with allergic response, e.g. hay fever, but is also thought to be involved in the destruction of parasites
	IgD	Maximum levels of this immunoglobulin are detected during childhood but its exact function is unknown

At birth the only antibodies present in the infant have been acquired from the maternal circulation; they are all IgG because this is the only immunoglobulin that can cross the placenta. Soon after birth, the infant begins to synthesise its own antibody so that by the time it is 1 year old it will be carrying adult levels of IgM. Adult levels of IgG will not be reached until between 5 and 7 years and IgA at between 10 and 12 years.

T lymphocytes

The T lymphocytes, derived from the thymus, are the second part of the specific immune response. Their role is to coordinate the immune response, being responsible for triggering and enhancing the activity of both B lymphocytes and macrophages. They also act as a form of surveillance against tumour cells, and play a major part in attacking microorganisms that are replicating inside cells of their host. Some microorganisms are intracellular parasites and can only replicate inside host cells, e.g. viruses; others are taken up by macrophages but multiply inside where they are protected from attack by antibodies, e.g. mycobacteria.

> The B lymphocytes are responsible for the production of antibodies and the T lymphocytes are responsible for destroying infected and tumour cells.

There are two types of T lymphocyte: the helper T cells regulate the activity of other cells and cytotoxic T cells which destroy infected cells and tumour cells. To effect these actions, T lymphocytes have to be able to distinguish healthy body cells from ones infected by microorganisms. They do this by recognising non-self antigens on the surface of infected cells. These antigens arrive on the surface of the cell because cells constantly degrade proteins into small peptide fragments. These fragments bind to molecules called the major histocompatibility complex (MHC), which then carry them to the surface of the cell. Most of these peptides will belong to the body's own proteins and will be ignored by circulating T cells. When the MHC displays a non-self peptide derived from an invading microorganism, a circulating T lymphocyte locks onto the combination of MHC and non-self peptide. This ensures that the T cell only recognises antigens that are on the surface of a body cell.

In the same way as B lymphocytes, each T lymphocyte is programmed at the time they are made to make a unique surface receptor and therefore each will recognise a specific antigen that best fits its shape. Once a T lymphocyte has attached to the two molecules, the antigen-presenting cell releases a soluble protein called interleukin, a lymphokine which activates the T lymphocyte to release other lymphokines and to divide rapidly to produce a large population of T lymphocytes all carrying the same surface receptor. Cytotoxic T lymphocytes are triggered to destroy the target cell by releasing lysosomal enzymes.

Lymphokines include a range of interleukins and interferon, which interact with other cells to coordinate the immune response. They attract macrophages to the site and increase macrophage antigen-presenting and killing activity. They also coordinate B lymphocyte activity, suppressing it if the invading organism is an intracellular pathogen and requires a cell-mediated response to attack it, but promoting B lymphocyte activity if the invasion is caused by a bacteria or bacterial toxin.

Memory lymphocytes

When both B and T lymphocytes are stimulated to divide, a proportion of the resulting cells become memory cells. These cells are primed to respond when the same antigen is encountered again, so that a large number of antigen-specific lymphocytes can be generated very rapidly. These cells protect against subsequent infection by the same pathogen and they are the reason why we can develop immunity after the first exposure to a particular infection. They also form the basis for immunisation as a means of protecting populations from infection by a wide range of infectious diseases (Ch. 13). The first time the body is exposed to a particular antigen, specific antibodies against it appear in measurable amounts in the blood after about 5 days, although the size of the response will depend on the type and amount of antigen. IgM will appear first and will be replaced after a few days by IgG. The levels of immunoglobulin peak after 2–3 weeks. As antigen is gradually removed, fewer lymphocytes are stimulated to produce antibody and the IgG (which has a half-life of 23 days)[1] is degraded.

A second exposure to the same antigen months or years later results in the immediate (within 1–3 days) appearance of specific antibodies and these are produced at a 10–15 times higher concentration than in the first response, even

---

[1]Half-life refers to the length of time taken for half of a substance to disappear from the body.

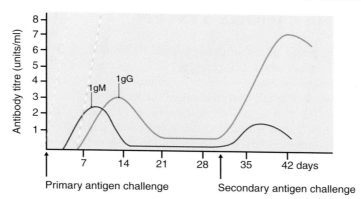

Fig. 14.6 *Primary and secondary antibody responses. In the primary response, IgM appears first. The secondary response is quicker and achieves higher antibody levels, mainly of IgG.*

if there is no detectable amount of antibody in the blood before the exposure to antigen. This rapid response is mediated by the memory B and T lymphocytes, which are able to stimulate IgG production almost immediately (Fig. 14.6).

> For both types of lymphocytes there are memory cells that respond rapidly to subsequent invasions of the body by specific foreign bodies.

INFLAMMATORY RESPONSE

Inflammation is the response, in the form of both vascular changes and cellular activity, made by the body to injury or invasion by a foreign substance. Cells damaged by injury or infection release prostaglandins, which increase the permeability of blood vessels in the area, allowing plasma proteins and white blood cells to pass through them into the tissues. IgE is firmly bound to mast cells and if the IgE encounters an antigen that fits its receptor, it triggers the release of granules from the mast cell. These contain vasoactive amines (Ch. 1), e.g. histamine, which stimulate local arterioles to dilate and the flow of blood to the area to be increased. These vascular changes cause the essential components of the immune response: phagocytic white blood cells, coagulation and complement proteins and lymphocytes to be concentrated in the area, confining and repelling the attack. Chemotactic substances released from dead cells and components of the complement system attract more immune cells to the area.

A dense mesh of fibrin is formed around the site of injury or invasion. This confines the infection, helping to prevent microorganisms escaping into other tissues. Killed bacterial cells, damaged tissue and white blood cells are liquefied by enzymes and form as pus. This can be absorbed by the tissues or discharged through the skin, but if it is trapped within the fibrin mesh it results in an abscess.

The visible signs of the inflammatory response can be seen on the surface of the skin following injury or after a surgical procedure; these include redness and heat caused by vasodilatation and swelling brought about by the influx of plasma and white blood cells. These effects may be accompanied by pain caused by pressure exerted by the swollen tissue on local nerve endings.

ORGANS OF THE IMMUNE SYSTEM

The response of the immune system to invaders is mounted from special lymphoid tissue, which is located in numerous parts of the body and particularly at points susceptible to invasion by microorganisms. These sites are connected by a network of small channels called the lymphatic system. Lymphocytes are recirculated from the blood to lymphoid tissues via these lymphatic channels. Lymphoid tissue is found in the liver, spleen, gut (Peyer's patches and appendix), tonsils and adenoids. It is also found in the lymph nodes, a series of small glands that occur at the junctions between lymph and blood vessels, which filter out and destroy circulating antigens.

The cells of the immune system originate from stem cells in the bone marrow (Ch. 9). They have a finite lifespan and therefore need to be constantly renewed. All types of blood cell originate from a single stem cell in the bone marrow, which undergoes several stages of differentiation to form other stem cells for red cells, white cells and platelets (Fig. 14.3).

Non-lymphoid stem cells

These cells remain in the bone marrow where they differentiate into several different lines producing red blood cells, platelets and the phagocytic cells, granulocytes and monocytes. Their proliferation is influenced by a variety of factors including interleukin and erythropoietin (produced in the kidneys in response to changes in levels of red blood cells).

Lymphoid stem cells

The lymphoid stem cells are responsible for the production of B and T lymphocytes. Some cells remain in the bone marrow where they differentiate several times before beginning the production of B lymphocytes. Other cells move to the thymus where they are influenced by factors in the local environment and differentiate into stem cells producing T lymphocytes. The thymus is a lobular gland, situated above the heart and extending around the base of the trachea. T lymphocytes live for a long time and their production diminishes with age. The thymus gland begins to atrophy soon after puberty. After production, T and B lymphocytes migrate to the lymphoid organs waiting to encounter microorganisms.

Response to invasion

When a microbe enters a lymph node or other lymphoid tissue, it is filtered out and trapped by phagocytes, mainly macrophages. The macrophages ingest the microbes and 'process' them, displaying the microbial peptides together with MHC molecules on their cell surface. T lymphocytes will recognise antigens located next to these self-marker MHC proteins, bind to them and activate the specific immune response against them and stimulate the B lymphocytes in the node to divide into antibody-producing plasma cells.

Lymphocytes from the node will also circulate around the body in search of the invader, but have a homing mechanism which means that they return the lymph organ from which they originated. After the infection has been repelled, memory B and T lymphocytes are distributed around the body in the lymph and blood vessels, ensuring that a rapid response can be mounted should the same antigen be encountered again.

RECOGNITION OF SELF

The body can only defend itself against an invader if it is able to distinguish between its own cells (self) and those of an invader (non-self). Each cell in the body carries on its surface the same distinct marker of 'selfness' called the major histocompatibility complex (MHC) marker. The structure of this group of molecules is peculiar to each individual, so that tissue introduced from another person, e.g. a transplant, has a different MHC marker and will therefore be recognised by the immune system as non-self and destroyed. Some people's MHC markers will be more alike than others, particularly those with shared genes such as members of the same family. Tissue typing is therefore used to identify donors whose MHC markers are very similar to those of the intended recipient. The genes coding for MHC markers are known to occur on specific points in the chromosome (Ch. 4) called human leucocyte antigen (HLA) loci. Genetic studies can be used to determine how similar are the donor and recipient markers.

A key feature of the immune system is its ability to recognise self against non-self cells. If the system does not recognise self cells this can lead to autoimmune disorders where the immune system begins to attack the cells of the body.

T lymphocytes are of major importance in recognising and eliminating non-self cells. During the development and differentiation of thousands of T lymphocytes in the thymus, a mechanism of selecting T cells that only recognise non-self markers and eliminating any that would recognise self markers occurs. The final set of T lymphocytes should therefore only contain cells that recognise non-self markers.

DISEASES OF THE IMMUNE SYSTEM

The activity of the immune system can be impaired by a range of disease processes, including abnormalities in genetic make-up, autoimmune disease, therapeutic agents and some viral infections.

Congenital disorders can result in various types of immune deficiency. Congenital immunoglobulin deficiency occurs when the stem cells in the bone marrow fail to differentiate into the B lymphocyte line. Affected infants cannot produce their own antibodies and are therefore susceptible to a variety of bacterial infections. They can be treated with preparations of human immunoglobulin and in the future it may be possible to correct the deficiency by gene therapy. Abnormal development of the thymus gland or defects in the T lymphocyte stem cells are rare. Children affected are susceptible to fungal and viral infections and often little can be done to protect them or to treat the deficiency. In severe combined immune deficiency syndrome (SCIDS), infants lack both T and B lymphocytes. They are therefore susceptible to bacterial, viral and fungal infections and most die whilst very young.

Hypersensitivity reactions

Sometimes, an immune system primed by an initial contact with an antigen produces an excessive reaction when exposed for a second time. This hypersensitivity to an antigen is often referred to as an allergic response and some people appear to be predisposed to them. Hypersensitivity reactions usually occur immediately, within minutes of a second exposure. Their effects can range from a mild local affect such as gastrointestinal upset in the case of food allergy or hay fever in pollen allergy, to a severe, often fatal, systemic anaphylactic reaction. The most common cause is insect stings, e.g. bees and wasps, in people who are highly sensitive. Exposure to the antigen on a second occasion causes rapid activation of IgE bound to basophils and mast cells, which triggers these cells to release vasoactive amines into the bloodstream. These increase local vascular permeability, causing oedema, and if released in excessive amounts into the bloodstream can cause hypotensive shock and cardiac and respiratory failure. Oedema in the upper airway can result in suffocation. Local anaphylaxis only causes an inflammatory reaction at the route of entry of the allergen: for example, pollen and animal fur is inhaled to cause asthma or hay fever, and allergenic foods are ingested and cause gastrointestinal upsets or skin reactions.

Some people develop a hypersensitivity reaction to components of antibiotics such as penicillin. When the drug is metabolised, components may bind to proteins and initiate an immune response from IgE. If the antibiotic is administered a second time it will bind to penicillin-specific IgE on mast cells causing a hypersensitivity reaction.

Other hypersensitivities are caused by antibody–antigen complexes and complement. For example, haemolytic anaemia occurs when a drug binds to red blood cells, inducing antibodies to bind to them, activating complement and subsequent lysis of the cells. The destruction of the red blood cells results in anaemia.

Some hypersensitivity reactions are delayed, occurring within 24–48 h of the exposure. These delayed hypersensitivity reactions occur as the result of the activity of helper T cells and macrophages and indicate defence against a second exposure to intracellular bacteria, e.g. mycobacteria. The tuberculin test, used to establish whether an individual has been previously exposed to *Mycobacterium tuberculosis*, is based on the delayed hypersensitivity reaction to the tuberculin antigen inoculated under the skin.

Autoimmune diseases

These diseases occur when the body's mechanism for recognising self cells is defective. These defects seem to have a genetic origin, frequently being associated with particular types of MHC and HLA genes. Antibodies can be formed to a variety of tissues. In juvenile-onset insulin-dependent diabetes mellitus, for example, the pancreatic islet cells that produce insulin are not recognised as self cells and are gradually destroyed, causing a progressive reduction in insulin production and eventually clinical diabetes. Other autoimmune diseases are listed in Table 14.2.

TABLE 14.2	Examples of Self-antigens Associated with Autoimmune Diseases
Autoimmune disease	Self-antigen recognised by T cells
Pernicious anaemia	Gastric parietal cells
Juvenile insulin-dependent diabetes	Pancreatic islet cells
Multiple sclerosis	Central nervous system myelin
Lupus erythematosus	DNA, red blood cells, lymphocytes, platelets
Rheumatoid arthritis	IgG

Acquired immune deficiency syndrome (AIDS)

Several viruses are able to cause immune deficiencies in a range of different species, e.g. human T-cell lymphotrophic viruses (HTLVs). The human immunodeficiency virus (HIV), which causes AIDS, has become a major pathogen of humans since it was first discovered in the early 1980s. This virus attaches to those cells in the body that carry a particular protein receptor called CD4. These include helper T lymphocytes and macrophages. The virus gradually damages the immune system by infecting and destroying T lymphocytes in the lymph nodes. The immune system may be able to control virus replication for many years, hence an infected individual can be asymptomatic for 10–15 years. HIV uses an enzyme called reverse transcriptase to convert its RNA genome into a double strand of DNA. This enzyme tends to make mistakes when it is copying so that the HIV genome varies considerably over several generations. New virus particles may therefore not be recognised by the same memory lymphocytes, providing the virus with an opportunity to invade more T cells until another immune response can be made. Gradually, the evolving HIV will deplete the T lymphocytes to such an extent that they are unable to mount a response to intracellular parasites such as mycobacterium, cryptosporidium and toxoplasma and viruses such as cytomegalovirus. In addition, certain malignancies that would normally be destroyed by T lymphocytes may develop, such as Kaposi's sarcoma, a tumour of endothelial cells.

IMMUNISATION

As described earlier in the chapter, immunity to a particular infection is conferred by memory lymphocytes, which are able to respond rapidly to reinfections by a microorganism that has been encountered previously. Natural immunity is acquired following the primary infection, but can also be induced artificially by vaccination.

The principles of immunisation were established in the 1800s with the pioneering work of Edward Jenner, who noticed that milkmaids were not susceptible to smallpox and suspected that they were protected from infection through exposure to cowpox, a similar infection that did not affect humans. He tested his theory by inoculating a boy with cowpox virus and then exposing him to smallpox. Fortunately, the vaccination did indeed protect the boy from infection.

The objective of vaccination is to induce immunity to a particular infection by priming a population of memory B and T lymphocytes, which can respond rapidly should the particular pathogen invade the body. It is most useful for protection against those infections that spread easily from person to person, because widespread vaccination can be used to protect the whole community. If sufficient people within the population are immune, the pathogen will not be able to find hosts in which to multiply and it will eventually die out.

Medicine is able to exploit the immune system by administering small or inactive doses of specific foreign bodies, such as bacteria or viruses, in order to trigger a protective immune response if the body is subsequently exposed to the foreign body.

The principle of vaccination is that the vaccine should not cause the actual disease it is aiming to protect against, but that it should contain sufficient antigen to induce a specific immune response. Vaccines can be made in several ways, as described below.

Killed organisms

Examples include typhoid, cholera and whooping cough vaccines. These can be made from whole cells that are killed, for example, by heat.

Live, attenuated organisms

Examples include polio, measles, mumps, rubella and BCG vaccines. The microorganisms have been altered so that whilst they behave like the original organisms, they are unable to cause disease. They are able to induce a better immune response than killed vaccines because the replication of the microorganism results in a much larger and more prolonged dose of antigen. Many can induce long-lasting immunity after just one dose, e.g. measles, mumps and rubella (MMR) vaccine. Because the live attenuated vaccines will multiply in the usual site of infection, they induce the correct response to ensure maximum protection should infection with the real pathogen occur: for example, polio vaccine multiplies in the gut and therefore induces an antibody response in both the blood and the epithelial lining of the gut.

Attenuated strains can be made by modifying their growth conditions: for example, by growing at temperatures above or below their optimum growth temperature or by taking out parts of their genome so that they are still active but unable to cause disease. The live, attenuated vaccine against *Mycobacterium tuberculosis*, BCG (Bacille, Calmette, Guérin), was discovered by accident by Calmette and Guérin in 1908 when they added bile to the medium they were using to culture the organism. Attenuated strains can also be strains of the infection which are only virulent in another species, for example the cowpox vaccine used by Edward Jenner.

Attenuated strains can revert to their virulent form and are associated with a small risk of complications, e.g. symptoms such as encephalitis, which occurs, rarely, after measles vaccination. However, the risk of such complications is much lower that that associated with the infection itself and it is important to balance the risk of complications with the risk associated with the disease.

Purified components

Toxins can be purified and inactivated with formaldehyde to produce a vaccine that will induce an antibody and complement immune response. The response is improved by adsorbing the toxin onto an adjuvant such as aluminium hydroxide, which prevents it from being dispersed from the site of inoculation too rapidly and stimulates the activity of macrophages.

Genetic recombination

Specific immunogenic antigens can be isolated, e.g. with monoclonal antibodies, and these can then be incorporated into an artificial vaccine. Genes for a particular antigenic protein have been inserted into the genome of a yeast, which can then be used to synthesise large quantities of the antigen. This is recovered, purified and made into a vaccine, e.g. hepatitis B vaccine.

Administration of vaccines

The Department of Health recommends a vaccination programme for all children (Table 14.3). Some vaccinations require several doses to achieve high levels of immunity whilst other, live, attenuated vaccines induce long-lasting immunity after just one dose, e.g. measles, mumps and rubella (MMR).

TABLE 14.3	Schedule for Routine Immunisation in the UK	
Vaccine	Age	Dose
Diphtheria, tetanus, pertussis (DTP),	2 months	1st dose
polio, Haemophilus influenzae (HIB)	3 months	2nd dose
	4 months	3rd dose
Measles, mumps, rubella (MMR)	12–15 months	1st dose
DTP		Booster
MMR		2nd dose
BCG (tuberculosis)	10–14 years	1st dose
DTP	13–18 years	Booster

Source: Department of Health, 1996.

Widespread immunisation programmes in developed countries have had a tremendous impact on levels of infant mortality. To be effective a minimum of 60% of the population must be immune and if the infection is particularly contagious and spreads rapidly then the percentage will need to be even higher.

Many viruses, for example those that cause colds and influenza, are difficult to vaccinate against because they continually change the structure of their surface antigens so that memory cells generated from a previous exposure may not recognise the modified antigens. These changes can be minor, mediated by single mutations in the viral genome (antigenic drift), or can involve swapping large sections of genetic material with similar viruses that have different animal hosts (antigenic shift). When an antigenic shift occurs, the population will have little immunity to the new strain and an epidemic of infection is likely to occur. Influenza vaccines are made annually by predicting which strains of the virus are likely to be most prevalent in a given year. Although they may not provide complete protection against the strains that finally emerge, they will usually considerably moderate its effect.

Passive immunity

Specific immunoglobulins can be used to provide temporary protection against an infection. If administered to an individual, they will bind to the antigen they are programmed to recognise and stimulate an immune response but will not be replaced at the end of their lifespan of a few weeks. Passive immunity occurs naturally during the first few months of a child's life when maternal antibodies (IgG) are transferred across the placenta and ingested in breast milk (IgA) to protect the newborn from infection whilst its immature system is developing.

Passive immunity can also be conferred artificially by collecting specific antibodies from the blood of people recently infected or who have high levels of antibody following vaccination. This type of immunisation is sometimes used to provide immediate protection to a susceptible individual who has been exposed to a particular pathogen: for example, hepatitis B immunoglobulin can be administered to a non-immune member of staff following a needlestick injury to prevent them acquiring the infection.

SUMMARY

The body has a range of defences that enable it to combat invasion by harmful microorganisms or foreign substances, called antigens. External defences, such as the skin or antibacterial secretions, provide physical barriers against the entry of microorganisms. Any which manage to bypass these defences are met by a series of internal defence mechanisms, known as the immune system. Phagocytic cells recognise microorganisms circulating in the blood or in tissue, ingest and digest them. A protein called complement stimulates the action of these phagocytic cells. B lymphocytes recognise an antigen and are triggered to produce large quantities of proteins called immunoglobulins, antibodies, which are able to bind specifically to the particular antigen. T lymphocytes also respond to specific antigens and both trigger and enhance the activity of B lymphocytes and phagocytes. They also attack microorganisms such as viruses, which replicate inside cells. After exposure to a particular antigen, memory cells are retained so that should the same antigen be encountered again, specific B and T lymphocytes can be generated rapidly. Immunity to infection can be artificially induced by inoculation of an antigen in the form of a vaccine.

The cells of the immune system originate in the bone marrow, but move to special lymphoid tissue distributed throughout the body. The lymphoid tissue is connected by a network of small channels called lymph vessels.

The immune system can be impaired by several disease processes. In some people, hypersensitivity occurs when an excessive response is induced after exposure to a particular antigen. Autoimmune diseases are caused by the immune system attacking cells within the body.

QUESTIONS

1. What is phagocytosis?

2. What functions do the lymphocytes play in protection?

3. List the different types of vaccines.

FURTHER READING

Hinchliff S (1996) Innate defences. In: Hinchliff S, Montague S, Watson R (eds) *Physiology for nursing practice, 2nd edn.* Baillière Tindall, London, pp 621–653

Betts A, Langelaan D (1996) Acquired defences. In: Hinchliff S, Montague S, Watson R (eds) *Physiology for nursing practice, 2nd edn.* Baillière Tindall, London, pp 654–678

Wilson J (1995) *Infection control in clinical practice.* Baillière Tindall, London

Watson R (1995) *Anatomy and physiology for nurses, 10th edn.* Baillière Tindall, London

15 Pharmacology

Jennifer Kelly

After reading this chapter you should be able to:
- understand what the subject of pharmacology is about
- explain how drugs can act on the body
- understand the factors which influence the distribution of drugs in the body.

INTRODUCTION

This chapter will examine the subject of pharmacology, which is the study of drugs and how they interact with the human body. As most people have taken drugs at some time in their life, if only an aspirin for a headache, drug therapy is something to which you can relate. Pharmacology will be used to illustrate some of the issues of cellular biology introduced in the previous chapters.

Before going any further it is necessary to define the term 'drug'. A drug can be defined narrowly as a single chemical substance that forms the active ingredient in a medicine. More broadly, it can be defined as any chemical that is used to modify or explore physiological systems or pathological states for the benefit of the recipient. The second definition includes conventional drugs such as aspirin, through vitamin tablets to foodstuffs. The second definition also suggests that it is not only the chemical itself that decides whether it is a drug, but also the intent of the prescriber. Thus heroin given to a patient in pain is a drug, but given with intent to kill is a poison.

The aim of drug therapy is to get the right drug to the right site in the body, in the right amount and for the right time. The achievement of this aim is brought about by the interaction of two processes, namely pharmacodynamics and pharmacokinetics. Pharmacodynamics is simply the process by which the drug interacts with the body to bring about its effects, and its study will form the focus of the first section. The second section looks at what the body does to the drug, i.e. the pharmacokinetics.

PHARMACODYNAMICS

Drugs exert their effects in one of two general ways: either they work by themselves mechanically or chemically, or they interact with cellular proteins and hence alter cell activities. Drugs are usually targeted at the physiological mechanisms of the body in an attempt to alter or control them. When treating infections and infestations the drugs used are, in effect, poisons. It is therefore necessary to find differences between the host's (i.e. your) body cells and the cells of the infecting organism, e.g. bacteria, in order that the drug will poison the infecting organism without poisoning you. You might like to look at bacterial cells and consider how they are different from your own cells, and therefore what possible targets there are for drug therapy (Ch. 13).

Mechanical/chemical agents

These drugs work simply as a result of their chemistry or mechanical properties. They make up some of the most commonly used drugs. Antacids are a good example of drugs that work through their chemistry. They include drugs such as magnesium hydroxide (Milk of Magnesia[1]), aluminium hydroxide (Aludrox) and calcium hydroxide. They are all alkalis and they are used to neutralise excess acid in the stomach, thereby preventing the formation of stomach and duodenal ulcers.

A group of drugs that act purely mechanically is the bulk laxatives. Bulk laxatives include methylcellulose and ispaghula (Fybogel). They work by increasing the volume of faecal material in the large intestine, and in so doing they stimulate the stretch detectors in the bowel, promoting peristalsis (Ch. 12) in the large intestine. Another group of laxatives is the osmotic laxatives and, if you think back to Section 1 to the definition of osmosis, you can deduce how they work (Ch. 1). Osmotic laxatives include magnesium salts (Epsom salts) and lactulose. They both exert an osmotic pressure and so retain fluid within the bowel. This fluid keeps the stool soft, and the increased bulk stimulates peristalsis.

Drugs interacting with cell proteins

The proteins of the plasma membrane include receptors, ion channels, enzymes and carriers. These proteins are all targets for drug therapy. They normally interact with the body's own chemicals, in particular with hormones and neurotransmitters (Chs 5 and 6).

Neurotransmitters

Neurotransmitters are chemicals such as noradrenaline, acetylcholine and dopamine, which are produced by nerve cells, or neurones. As you know, nerves carry information throughout the body using electrical impulses. However, where one nerve meets, or a group of nerves meet, there is a gap called a synapse. In order for the signal to pass across the gap, or synaptic cleft as it is called, the presynaptic membrane releases packages or vesicles of neurotransmitter into the gap (Ch. 5). The neurotransmitter diffuses across the space and binds to receptors on the other side where it can initiate a new electrical impulse (Fig. 15.1).

You might be wondering why we need synapses if all they do is pass the mes-

---

[1]Drugs tend to have at least two names. One is the generic name, e.g. magnesium hydroxide, which is the name of the active ingredient, while the other, e.g. Milk of Magnesia, is the brand name. In this text the generic name will be used, with the brand name in parentheses where appropriate.

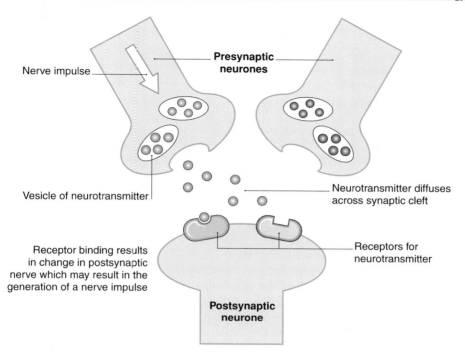

Fig. 15.1   *Synapsing of neurones.*

sage across the gap. Why not just have longer nerves? The reason is that some nerves are excitatory and some are inhibitory. Thus, when several nerves meet at a synapse, both excitatory and inhibitory neurotransmitters can be released. Thus, whether the postsynaptic neurone generates a nerve impulse will depend on the balance between excitatory and inhibitory neurotransmitters arriving at the postsynaptic membrane.

The initial binding of neurotransmitter and receptor conveys a primary signal to the cell. This primary signal has to be translated into some kind of event, and this translation is called signal transduction. Many of the nerve cells have receptors that control a 'gate' across a channel through the cell membrane. Normally the channel is closed, but after binding the neurotransmitter there is a structural change and the 'gate' opens, allowing small ions such as sodium and chloride to pass through the channel and into the cell. It is the movement of these ions into the neurone that generates the nervous impulse.

Some neurotransmitters such as noradrenaline do not use ion channels, but instead the binding of the neurotransmitter to the receptor causes the release of secondary messengers, for example cyclic adenosine monophosphate (cyclic AMP). The secondary messenger leads to a cascade of events finally resulting in activation or inhibition of key enzymes. These receptors that do not involve ion channels are true receptors, and we will look at them first in relation to drug therapy.

Many drugs act by interfering with the natural interaction between chemicals in the body such as neurotransmitters and their receptors.

Receptors

Drugs that interact with receptors can work in two main ways. They can act as agonists or as antagonists.

Agonists

Agonists are molecules that bind to a receptor and produce the appropriate response, i.e. the response that the normal chemical in the body would produce. This means that all the hormones and neurotransmitters in the body can be classified as agonists. For example, adrenaline is an agonist at adrenoreceptors (adrenaline receptors). If you are injected with a syringe full of adrenaline the drug will bind to its receptors, including those on the heart, and will cause the heart to beat faster. The same effect is experienced if you are frightened when watching a horror movie – your body produces adrenaline in response to your fear, and your heart beats faster.

However, a frightened person not only has palpitations but also goes pale and sweaty, for example. The adrenaline binds to many different cells around the body – not just heart cells – and brings about many different symptoms. Thus, if adrenaline is given to speed up the heart rate, it will also constrict the blood vessels to the skin (causing paleness), which is a side-effect of the drug, i.e. it is an unwanted effect. However, if bleeding heavily, a compress of adrenaline applied to the skin will cause the blood vessels supplying the skin to shut down. This is the goal, and the increased heart rate now experienced will become the side-effect. This demonstrates a very important principle of drug therapy. Drugs usually have a variety of effects, and what is the therapeutic effect of a drug and what is a side-effect is purely dependent upon the intention of the prescriber.

Receptor subtypes

Research has found that all the receptors for a particular hormone or neurotransmitter are not identical, and that there are receptor subtypes. Figure 15.2 demonstrates the case for histamine, a chemical that is both a neurotransmitter and a localised hormone. When histamine receptors are examined by molecular biologists they are found to differ slightly from each other, and they are classified accordingly as H_1, H_2 and H_3. Histamine binds to all these receptors and brings about its appropriate biological response, as indicated. Drug companies can use the different shapes of the receptors to produce drugs to minimise unwanted effects from drugs.

This is achieved by producing drugs that fit into one receptor subtype, but not another. For example, if you wanted for some reason to cause the stomach to produce more acid you could give an H_2-agonist that will bind to H_2 receptors but not to H_1 receptors. Thus, you would get the effect you wanted – production of stomach acid without the side-effects, i.e. an allergic response. As more receptor subtypes are identified, drug companies can produce increasingly more-specific drugs.

You might think that all agonists are simply the endogenous (own) chemicals of the body given as drugs, but this is not entirely true. Morphine is an example of an agonist that has been used to relieve pain for thousands of years. However, until recently it was not known how morphine worked.

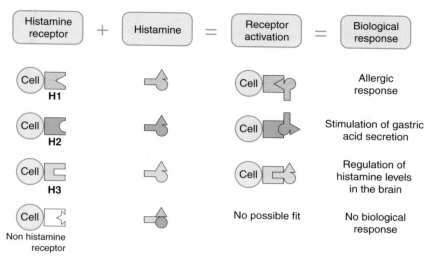

Fig. 15.2   *Receptor subtypes.*

Eventually, receptors were found in the brain and spinal cord to which morphine bound. Scientists argued that if the body had receptors for morphine, then the body must produce endogenous chemicals that normally bind to these receptors, and these were eventually found in 1975. They are called endogenous opioid peptides and consist of three groups: endorphins, enkephalins and dynorphins. They are the body's own painkillers and are produced in response to stress.

Antagonists

Antagonists are drugs that prevent an agonist from binding to a receptor. Antagonists do not themselves have any pharmacological actions mediated by the receptors; they simply work by preventing the endogenous chemical from working. Consider our earlier example of histamine. Normally one would not want to stimulate gastric acid secretion, but instead would want to suppress its secretion to prevent patients from developing stomach ulcers. This can be achieved by a drug called cimetidine (Tagamet), which is an H_2-antagonist. It blocks the histamine receptors on the stomach involved with gastric acid secretion, but has a minimal effect on the other receptor subtypes.

> Agonists mimic the effect of a natural neurotransmitter or hormone in the body and antagonists oppose this action.

Another example of an antagonist is propranolol (Inderal), which is an antagonist at adrenoreceptors. A doctor might prescribe propanolol for a patient with symptoms of stress before taking an examination. This will bind to adrenoreceptors and stop the adrenaline from having its effect, i.e. it will stop palpitations and feelings of stress. However, an individual that is not stressed and is very relaxed about taking examinations will not release any endogenous adrenaline or noradrenaline and so the drug will have no effect. This is an important property of antagonists; they will only have an effect if there is endogenous chemical trying to bind to receptors that they can block.

Another example of an antagonist is the drug tamoxifen (Tamofen). This is used to treat breast cancer. It binds to receptors *in* the cytoplasm of breast cells. Not all receptors are in the cell membrane; some are in the cytoplasm itself. Drug molecules have to pass through the cell membrane. They must be lipid-soluble, like the group of hormones called steroids, of which oestrogen is an example. Tamoxifen binds to receptors in breast tissue and blocks the oestrogen that normally binds to the receptor. As the oestrogen is important in stimulating the breast cell to grow and multiply, the blockage of the receptor slows the growth of the cancer.

To check your understanding of receptors, try to work out which of the drugs listed in Table 15.2 would be most sensible to give to the patient described in the scenario below. Remember that your aim, as with all drug therapy, is to maximise the therapeutic effect of the drug and minimise the side-effects.

You are in a position where you can prescribe drugs. Billy has recently been suffering from breathlessness and has been diagnosed as suffering from asthma. One of the main problems in asthma is that the smooth muscle of the bronchus (or windpipe) contracts, narrowing the lumen of the windpipe. The problem is made worse by a type of white blood cell, called a mast cell, which releases histamine, causing the tissues lining the airway to become swollen and so narrowing the windpipe further. Use Table 15.1 to identify which of the four adrenoreceptor subtypes you want to target, and then choose the appropriate drug from Table 15.2.

The best drug to prescribe Billy is salbutamol. The problem Billy has is with

TABLE 15.1   *Effects Mediated by Adrenoreceptor Subtypes*

Tissue	α_1	α_2	β_1	β_2
Heart muscle			Increases rate and force of contraction	
Blood vessel smooth muscle	Constricts	Constricts		Dilates
Smooth muscle of bronchi	Constricts			Dilates
Uterine smooth muscle	Contracts			Relaxes
Skeletal muscle				Tremor
Adipose tissue			Fat breakdown	
Liver	Breakdown and release of sugar stored in the liver			Breakdown and release of sugar stored in the liver
Mast cells				Inhibition of histamine release

TABLE 15.2		*Effects of Agonists and Antagonists at Different Adrenoreceptor Subtypes*		

	Adrenoreceptor			
	α_1	α_2	β_1	β_2
Agonists				
Noradrenaline	+++	+++	++	+
Adrenaline	++	++	+++	+++
Isoprenaline	–	–	+++	+++
Salbutamol	–	–	+	+++
Antagonists				
Propranolol	–	–	+++	+++
Atenolol	–	–	+++	+

+, small effect; ++, moderate effect; +++, large effect; –, no effect.

the smooth muscle of his bronchial tree or windpipe, which is too narrow because the muscle is contracting. This problem can be dealt with in one of two ways. Just like stopping a car, you can either take your foot off the accelerator or put it on the brake. The equivalent in this scenario is to either stop the constriction of the bronchial smooth muscle or promote its dilatation. You see from Table 15.1 that α_1 adrenoreceptors constrict the bronchi, so an antagonist could be used to stop this constriction. From Table 15.2 you will see that there is not an antagonist listed that works on α_1 receptors. Going back to Table 15.1 and the bronchial smooth muscle, you will see that β_2 receptors have a dilatory effect, which you could promote by using an agonist. Looking at Table 15.2, there are four agonists from which to choose.

Adrenaline and noradrenaline have an agonistic effect on α_1 receptors, and will cause constriction of the bronchial smooth muscle, so they are not very useful. That leaves isoprenaline and salbutamol (Ventolin). Isoprenaline has a strong agonistic effect on both β_1 and β_2 adrenoreceptors. If you look again at Table 15.1 you will see that a β_1 agonist will increase the heart rate, giving Billy palpitations, which he does not want. In the days before salbutamol was available, isoprenaline was used to treat asthma, and several people died from their palpitations. Thus the best drug in Table 15.2 is salbutamol. If you look again at Table 15.1 you will see that there is an added bonus of using a β_2 agonist, because it also inhibits histamine release by mast cells. Salbutamol will therefore help Billy in two ways: it will dilate his bronchial smooth muscle and inhibit histamine production.

Salbutamol is not the 'ideal' drug to give Billy because it does have some effect on β_1 receptors, although much less than isoprenaline. Drug companies are working towards producing the ideal drug to treat asthma. The ideal drug would be an agonist at β_2 adrenoreceptors that has no effect on β_1 receptors.

Ion channels

Ion channels are proteins in cell membranes. They allow the movement of ions, or small charged particles, through them in response to the binding of a molecule to a binding site or receptor on the ion channel. One way to affect ion channels with drugs is to block the mouth of the channel so that the ions cannot move through, i.e. to use a blocker.

Blocker

Examples of blockers of which you might have had experience if you have ever had any dental work done are lignocaine (Xylocaine) or novocain. These are both local anaesthetics.

Chapter 5 looked at how nerves conduct a nervous impulse. The formation of a nerve impulse depends on sodium ions entering through ion channels. If you are given lignocaine, the drug diffuses into the nerve and blocks the ion channels that allow the sodium ions to move into the nerve. When the dentist comes to drill your teeth the sodium ions are unable to enter the pain nerves. The nerves can therefore not send messages to your brain telling it that your mouth is hurting. You might be wondering why the pain nerves are affected but not your motor nerves (the ones that control movement). You might even have had the experience after a trip to the dentist of chewing the inside of your own mouth without feeling it. The reason for the discrepancy is that motor nerves have a thicker sheath around them than the nerves that conduct pain messages. Thus the lignocaine is unable to diffuse into them as easily as it can into the pain nerves.

Modulator

The second way in which drugs can interact with ion channels is as modulators. This means that the drug either increases or decreases the ease with which ion channels open. This effect can be illustrated with the example of diazepam (Valium). This well-known drug is a tranquilliser that interacts with a neurotransmitter called GABA (gamma-amino butyric acid). GABA is an example of an inhibitory neurotransmitter. This means that when it is released at a synaptic junction it tends to diffuse across the synaptic cleft and to inhibit the postsynaptic nerve from conducting a nervous impulse (Fig. 15.3).

As Figure 15.3 shows, when GABA is released from a nerve terminal it diffuses across the synaptic gap and binds to a binding site on the ion channels on the postsynaptic membrane. This causes the ion channels to open and chloride ions to enter. If a patient has taken some diazepam, this binds to another binding site on the ion channel. In so doing the diazepam makes it easier for the GABA to bind to its binding site, and therefore more likely for chloride ions to enter the nerve. If more chloride ions move into the postsynaptic nerve, it becomes inhibited and this general inhibition of the nervous system brings about the tranquillising effects of diazepam.

Enzymes

Enzymes are proteins found both inside cells and in tissue fluids that act as biological catalysts. This means that they speed up the rate of chemical reactions. By using drugs that interact with enzymes, many important bodily processes can be controlled.

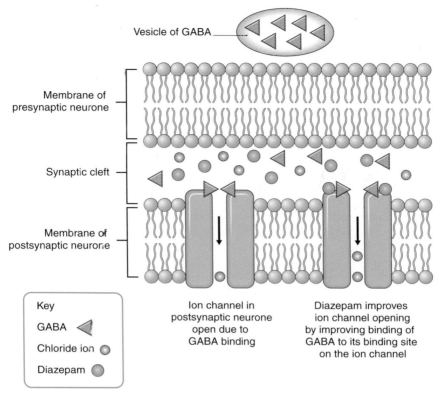

Vesicle of GABA

Membrane of
presynaptic neurone

Synaptic cleft

Membrane of
postsynaptic neurone

Key

GABA

Chloride ion

Diazepam

Ion channel in
postsynaptic neurone
open due to
GABA binding

Diazepam improves
ion channel opening
by improving binding of
GABA to its binding site
on the ion channel

Fig. 15.3   *Modulation by diazepam of the effect of GABA on its ion channel.*

Inhibitor

One way that drugs can interact with enzymes is as an inhibitor, which works
by binding to the active site of the enzyme. A good example of this is the drug
aspirin.

When tissue is damaged, a chemical called arachidonic acid is produced. This
is converted to prostaglandins by the enzyme cyclo-oxygenase. Prostaglandins
are a complex group of chemicals that have a variety of effects. One of their
functions is to cause the symptoms of inflammation, i.e. redness, swelling, pain
and fever. A drug that can inhibit the enzyme cyclo-oxygenase can prevent
prostaglandins being formed and thus reduce the symptoms that they evoke.
This is in fact what aspirin and related drugs such as paracetamol and ibuprofen
(Nurofen) do – they block the enzyme, prevent the formation of prostaglandins
and so reduce pain and fever.

Pro-drug

Drugs do not just interact with enzymes by inhibiting them. Another use is to
give a patient an inactive drug, called a pro-drug, and use enzymes in the body
to activate it. This might seem a strange thing to do – why not give the active
drug in the first place? The ingenuity of this method of treatment can be demonstrated in the management of Parkinson's disease. This condition is caused by a

lack of dopamine in a part of the brain (the basal ganglia) that controls movement. The patient with Parkinson's disease has stiff, sluggish, uncontrolled movements and often has difficulty speaking because of poor control of the muscles of speech.

The obvious way to treat Parkinson's disease would be to be given dopamine. This does not work, however, because the dopamine cannot be absorbed into the brain. This is because the brain is protected by what is termed the blood–brain barrier. This means that the capillaries supplying the brain are relatively impermeable, making it difficult for certain chemicals to pass out of the blood into the brain. As dopamine cannot be given, the pro-drug levodopa is given. This can enter the brain, where an enzyme (dopa decarboxylase) converts it into dopamine. This would appear to solve the problem because there is now dopamine in the brain where it is needed and the symptoms of Parkinson's disease are ameliorated. Unfortunately, dopa decarboxylase is also found in the rest of the body and so dopamine is also made in the periphery. There is now an excess of dopamine in the peripheral tissues, and this results in involuntary choreiform movements. This can be prevented by giving a decarboxylase inhibitor that is unable to cross the blood–brain barrier, e.g. carbidopa. Thus by giving a mixture of levodopa to replace the missing dopamine in the brain, and carbidopa to prevent the formation of dopamine in the peripheral nerves, the symptoms of Parkinson's disease can be reduced and the side-effects minimised. Sinemet is an example of this drug combination.

> The treatment of Parkinson's disease is a classic example of the administration of a pro-drug, which is taken up by the brain and converted to the active drug rather than the administration of a drug that will not cross the blood–brain barrier.

Carriers

Carriers, or transporters, are proteins in the cell membrane that transport specific substances, e.g. amino acids, across the membrane by changing shape. Carriers can move molecules with their concentration gradient in a process termed facilitated diffusion, or against their concentration gradient by active transport. They form an important target for drug therapy with the drugs acting in one of two ways: as inhibitors or as false substrates.

Inhibitor

An inhibitor, as its name suggests, prevents a carrier from doing its job. A good example of a drug that is an inhibitor is omeprazole (Losec), which is used to prevent stomach ulcers. The history of the drug management of stomach ulcers is fascinating, and reflects the general history of drug therapy.

The problem with stomach ulcers is that too much acid is produced in the stomach and this damages the stomach lining. The initial response to the problem was to give the patient alkalis to neutralise the acid. Management then became a little more sophisticated, when it was discovered that the acid-producing cell (the parietal cell) had receptors on its surface for the neurotransmitter acetylcholine, as well as for histamine. Thus, drugs were developed to block the binding of these endogenous molecules to their receptors.

These blocking drugs are antagonists. They consisted of pirenzepine (Gastrozepin), which antagonises acetylcholine, and cimetidine (Tagamet), which antagonises histamine at H_2 receptors. The problem with pirenzepine is that it antagonises acetylcholine, which is used extensively throughout the nervous system, so the drug has many side-effects. Conversely, H_2 receptors appear to be specific to the stomach and so cimetidine has become a popular drug in the treatment of stomach ulcers. However, the use of antagonists does not treat the supposed root of the problem – the carrier in the parietal cell that is pumping hydrogen ions into the stomach. This is where omeprazole comes in, by blocking the pump and so preventing the acid being released into the stomach. This is an example of the magic 'silver bullet' that drug companies are looking for – a drug that deals with the problem itself rather than a step divorced from the problem. The advantage of the 'silver bullet' is that there are minimal side-effects. Unfortunately for the manufacturers of omeprazole, the drug has not proved to be the wonder drug that was hoped for. This is because it now appears that the root cause of stomach ulcers is infection, which can easily be treated with antibiotics.

False substrate

The second way in which drugs can interfere with carriers is as false substrates. In this case, the drug appears to be very similar to the normal molecule that the carrier moves across the cell membrane. By this deception it causes the carrier to move it across the membrane instead of the normal molecule. This is how amphetamines work (Fig. 15.4).

After a neurotransmitter has been released into the synaptic cleft, it is inactivated, either by being broken down by enzymes in the synaptic gap or by being taken up by carriers on the synaptic membrane. In the case of neurones using the neurotransmitter noradrenaline, carriers are used to take up the chemical into the presynaptic neurone. Here it is stored in vesicles until the nerve is next stimulated and needs to release the transmitter. Amphetamine fools the carrier into taking it into the nerve terminal. In the presynaptic neurone the amphetamine displaces noradrenaline from its storage vesicle, causing it to be released into the synaptic cleft where it diffuses across and binds to the postsynaptic receptors. The stimulant effects of amphetamines thus result from excess release of noradrenaline in the central nervous system.

PHARMACOKINETICS

Pharmacokinetics is the study of what the body does to a drug over time. It explores the processes of absorption, distribution, metabolism and excretion. Each of these processes will occur at a specific rate characteristic for that drug, and the overall action of the drug will be dependent on these processes. The remainder of the chapter will examine each of the four processes in turn.

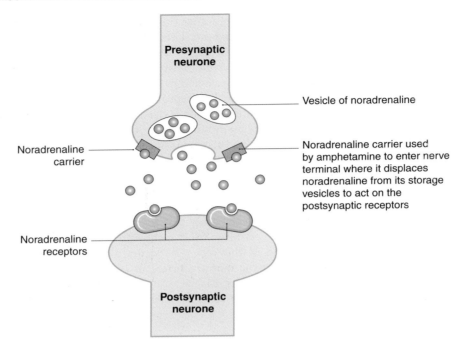

Fig. 15.4   *Amphetamine as a false substrate.*

Absorption

Absorption can be defined as the passage of a drug from the site of administration into the blood or plasma. As most drugs are taken orally they must pass through the gut wall and enter the blood. The effects of a drug will depend on its rate of absorption, because this will determine its peak effect. For example, an antibiotic that is very slowly absorbed when taken orally might be excreted as fast as it is absorbed. This means that the blood concentration of the drug will never be very high, and it may not be high enough to kill the bacteria that are causing the infection.

As well as rate of absorption, drugs vary in their bioavailabilty or extent of absorption. Thus, if a drug is poorly absorbed from the gut, most of it will simply pass out of the body with the faeces. If that drug is an antibiotic it will have no effect on the bacteria causing, for example, a chest infection. However, this property of a drug can also be put to good use. The antibiotic neomycin is poorly absorbed from the gut, but it is used very effectively to cleanse the gut of bacteria before gastrointestinal surgery.

Absorption is affected by a wide variety of factors, of which we will look at just a few. Firstly, the drugs themselves can affect absorption. Tablets do not just contain the active drug but also various other chemicals to hold the tablet together, give it bulk and make it taste pleasant, for example. In 1968 the manufactures of the anti-epileptic drug phenytoin changed one of the bulking agents in their tablets from calcium sulphate to lactulose, for reasons of convenience. The result was that several patients taking the medication suddenly started to show signs of toxicity, e.g. poor coordination and fits. The reason for these effects was that the calcium sulphate in the original tablets inhibited absorption of the drug. When this was changed to lactulose, more drug was absorbed, giving the patients the equivalent of an overdose.

Most drugs are taken orally and they have to contend with the adverse conditions of the gut, which can have major effects on their absorption. Many drugs that are protein in nature, e.g. insulin, cannot be taken orally because they are digested by the gut and hence absorbed as amino acids (Ch. 2) rather than active drug. Similarly, the strong acidity of the stomach affects some drugs such as the antibiotic benzylpenicillin and inactivates them.

Other foods in the gut also have an effect. For example, many antibiotics such as tetracycline should not be taken with food because the drug binds to the food and is not properly absorbed. The motility of the gut will also affect absorption. Thus, if you have an increased rate of peristalsis, drugs may pass through the gut too rapidly to be effectively absorbed. This is why women taking the oral contraceptive pill are advised to take extra precautions if they have diarrhoea.

The final factor that we will consider in relation to absorption is blood flow to the area. In casualty departments people are often brought in who are in considerable pain. To relieve that pain they are given an injection, into their buttock muscle, of a strong painkiller such as morphine. However, this does not always control the pain. Casualty patients are often in a lot of pain because they have sustained serious injuries, and they are often bleeding. When you bleed, the blood that is left in your circulatory system is sent to the vital centres, and your buttock muscle is not a vital area. Consequently, the muscle gets very little blood supply, the drug is not absorbed, and the patient is left in pain.

Drug distribution

Drug distribution is the movement of the drug from the blood to the site of action. Tissue distribution depends on a variety of factors, including regional blood flow. Thus organs that normally get a good blood supply, e.g. the liver and lungs, will get a lot of drug. Tissues with a poor blood supply, e.g. bone, do not get much drug and so treating bone infections such as osteomyelitis can be very difficult.

A very important factor that affects drug distribution is the binding of plasma protein. Drugs transported in the blood are often carried attached to protein molecules. While the drug is bound to the plasma protein it cannot interact with the tissues and exert its effect. When it is no longer bound, it carries out its function, such as binding to receptors or enzymes. If a patient takes two drugs that are both carried by the same plasma protein, the drugs will both compete for the same binding site, in the same way that people compete to get on to a London underground train at rush hour. The competition will result in one drug being displaced by the other. This means that there will be more active, i.e. non-bound, drug available to interact with the tissues, giving the effects of an overdose. The case study in Box 15.1 illustrates this issue.

Metabolism

Metabolism describes the chemical transformations that drugs undergo.

| BOX 15.1 | *Case Study* |

While on holiday, Mr Small developed severe pain in his right leg, which became hot and swollen. The local general practitioner (GP) saw him and had Mr Small admitted to hospital because he believed that Mr Small had a blood clot (deep vein thrombosis) in his right leg. To prevent the clot getting any larger the hospital doctor prescribed Mr Small heparin, which was given intravenously by a pump. After a few days Mr Small's treatment was changed to warfarin, another anti-clotting drug, which has the advantage that it is absorbed when taken orally. Mr Small was discharged home on warfarin. He was given an appointment to attend his local anticoagulant clinic for check-ups, to ensure that his blood was not becoming too 'thinned', which could result in haemorrhage.

A few weeks after discharge Mr Small developed a chest infection. He went to see his regular GP who had not received a letter from the hospital and so did not know that Mr Small had been in hospital, or that he was taking warfarin. Mr Small was no longer getting any pain from his leg, so he did not think to tell his doctor that he had been in hospital. The GP prescribed a sulphonamide for the chest infection. A few days later Mr Small vomited fresh blood and was rushed to hospital. What had gone wrong?

The warfarin Mr Small was prescribed is carried around the body on plasma proteins. The dose was adjusted, prior to his leaving hospital, to ensure that he was receiving just the right dose so that his clot did not reoccur but neither did he start bleeding. Sulphonamides use the same plasma protein as the warfarin for distribution around the body. When Mr Small started taking the sulphonamide, it displaced the warfarin. There was now more unbound warfarin free to interact with the tissues. This it did, inhibiting an enzyme responsible for the synthesis of clotting factors, and hence causing Mr Small to haemorrhage.

Metabolism changes drugs in two principal ways. Firstly, it makes a drug progressively more water soluble so that it can be eliminated in the urine, and secondly it alters the biological behaviour of the drug. There are three ways that the activity of a drug can be altered. Firstly, and the case for most drugs, metabolism converts a pharmacologically active substance into an inactive substance. Alternatively, metabolism can result in the conversion of a pharmacologically active substance to another active substance: for example, the painkiller codeine is metabolised to morphine, itself a powerful painkiller. Thirdly, a pharmacologically inactive drug, or pro-drug, can be converted to an active substance. For example, benorylate (Benoral) found in many cough remedies is converted to salicylic acid (a relation of aspirin) and paracetamol (Panadol).

Several tissues, including the kidney, gut, lung, and skin, metabolise drugs, but the liver is the most important organ in this respect. The cells of the liver contain many hepatic enzymes that are found on the smooth endoplasmic reticulum (Ch. 4). Metabolism is affected by several factors, including the route of administration. Any drug that is swallowed is absorbed from the gut and taken directly to the liver by the blood. Here the hepatic enzymes start to break the drug down before it ever gets to the tissues where it is going to act. A good example of this process is glyceryl trinitrate, which is taken for chest pain. If the tablets of this drug are swallowed, rather than allowed to dissolve under the tongue, they are taken to the liver where they are completely metabolised. This leaves no active drug to work on the heart. If the tablets are allowed to dissolve in the mouth, however, the drug will be absorbed directly from the mouth into the blood. The blood from the mouth does not go directly to the liver, but around the body first. This gives the glyceryl trinitrate a chance to have an effect on the heart before it is broken down by the liver.

Another aspect of metabolism is the enterohepatic recirculation. A drug such as the combined oral contraceptive, i.e. the 'pill', is absorbed from the gut and taken to the liver. Some of the drug will be broken down by the liver, and some will enter the systemic circulation and will prevent an egg being released into the fallopian tubes. The broken down drug is excreted into the bile, which in turn is secreted into the gut by the gall bladder. In the gut there are bacteria which act on the metabolised oral contraceptive and reactivate it. The reactivated drug is then reabsorbed into the blood; it travels to the liver where again some of the drug is broken down and some of it enters the systemic circulation where it continues to prevent ovulation. This cyclical recirculation of the drug ensures that the woman is protected from becoming pregnant. However, broad-spectrum antibiotics will disturb this cyclical process. The antibiotics kill the bacteria in the gut that are reactivating the contraceptive. Thus the effect of the contraceptive is lost after the first cycle through the liver, with the possibility of the drug failing and pregnancy ensuing.

Metabolism is a process involving enzymes. Several things can happen to the enzymes and these in turn can have effects on metabolism. The first effect is termed dose level saturation, where the enzymes that break down the drug cannot deal with the amount of drug put into the system. As a result an alternative pathway is found. This is safe provided the new pathway does not result in the production of harmful metabolites, which is what happens with an overdose of paracetamol (Panadol). Under normal conditions, 90% of a dose of paracetamol is converted to the inactive sulphate and glucuronide of the drug. The other 10% is converted to a reactive intermediate, which is quickly inactivated by the addition of glutathione. In the case of an overdose, more drug goes through the second pathway and the enzyme adding the glutathione cannot cope. The reactive intermediate is therefore not removed rapidly and instead interacts with the liver cells causing permanent liver damage that can be fatal.

The ability of the body to metabolise drugs can be altered by the drugs themselves. In the process of enzyme induction there is an increase in enzyme amount and activity following exposure to chemicals such as tobacco smoke, alcohol, barbecued meats and some drugs. Induction is relevant to drug therapy because it can lead to clinically important drug interactions. For example, patients taking anti-epilepsy drugs or rifampicin, which is used to treat tuberculosis, are advised not to rely on the 'pill' as a contraceptive. The reason for this is that both the anti-epilepsy drugs and rifampicin induce the enzymes that break down the oral contraceptive, thus preventing it from fulfilling its function.

Enzyme induction may also partially explain drug tolerance. Tolerance to drug therapy is sometimes seen with drugs such as heroin, or diamorphine as it is also known. The person using the drug, either for pain relief or for pleasure, requires more and more of the drug to get the same effect. One explanation is that their body is adapting to the drug, producing more enzymes, and so breaking the drug down faster.

Enzyme inhibition is the opposite of enzyme induction. Here, one drug can inhibit the metabolism of a second drug and hence can lead to toxic effects. For example, the antibiotic chloramphenicol inhibits the metabolism of the anti-diabetic drug tolbutamide (Rastinon). The danger here is that the tolbutamide is not broken down and continues to be active. Because tolbutamide lowers the patient's blood sugar level, its failure to be broken down can precipitate a hypoglycaemic (low blood sugar) coma.

Other factors that can interact with metabolism are diseases and genetics. The most obvious diseases that affect metabolism are diseases of the liver, such as inflammation of the liver (hepatitis) and hardening of the liver (cirrhosis, often produced by excessive alcohol consumption). The damaged liver will have inadequate enzymes to break drugs down and so metabolism will be slowed, with the result that the drugs can build up to toxic levels.

Genetic abnormalities can affect metabolism. Suxamethonium (Scoline) is a short-acting muscle relaxant frequently used for clients undergoing surgery. It is metabolised and inactivated in the blood by an enzyme called plasma cholinesterase. Some people lack this enzyme and so are very slow at metabolising the drug. Thus, whereas suxamethonium usually only lasts for about 5 min, in people lacking the enzyme the drug works for several hours. While it is working, the patient's muscles are paralysed and so they cannot breathe. Consequently, they have to be nursed on a ventilator until the effect of the drug eventually wears off.

Drug elimination

Drug elimination is the removal of the drug from the body. The drug can be excreted via any body fluid, including urine, bile, sweat, saliva, faeces, breast milk, and across the placenta. Some drugs such as anaesthetic gases are eliminated in respired air. However, elimination is mainly via the kidneys and liver. Depending on metabolism the excreted drug may or may not be active. If the drug is still active then elimination is important in getting rid of the drug and preventing it from building up in the blood and becoming toxic. If the drug is in an inactive, non-harmful state then the process of elimination is not quite so crucial.

The term 'clearance' is used to express removal of a drug from the blood, and is usually associated with the kidney. Renal clearance is dependent on three factors. The first is filtration, which is the main process by which urine is made (Ch. 11). The process of filtration decreases, not surprisingly, with renal disease but also quite considerably with age. Thus, the elderly have a reduced ability to clear drugs from their body, which partly explains why this age group is particularly prone to developing side-effects from drugs. The problem in the elderly is complicated by the fact that many of the drugs which they take have what is termed a narrow therapeutic window. This means that the difference between the therapeutic or helpful dose of the drug and the toxic dose is small. Thus, a small decrease in metabolism or excretion can result in the rapid development of side-effects.

The second factor that affects renal clearance is passive diffusion. Once the blood has been filtered, some of the materials in the kidney tubule will return to the bloodstream, including drugs (Ch. 11). If the kidney tubule is freely permeable to the drug then about 99% of the filtered drug will return back to the blood. This means that getting rid of a drug could take a long time. One way of speeding up the process of elimination, which is used for cases of drug overdose, is to change slightly the pH of the urine. The administration of sodium bicarbonate will make the urine more alkaline and this will hold acidic drugs, such as aspirin and barbiturates, in the kidney tubule and prevent them being reabsorbed. Similarly, acidification of the urine will speed up the excretion of alkaline drugs such as amphetamines. This process is called forced diuresis.

The third process that affects renal clearance is active transport. This is an energy-requiring process performed by the cells lining the kidney tubule. Active transport allows the body to excrete normal waste products such as creatinine more effectively. Although there are no active transport mechanisms designed by the body to get rid of specific drugs, the proteins that carry out the shunting process can be 'hijacked' by drugs. Thus, for example, penicillin uses these carrier proteins, which speeds up its elimination from the body. When penicillin was first discovered in 1928, this was a problem. Initially the penicillin could not be produced in sufficient quantities to meet demand, even though the urine of patients treated with the drug was collected and the drug extracted. One solution to this problem was to give the drug probencid, which is used to treat gout. This drug uses the same transport molecule as penicillin, and so the probencid molecules and penicillin compete for sites on the transport molecule, with the result that less penicillin is excreted. Thus, smaller doses of penicillin are required to achieve the same therapeutic effect. Probencid penicillin is still available today.

Half-life and steady state

The four components of pharmacokinetics do not work alone, but in concert. Two examples will illustrate this fact. Firstly, metabolism and excretion work together to affect the half-life of a drug. Half-life is the time taken for the concentration of a drug in the blood to fall by half. What this term actually means is illustrated by the example in Box 15.2.

BOX 15.2	

A frog is sitting on a lily pad in the middle of the pond. It can jump half the distance to the edge of the pond with each leap. How many leaps will it need to get on to dry land?

The answer is an infinite number of leaps, or that it will never get out of the pond. The reason for this is that each jump is smaller than the last. This can be seen if we put some numbers into the problem. If the lily pad is 4 metres (m) from the bank the first jump will be 2 m. The frog is now 2 m from the bank and so can jump half that distance, i.e. 1 m. The next jump will be half of 1 m, and the next a quarter of 1 m, and so on.

The relevance of half-life is that drugs with long half-lives have the potential to accumulate and reach toxic levels. This is very worrying with drugs such as digoxin (used to slow the heart rate), which already have narrow therapeutic windows. Any increase in the half-life can quickly turn a therapeutic dose of drug into a toxic dose.

The level of a drug in the bloodstream and in the body as a whole depends on the relative rates of absorption of the drug and its elimination. If drug is administered faster than it is eliminated, it will accumulate as time goes by. The concentration increases until a steady state is attained. The concentration does not carry on rising indefinitely because the body reacts to the increasing blood levels and increases metabolism and excretion. Steady state may take several weeks in the case of drugs such as the anti-epileptic drug phenytoin (Epanutin). This means that there is no point in frequently changing drug doses if they do not have an effect immediately.

The idea of steady state underpins the modern approach to pain control. After major surgery, patients tend to have considerable pain, for which they are given strong analgesia. If this is given every 4–6 h by intramuscular injection, the patient has to wait for the drug to be absorbed before experiencing any benefit. Thus, peaks and troughs are experienced in pain control, as shown in Figure 15.5. If the patient is given the same drug by intravenous infusion then the drug does not have to be absorbed because it is already in the blood. Furthermore, if a very small dose of the painkiller is infused continuously, drug levels remain at a steady state and the pain is effectively controlled with minimal side-effects (Fig. 15.6).

SUMMARY

This chapter has looked at how drugs interact with the body to bring about their effects. It looked briefly at drugs that exert their effect purely as a result of

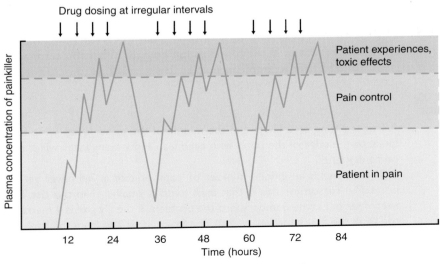

Fig. 15.5 *Peaks and troughs in pain control with irregular injections of painkillers.*

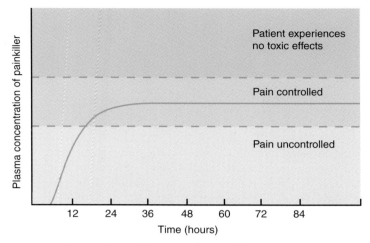

Fig. 15.6 *Good pain control and minimal toxic effects when the painkiller is continuously infused.*

their chemistry or mechanical properties, as well as examining drugs that interact with cellular proteins. In particular, the chapter examined receptors, ion
channels, enzymes and carriers. The chapter also considered how the body acts
on drugs. It outlined the four processes of absorption, distribution, metabolism
and elimination, and looked at how these processes affect drug activity.

QUESTIONS

1. What is a receptor and how may drugs act at receptors?

2. Explain the factors which influence the uptake of a drug into the body and
    its subsequent levels in the body.

3. What is the half-life of a drug?

FURTHER READING

Trounce J, Gould D (1997) *Clinical pharmacology for nurses, 15th edn.*
Churchill Livingstone, Edinburgh

INDEX

Index

Note: page numbers in *italics* refer to figures, tables and boxed material